Molecular Signaling in Spermatogenesis and Male Infertility

T0230632

Molecular Signaling in Spermatogenesis and Male Infertility

Edited by
Rajender Singh

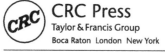

CRC Press
Taylor & Francis Group
Boca Raton London New York

CRC Press is an imprint of the
Taylor & Francis Group, an **informa** business

CRC Press
Taylor & Francis Group
6000 Broken Sound Parkway NW, Suite 300
Boca Raton, FL 33487-2742

First issued in paperback 2021

© 2020 by Taylor & Francis Group, LLC
CRC Press is an imprint of Taylor & Francis Group, an Informa business

No claim to original U.S. Government works

ISBN-13: 978-0-367-19930-2 (hbk)
ISBN-13: 978-1-03-208573-9 (pbk)

This book contains information obtained from authentic and highly regarded sources. While all reasonable efforts have been made to publish reliable data and information, neither the author[s] nor the publisher can accept any legal responsibility or liability for any errors or omissions that may be made. The publishers wish to make clear that any views or opinions expressed in this book by individual editors, authors or contributors are personal to them and do not necessarily reflect the views/opinions of the publishers. The information or guidance contained in this book is intended for use by medical, scientific or health-care professionals and is provided strictly as a supplement to the medical or other professional's own judgement, their knowledge of the patient's medical history, relevant manufacturer's instructions and the appropriate best practice guidelines. Because of the rapid advances in medical science, any information or advice on dosages, procedures or diagnoses should be independently verified. The reader is strongly urged to consult the relevant national drug formulary and the drug companies' and device or material manufacturers' printed instructions, and their websites, before administering or utilizing any of the drugs, devices or materials mentioned in this book. This book does not indicate whether a particular treatment is appropriate or suitable for a particular individual. Ultimately it is the sole responsibility of the medical professional to make his or her own professional judgements, so as to advise and treat patients appropriately. The authors and publishers have also attempted to trace the copyright holders of all material reproduced in this publication and apologize to copyright holders if permission to publish in this form has not been obtained. If any copyright material has not been acknowledged please write and let us know so we may rectify in any future reprint.

Except as permitted under U.S. Copyright Law, no part of this book may be reprinted, reproduced, transmitted, or utilized in any form by any electronic, mechanical, or other means, now known or hereafter invented, including photocopying, microfilming, and recording, or in any information storage or retrieval system, without written permission from the publishers.

For permission to photocopy or use material electronically from this work, please access www.copyright.com (http://www.copyright.com/) or contact the Copyright Clearance Center, Inc. (CCC), 222 Rosewood Drive, Danvers, MA 01923, 978-750-8400. CCC is a not-for-profit organization that provides licenses and registration for a variety of users. For organizations that have been granted a photocopy license by the CCC, a separate system of payment has been arranged.

Trademark Notice: Product or corporate names may be trademarks or registered trademarks, and are used only for identification and explanation without intent to infringe.

Library of Congress Cataloging-in-Publication Data

Names: Singh, Rajender (Scientist) editor.
Title: Molecular signaling in spermatogenesis and male infertility / [edited] by Dr. Rajender Singh.
Description: Boca Raton : CRC Press, [2020] | Includes bibliographical references and index. |
Summary: "Spermatogenesis involves the coordination of a number of signaling pathways, which culminate into production of sperm. Its failure results in male factor infertility, which can be due to hormonal, environmental, genetic or other unknown factors. This book includes chapters on most of the signaling pathways known to contribute to spermatogenesis"-- Provided by publisher.
Identifiers: LCCN 2019030763 (print) | LCCN 2019030764 (ebook) | ISBN 9780367199302
(hardback : alk. paper) | ISBN 9780429244216 (ebook)
Subjects: MESH: Signal Transduction--physiology | Spermatogenesis--physiology | Spermatozoa--physiology |
Infertility, Male--etiology
Classification: LCC QP255 (print) | LCC QP255 (ebook) | NLM WJ 834 | DDC 612.6/1--dc23
LC record available at https://lccn.loc.gov/2019030763
LC ebook record available at https://lccn.loc.gov/2019030764

Visit the Taylor & Francis Web site at
http://www.taylorandfrancis.com

and the CRC Press Web site at
http://www.crcpress.com

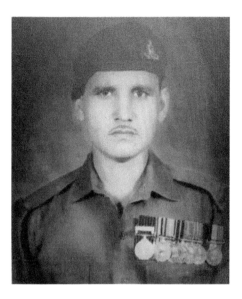

In loving memory of my father, the Late Sep. Phool Singh

Life is what you make of it; yes, indeed he proved it. I was born into a large, lower-income family with tight financial circumstances. No transportation in the village and no good schools were big hurdles that added to the complexity of the situation. My father was a great admirer of education and motivated me from childhood. Despite the lack of resources, he stood firm and sent me to the best college available in my area. This simply meant a huge expenditure, way above what he could afford. But he maintained his decision in an assertive military way, and this was the most transformative decision that would twist my career 360 degrees. He knew little about what I could become by studying a particular subject, but he knew very well what I could become by getting a good education. This provided me the platform from which to rise up the ladder of a career steadily and swiftly. Thank you, Dad, for your high-thinking that kept my aspirations high.

I remember every teaching he offered in various vocal and silent ways. I did not find the word "impossible" in his dictionary. He taught honesty, hard work, dedication and sincerity. He would often tell tales of heroism, sheer dedication to the duties and importance of education in human life. One of his quotes that I always carry with me came from his army background. For any arduous task, he would say *dushman to maarne se marega* ("the enemy would die only if you kill him"). This may have been their popular military phrase that would give them strength to fight. It gave me the courage to take on anything head-on. As he would do, I never let the difficult tasks take on me; rather, I took on them. Nothing is impossible—it may be hard to achieve, but it can be achieved. Thank you, Dad, for making me strong enough to win over my challenges.

It is so hard to accept that he is no longer with us. In early 2018, he reported difficulty in standing and walking. The disease crept in too slowly and silently for us to immediately recognize it. A firm diagnosis came after some initial check-ups, and to hear the doctor saying, "it is the motor neuron disease (MND)," was the saddest moment for me. I knew what MND meant. Unfortunately, there is not yet any medicine that can cure MND. Riluzole is the only medicine approved for MND, which may slow the progression (barely by 2–3 months) but cannot cure it. Riluzole was not available anywhere close by, and I procured it from Jammu and Kashmir. The medicine may have helped him survive a little longer, but it could not perform a miracle. Ultimately, he left us on August 15, 2018, for his further duties. An army fighter had to lose the battle of life to motor neuron disease. I will miss his love, dedication and inspiring and strong ways all through my life.

Dr. Rajender Singh

Contents

Foreword

Starting my career as a biochemist, I never thought I would end up being a reproductive biologist addressing male reproduction. In my opinion, contraception was the biggest problem for reproductive biologists around the globe, especially male contraception, where the challenge was to stop almost every single sperm among the millions being produced by men every day from doing what nature had designed them for. At mid-career, Rajender joined as a faculty member with me, and he introduced me to an equally challenging area of male infertility, where every single, fertile sperm was important. Sitting in adjacent offices, we often met to discuss the targets that seemed to be common for both the tasks. Being a biotechnologist and geneticist by training, Rajender could bring about a paradigm shift in my thoughts. We were soon discussing polymorphisms, microRNAs and genes.

What I like about this book is that it addresses the basic biology of spermatogenesis in mammals (which has been my favorite subject) with respect to the cell signaling cascades that seem to govern most of the biological processes in our body. Rajender has beautifully edited the chapters to highlight how aberrant cell signaling leads to male infertility. Most of the chapters are comprehensive, yet focused on the core theme. This book promises to answer almost every query about male fertility and fecundity, catering to the curiosities of experts as well as students.

I would like to end this foreword with a word of gratitude to Rajender who introduced me to an entirely new world of personalized medicine and diagnostics. As a modern medicine man, Rajender has a lot to offer to the society and the world.

Gopal Gupta
Senior Principal Scientist
Reproductive Biology Group
CSIR-Central Drug Research Institute, Lucknow

Preface

Male infertility is on the rise in the modern era, owing to a number of poor lifestyle and environmental factors. We recently published a book, *Male Infertility: Understanding Causes and Treatment*, which was a collection on the basics of spermatogenesis, its causes, and the methods of treatment. The treatment of infertility remains the most important challenge, pending the identification of molecular targets that can be intervened to reverse infertility. Significant advancements have been made in understanding molecular signaling via a number of pathways that operate in a complex yet uniquely orchestrated way to make it possible to incessantly produce sperm and upkeep fertility. There was no book on the molecular signaling aspects in spermatogenesis and male infertility. Hence, I made an effort to put forth a collection of information on molecular signaling pathways that operate in the tiny organs to contribute to the making of the generations to come.

Molecular signaling in the testis is so intricate that it is not possible to see each signaling pathway in isolation. This book includes chapters dedicated to specific signaling pathways, which undoubtedly cross over with others to program the process of cell division, meiosis and differentiation that converts diploid germ cells into haploid motile spermatozoa. Some authors have in fact discussed the possible interconnections among various pathways. There are at least two unique phenomena in the testis that make it very interesting

for molecular investigations. Meiosis in the whole male body takes place in the testis only, making it mandatory to dissect the testes to understand the molecular players in meiosis. Spermatozoa are the only motile cells in the human body that can actively travel. A spermatozoon can travel up to one lac times of distance of its own length. This is equivalent to a 6-foot-tall man swimming up to 56 km. Isn't it marvelous? I believe this book will be a helpful resource to those interested in investigating the molecular players participating in these interesting events.

The compilation of this book had the direct and indirect participation of my laboratory members. I am grateful to Meghali Joshi for helping in sending out the invitations and following them up. Special thanks to Poonam Mehta for drawing the cover image. The help of Rahul Vishvkarma in checking the chapters for plagiarism, spellings and grammar is highly appreciated. I am thankful to all the contributors for readily accepting to contribute to this book and delivering their chapters in a timely manner. This has added to the diversity of the content. Further, since all the chapters were externally peer reviewed, I am grateful to the peer reviewers for their time in helping improve the quality of the manuscripts.

Dr. Rajender Singh

Editor

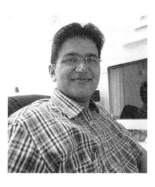

Rajender Singh, PhD, is a principal scientist at the CSIR-Central Drug Research Institute, Lucknow. He received a Bachelor of Science degree from Kurukshetra University in the field of medical sciences. During Master of Science courses in Biotechnology from Guru Nanak Dev University, Amritsar, he received a fellowship from the Department of Biotechnology, Government of India. He received a research fellowship from the Council of Scientific and Industrial Research (CSIR) to pursue a PhD in reproductive genetics from the Centre for Cellular and Molecular Biology (CCMB), Hyderabad. Immediately upon completion of a PhD, Singh joined the CSIR-Central Drug Research Institute, Lucknow, as a scientist.

His research interests include understanding the causes of and developing modalities for the treatment of male infertility. His recent research work has identified DNA methylation–based markers that can differentiate fertile sperm from infertile sperm. This would help in sperm selection in infertility clinics and also explain the etiology of infertility in a number of couples whose infertility remains idiopathic. After exhaustive work on the genetics of infertility, he has come up with an infertility genetic diagnostic kit, which will assist in the treatment of infertility in *in vitro* fertilization (IVF) clinics and in the assessment of infertility risk early in life. He has also identified a number of miRNAs and mRNAs in sperm that show a strong linkage with infertility.

Dr. Singh has published more than 100 research articles and 19 book chapters. He is on the editorial boards of *Reproductive Biology and Endocrinology, Andrologia, World Journal of Meta-Analysis, Research Reports* and *Polymorphism*. His work has been recognized by a number of prestigious scientific bodies in the form of the Haryana Yuva Vigyan Ratna Award (2018), the INDO US Postdoctoral Research Fellowship at the University of Alabama at Birmingham (2017), the Innovative Young Biotechnologist Award from the Department of Biotechnology (2015), the Young Scientist Award from the Council of Scientific and Industrial Research (2014), the Young Scientist Award from the Indian Science Congress Association (2012), the Young Scientist Award from the Indian National Scientific Academy (2011) and the Young Scientist Award from the Indian Society of Human Genetics (2006).

Contributors

Sandhya Anand
Stem Cell Biology Department
National Institute for Research in Reproductive Health
Mumbai, India

Mohamed Arafa
Hamad Medical Corporation
Doha, Qatar

and

Department of Andrology
Cairo University
Cairo, Egypt

and

Weill Cornell Medicine
Education City, Qatar

Sandeep Kumar Bansal
Reproductive Biology
CSIR-Central Drug Research Institute
Lucknow, India

Deepa Bhartiya
Stem Cell Biology Department
National Institute for Research in Reproductive
Health
Mumbai, India

Carmine Bruno
Operative Unit of Endocrinology
Fondazione Policlinico Universitario Agostino Gemelli
Università Cattolica del Sacro Cuore
Rome, Italy

Arijit Chakraborty
Department of Molecular and Human Genetics
Banaras Hindu University
Varanasi, India

Archana Devi
Reproductive Biology
CSIR-Central Drug Research Institute
Lucknow, India

Haitham Elbardisi
Urology Department
Hamad Medical Corporation
Doha, Qatar

and

Urology Department
Weill Cornell Medicine
Education City, Qatar

Elena Giacchi
Center for Study and Research on Natural
Fertility Regulation
Università Cattolica del Sacro Cuore
Rome, Italy

Gopal Gupta
Reproductive Biology
CSIR-Central Drug Research Institute
Lucknow, India

Meghali Joshi
Reproductive Biology
CSIR-Central Drug Research Institute
Lucknow, India

Ankita Kaushik
Stem Cell Biology Department
National Institute for Research in
Reproductive Health
Mumbai, India

Pradeep G. Kumar
Division of Molecular Reproduction
Rajiv Gandhi Centre for Biotechnology
Kerala, India

Bhavana Kushwaha
Reproductive Biology
CSIR-Central Drug Research Institute
Lucknow, India

Antonio Mancini
Operative Unit of Endocrinology
Fondazione Policlinico Universitario Agostino Gemelli
Università Cattolica del Sacro Cuore
Rome, Italy

Poonam Mehta
Reproductive Biology
CSIR-Central Drug Research Institute
Lucknow, India

Andrea Palladino
Operative Unit of Endocrinology
Fondazione Policlinico Universitario Agostino Gemelli
Università Cattolica del Sacro Cuore
Rome, Italy

John J. Parrish
Department of Animal Sciences
University of Wisconsin–Madison
Madison, Wisconsin

Hiren Patel
Stem Cell Biology Department
National Institute for Research in Reproductive Health
Mumbai, India

Rita Payan-Carreira
CECAV-UTAD and Department of Veterinary Medicine
Universidade de Évora
Évora, Portugal

Sreepoorna Pramodh
College of Natural and Health Sciences
Zayed University
Dubai, United Arab Emirates

Mahitha Sahadevan
Division of Molecular Reproduction
Rajiv Gandhi Centre for Biotechnology
Kerala, India

Dario Santos
CITAB and Department of Biology and Environment
Universidade de Trás-os-Montes e Alto
Douro (UTAD)
Vila Real, Portugal

Saumya Sarkar
Reproductive Biology
CSIR-Central Drug Research Institute
Lucknow, India

Pallav Sengupta
Department of Physiology, Faculty of Medicine
MAHSA University
Jenjarom, Malaysia

Bineta Singh
Reproductive Biology
CSIR-Central Drug Research Institute
Lucknow, India

Kiran Singh
Department of Molecular and Human Genetics
Banaras Hindu University
Varanasi, India

Rajender Singh
Reproductive Biology
CSIR-Central Drug Research Institute
Lucknow, India

Vertika Singh
Reproductive Biology
CSIR-Central Drug Research Institute
Lucknow, India

Edoardo Vergani
Operative Unit of Endocrinology
Fondazione Policlinico Universitario Agostino Gemelli
Università Cattolica del Sacro Cuore
Rome, Italy

1

Primordial germ cells: Origin, migration and testicular development

SAUMYA SARKAR AND RAJENDER SINGH

HIGHLIGHTS

- Primordial germ cells (PGCs) are predecessors of sperm and oocytes, which undergo complex developmental process to give rise to the upcoming generations.
- Germ cell–specific genes and many other proteins, like BMP and SMAD, are responsible for the proper growth of PGCs.
- After specification, germ cells enter the migratory phase where they relocate themselves to constitute the gonadal ridge.
- This migration phase is crucial for the PGC development where various pathways, mechanisms and proteins exert their actions.
- The gonadal ridge undergoes extensive morphological and molecular developmental changes, where it attains its ability to produce and nurse the germ cells.

1.1 INTRODUCTION

Primordial germ cells (PGCs) are the precursors of sperm and ova, which are specified during early mammalian postimplantation development. These entities have the full potential to generate an entirely new organism by undergoing specific genetic, epigenetic and molecular programming. Studies on the PGC development revealed surprising control and regulation patterns in the process of migration, which are conserved across many species. The testis and ovary arise from a common primordial structure but are functionally analogous in nature. Very specific programs of gene regulation and cellular organization drive the development of the genital ridge into the testis.

1.2 ORIGIN OF PRIMORDIAL GERM CELLS

During development at the early gastrulation stage, a scanty population of pluripotent epiblast cells "set aside" to become spermatozoa and oocytes are described as the primordial germ cells (PGCs) (Figure 1.1). These PGCs originate from pregastrulation postimplantation embryos

1

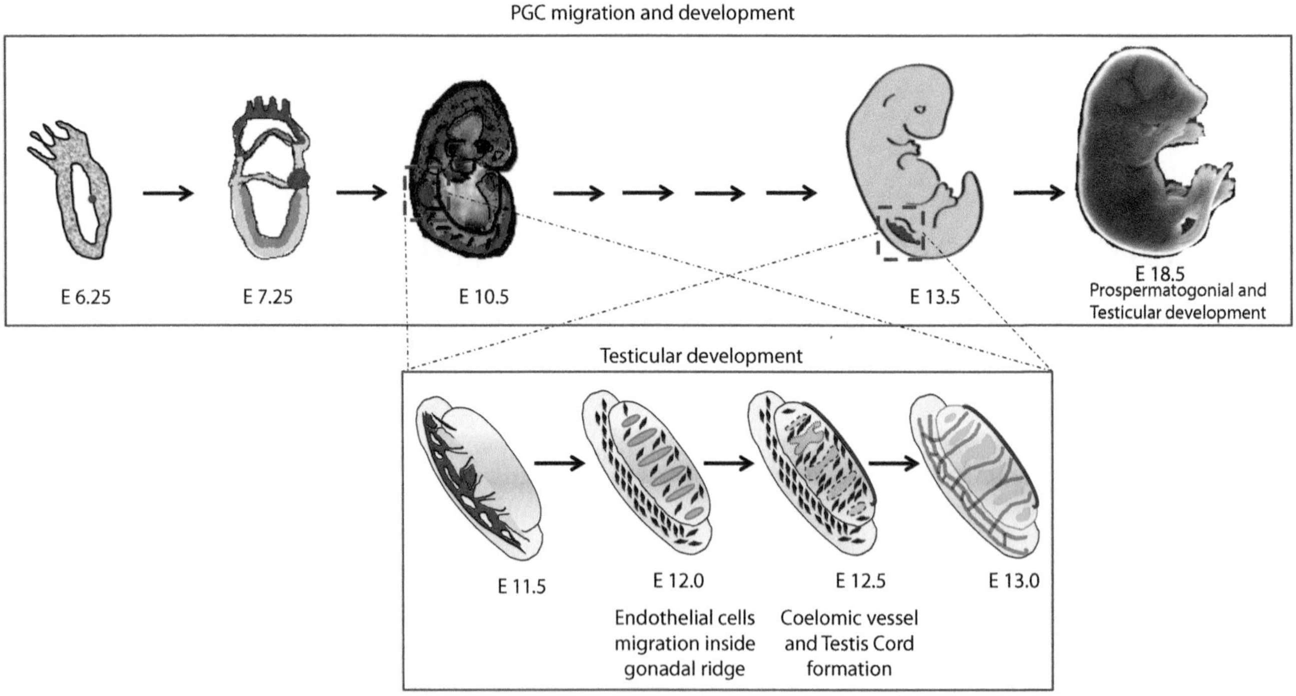

PGC migration and development

Testicular development

E 11.5   E 12.0   E 12.5   E 13.0

Endothelial cells   Coelomic vessel
migration inside   and Testis Cord
gonadal ridge   formation

Figure 1.1 The timeline of the PGC origin, migration and gonad formation. The gonadal ridge transforms itself into male testis until the E13.0 stage, where Sertoli cell differentiation along with testis cord formation takes place.

and play a uniquely important role of transmission (after meiotic recombination) of genetic information from one generation to the next in every sexually reproducing animal and plant. The production of sperm and ova by the process of spermatogenesis and oogenesis, respectively, has been intensively studied by the reproductive biologist in various species of both vertebrates and invertebrates. In 1954, Duncan Chiquoine identified PGCs for the first time in mammals by their high alkaline phosphatase (AP) activity and capability of generating both oocytes and spermatozoa (1). He found these cells at the base of the emerging allantois in the endoderm of the yolk sac of mouse embryos at E7.25 immediately below the primitive streak. However, the origin of human PGCs (hPGCs) was less well studied because of the ethical and technical obstacles. Recent studies by simulation *in vitro* models using human pluripotent stem cells with nonrodent mammalian embryos have given us the first ever insights on the probable origin of hPGCs, suggesting the posterior epiblast in pregastulation embryos as the source (2). The investigations on the presence of AP across different studies have observed different origin sites for the PGCs, for example, the posterior primitive streak (2–4), the yolk sac endoderm (2) and the extraembryonic allantoic mesoderm (5). However, it was suggested that allantoic tissue cannot give rise to embryonic body tissues, including the germ cells at the E7.25 stage (6). A study using transgenic mice expressing green fluorescent protein (GFP) under a truncated Oct4 promoter visualized living PGCs as a dispersed population in the posterior end of the primitive streak (7).

1.2.1 Molecular mechanisms during the origin of PGCs

Speciation of the PGCs requires specific molecular changes, and to understand these, a few studies have suggested a method to identify key determining factors for germ cell fate. The embryonic region containing the founder germ cells shows a difference in the expression of two germ cell–specific genes, *Fragilis* and *Stella*. The expression pattern of *Stella* is restricted to those cells that are going to be PGC with the universal expression of *Fragilis*. Therefore, both genes appear to play important roles in germ cell development and differentiation (8). Bone morphogenic proteins (BMPs) also play a vital didactic role in PGC speciation and formation at the time of their origin. BMP2, BMP4 and BMP8B are the players that act through SMAD1 and SMAD 2 signaling. This provocative nature of BMPs is well studied. It is suggested that the response of the epiblast cells to PGC specification is dose dependent in nature *in vivo*, as BMP2 and BMP4 alleles decrease, the proportion of PGC also goes down (9). Whereas, *in vitro*, only BMP4 is required for PGC induction, along with WNT3, which is required to induce competence for PGC fate and proper cross talk to BMP signaling for PGC specification (10). Every cell of postimplantation epiblast at this stage is capable of becoming a PGC, but it is only due to selective gradients of BMP signaling and inhibitory signals of Cerberus 1 (CER1), dickkopf 1 (DKK1) and LEFTY1 from distal and anterior visceral endoderm that a few attain PGC fate (10,11). Along with developmental pluripotency-associated 3 [Dppa3 (previously Stella) BLIMP1, a positive regulatory (PR) domain zinc-finger protein product of Prdm1 acts as a key regulator of PGC specification (12–15). BLIMP1 expression in the proximal epiblast cells at ~E6.25 marks the onset of the PGC specification (16). BLIMP1 represses the incipient mesodermal program, which distinguishes germ cells from the neighboring somatic cells (13,14,17). Mutations in BLIMP1 and Prdm14 resulted in aberrant PGC-like cells at ~E8.5 and ~E11.5, respectively (14). Prdm14-null cells were deprived of Dppa3 and Sox2 expression at ~E8.5, thus impairing the PGC specification (18,19). Another protein named AP2γ encoded by the Tcfap2c gene also plays an important role in PGC specification, as a mutation in this gene resulted in early loss of PGC since this is a direct modulator for BLIPM1 (17,20,21). BLIMP1 also binds repressively to all four Hox gene loci (HoxA, HoxB, HoxC and HoxD) in order to safeguard PGCs, which are pluripotent in nature, from responding to various extrinsic signals as they migrate toward gonads (22). WNT signaling has also been implicated in playing an essential role in PGC fate, suggesting its action on BMP signaling post-transcriptionally (10). WNT signaling helps to avert degradation of Smad1 by inhibiting GSK3-mediated phosphorylation of its linker region, which is important for PGC (23) along with the tyrosine-kinase receptor c-kit and its ligand that are essential for the organization of PGCs in both sexes (24). A zinc finger protein called Sall4, which is critical for embryonic stem cell pluripotency, is also found to be essential for PGC specification. In association with Prdm1, Sall4 activates the histone deacetylase repressor complex in order to suppress the somatic cell program and, hence, enables PGC specification (25). These observations together suggest the presence of a highly controlled interdependent pathway for PGC fate determination.

1.3 MIGRATION OF PGCs

The outset of mouse PGC migration is characterized by cellular movements from the posterior primitive streak to the endoderm at the E7.5 stage (Figure 1.1). *Tnap*-positive PGCs start their travel within the growing hindgut epithelium and exit mesentery followed by bilateral migration to colonize the developing gonads by E11.5 (8). Only after this point in time, PGCs undergo a sex-specific process by getting mitotically arrested in case of males and entering into meiosis in case of females (26,27). PGCs during migration experience a great deal of genome and epigenome reprogramming, such as changes in DNA methylation and histone modifications, and the global erasure of gene imprinting essential for germ cell lineage totipotency reestablishment (26). The mammalian PGC population actively proliferates at the time of their migration with a doubling time of 16 hours, increasing in size from approximately 45 cells at E7.5 to ~200 at E9.5 (8, 28,29), ~2500 at E11.5 (30) and around 25,000 at E13.5 (31). This characteristic of mammalian PGC is totally different from PGC in another organism where proliferation starts after the migration (32–34). Currently, there is no evidence for sex-specific differences in germ cell migration in any organism.

1.3.1 Molecular mechanisms during PGC migration

PGC migration is a very complex process with a myriad of cellular and biological processes taking place simultaneously with proliferation, survival and epigenetic reprogramming (35). Various proteins and transcription factors have been investigated for the maintenance of PGC migration and development. Knockdown of the Sox17, a SRY (sex-determining region Y)-box 17 transcription factor caused failure in PGCs' migration to the genital ridge and instead resulted in their scattering in the extra-embryonic endoderm. The removal of Sox17 also caused improper development of hindgut endoderm in mice (36). Previous research has also suggested the need for Sdf-1 and its receptor CXCR4 as important factors for mouse PGC survival and proliferation. The expression of SDF-1 at the genital ridges in the surrounding mesenchyme and CXCR4 expression within the PGCs provide chemotactic and survival signals to the PGCs. This signaling pathway seems to be specific for the later stages for PGC migration only. The absence of either SDF-1 or CXCR4 leads to a diminished number of PGCs, while insufficient expression of SDF-1 causes inefficient PGCs colonization within the gonads (37,38). The c-Kit and its ligand Steel were well known for their roles in PGC proliferation, migration and survival. Recently, very specific roles of these two factors have been identified during the migration stage. Steel and c-Kit were seen to be responsible for the regulation of general PGC motility, as knockout of Steel leads to a very slow-paced migration of PGCs without any impairment to their direction of migration (39). Consistent with their roles in PGC motility throughout all stages of migration, c-Kit protein and Steel show expression in the PGCs and surrounding somatic cells, respectively (39). The noncanonical form of Wnt signaling also plays a crucial role in PGC migration, as Wnt5a receptor Ror2 was observed to be responsible for the control of motility in migrating PGCs (30). Complete functional loss and/or cKO mutant of the receptor resulted in an accumulation of a large number of germ cells outside the gonadal ridge at the end of the migration phase (30,40). Another autonomous function for Ror2 is in the regulation of PGC proliferation, as aberrantly high rates of cycling PGCs were found in the hindgut of both ubiquitous and PGC-specific mutants (40). Apart from signaling pathways, cell adhesion molecules also have a role in mammalian PGC migration. E-cad expression is observed in PGCs, disruption of which causes problems with PGC-PGC adhesion, resulting in impaired colonization inside the gonads (41,42). Integrin β1 is also required for proper PGC migration as it is responsible for the exit from the hindgut into the genital ridges (43).

1.3.2 Migration stoppage of PGCs

The completion of PGC migration is characterized by the loss of cell motility and association of PGCs with the surrounding somatic cell population to constitute the gonad as evidenced from the *Drosophila melanogaster* model, in which PGCs become nonmotile with the formation of tight contacts with each other and the surrounding somatic cells (44). Not all migrating PGCs colonize within the gonadal ridge, as it has been observed that about 5% of the cells that failed to reach the gonads were eliminated by apoptosis (30). Upon arrival in the gonad, PGCs need germ cell–specific RNA binding protein DAZL (deleted in azoospermia-like), a translational enhancer for their development (45). Knockout studies for DAZL binding partners (Mvh, Scp3 and Tex19.1) and DAZL itself resulted in severe phenotypic changes and the developmental failure of germ cells beyond the PGC stage, suggesting additional roles of DAZL during the mammalian PGC development (46–48). DAZL also regulates apoptosis in the PGCs by controlling the expression of Caspases, which prevents unmigrated or uncolonized PGCs from forming into teratomas (49). Understanding of the underlying mechanism behind the cessation of PGC migration came from *D. melanogaster* and Zebrafish models, which suggests that the site of highest attractant expression is the place where PGCs lose their motility. In *D. melanogaster* and Zebrafish, the site of the highest expression of Hmgcr and SDF-1a, respectively, dictates the stoppage of PGC migration (50,51). This suppression of inherent motility behavior seems to be essential for proper gonad formation. However, the entire molecular mechanism behind suppression is still unclear in nature. PGCs attain their sex-specific morphologies only after they stop migration and associate with somatic cells of the gonad. A subset of germ cells in the gonad acquires the ability to function as germline stem cells, which undergo meiosis to produce sperm and ova and promote the next generation of embryonic development and PGC migration.

1.4 GONAD AND TESTICULAR DEVELOPMENT

The gonads initially develop from the mesothelial layer of the peritoneum and are a part of the prenatal development of the reproductive system that eventually forms the testes in males and the ovaries in females. Although the testis and ovary arise from a common primordial structure, the genital ridge, they are remarkably analogous to each other, with distinct mechanisms of gene regulation and cellular organization for their development. Here we focus only on the development procedure of the testis. After migration, the germ cells get covered by surrounding somatic cells, which eventually become the testicular cord by the process of testicular differentiation. This process has to be perfectly regulated and synchronized so that this happens only after the germ cell localization to the gonadal ridge but not before that. Few studies have pointed out that the initiation of testicular development is not entirely dependent on the localization of gonocytes, as many germ cell–deficient mouse models have successfully developed normal testis with adequate endocrine function (52–55). The exact mechanism behind the commencement of testicular development is still

elusive in nature. However, the process of transformation of a group of cells to a specific organ in a very short span of time is known to involve three major steps: (a) Sertoli cell specification and expansion, (b) testis cord formation and compartmentalization, and (c) formation of seminiferous tubules from testis cords.

1.4.1 Sertoli cell specification and expansion

Research in the 1990s suggested that the Sertoli cells are exclusively present in the XY type of gonadal ridge, suggesting an XY-specific cell-autonomous action of the testis-determining gene for their development. Sertoli cells emerge possibly from one type of "supporting cells," but by two sources: (a) from a subpopulation of coelomic epithelium progenitor cells expressing steroidogenic factor-1 (SF-1) that preexists in the gonads and (b) from a single layer of coelomic epithelium cells that covers the entire coelomic cavity and the genital ridge. Cell lineage studies have suggested that these progenitor coelomic epithelial cells pass into the XY gonad, and this results in the formation of Sertoli as well as interstitial cell types by activation of testis-determining factor *Sry* (56,57). Coelomic epithelial cells can give rise to the Sertoli cells only within a 2-hour window from 11.2 to 11.4 dpc beyond which it has the ability to form interstitial cells only (56,58–61). The expression pattern of Sry is observed first in the middle of the gonadal ridge and later tends to expand toward the poles, which suggests its dependency on various transcription factors present differentially in the gonads (57,62). However, it is still unclear how the expression of *Sry* spreads in the center-to-pole pattern, but it certainly shows the gradual differentiation of Sertoli cells in gonads (63). Transcription factor SRY box9 (Sox9), known as the first to be targeted by Sry, upregulates many additional genes important for Sertoli cell differentiation, like prostaglandin D synthase (*Ptgds*) and fibroblast growth factor 9 (*Fgf9*) (64,65). Mice lacking Fgf9 failed to maintain Sox9 levels that caused abnormalities in Sertoli cell differentiation (66). Sox9 mRNA levels were seen to be reduced in mice lacking prostaglandin D2 producing enzyme as compared to controls along with impairment in Sertoli cell differentiation and testis cord formation (67). The activation of Sox9 expression requires a certain level of Sry expression, but it is not always sufficient. In ovo-testis phenotype, where testicular structure develops at the center and ovarian qualities at the poles, it is observed that despite Sry expression in the entire gonad, Sox9 expression is limited only to the center (68,69). Further, ectopically induced expression of Sry in XX gonads did not initiate the expression of Sox9 (70). Soon after the setup of Sertoli cell differentiation, the subsequent change that XY gonads experience is the increase in somatic cell proliferation, which starts around 11.5 dpc (58,71). This increased rate of proliferation is due to Sry expression and results in an amplification of Sox-9 positive cells with respect to the negative ones. However, recent studies on *Cbx2* mutant mouse gonads uncoupled the

Sry-dependent increased proliferation of pre-Sertoli cells from the observed increased growth rate of testes relative to ovaries, suggesting that other genes, mechanisms, and perhaps cell lineages contribute to gonadal size determination (72). The XY gonad copes with this extravagant proliferative surge by rapidly increasing in size, doubling every 24 hours. This proliferation surge is essential for the growth of the fetal testis and for Sertoli cell lineage maintenance. Fetal testes upon exposure to proliferation inhibitors like 5-fluorouracil (5-FU) or methotrexate (MTX) exhibited reduction in Sertoli cell numbers along with failure to form the testis cord during 10.8–11.2 dpc (71).

1.4.2 Testis cord formation and compartmentalization

Testis cord formation, which later constitutes the seminiferous tubules, is one of the most important episodes in testicular development, as they will eventually result in two main functions of the testis: androgen production and spermatogenesis. These structures also protect the gonocytes from retinoic acid action, which if not done will cause the gonocytes to undergo meiosis well ahead of time (73). Soon after Sox9 activation, the cells from the coelomic epithelium and mesonephros start migrating into the fetal testis to accumulate around clusters of germ cells and form cords, at which point they are referred to as the Sertoli cell. The migration of these cells is coincident with pre-Sertoli cell proliferation, which occurs at around 11.5 dpc (56). Testis cord formation is dependent on many genes for its execution. Neurotrophic tyrosine kinase receptors (NTRKs) and their ligands are expressed at the onset of testis cord formation as Ntrk3 and NTRK ligand. NTF3 seems to have a significant role in the formation of adhesive cellular junctions (74–76). Knockout studies on Ntrk3 and Ntrk1 showed disruptive seminiferous tubule formation; however, a complete absence of it was not seen (75). Testis cord formation is a synchronous process despite the fact that Sry and Sox9 expression is nonsynchronous in nature, moving from the center to poles. When gonads were segmented and cultured, the polar part did not show initiation of testis cord formation until a protein called Fgf9 was supplied exogenously. This experiment implicated Fgf9 to be important for cord formation in fetal testis (77). Additional to these factors, Sertoli cells also produce a number of chemotactic signals like platelet-derived growth factor alpha (PDGF-α), nerve growth factor (NGF), anti-Müllerian hormone (AMH), and the transforming growth factor beta (TGF-β) family members activin A and B (55,75,78) that mediate cord formation by prompting mesonephric cell movement inside fetal testis. Vascularization at 12.5 dpc is characterized by the development of toroid-like structure controlled by Sry. The first step in this process is the breakdown of mesonephric vascular plexus (MVP) into individual cells that goes into the distal edge of the coelomic domain to form the coelomic vessel, which is also regarded as proto-cords (79). Blockage to this movement has severe implications in cord

formation (79,80). The first entry of MVP cells into the coelomic domain is controlled by the vascular endothelial growth factor (VEGF), which is expressed solely in the testis interstitium. XY gonads in the presence of VEGF inhibitors failed to develop the coelomic domain and initial protocords (81). Further evidence of the presence of VEGF receptors (FLK-1 and NRP1) in the endothelial cells of gonads also suggested the importance of VEGF in vascularization (81). As the cord starts to elongate, the Sertoli cells continue their proliferation and establish an even more robust connection with the germ cells (82). Signal molecule Wnt4 also provided molecular mechanisms based on evidence for the control of endothelial cell migration in testis development. Wnt4 with its target follistatin (Fst) represses endothelial cell migration and vascularization in the fetal ovary. This repression caused ectopic testis-like structure formation in the fetal ovary (83,84). The WNT4/FST pathway is necessary for ovarian structure development, as activin B is repressed by Wnt4 and Fst both, which is necessary for testis vasculature (84,85). Both molecular and physical factors help in the making of toroid testis cords. At 13 dpc, the Sertoli cells also mature to an epithelial-like morphology (82), and the testis cords develop an outer layer of peritubular myeloid cells (PMCs) and an extracellular matrix (ECM). Testicular compartmentalization is the penultimate process in which PMC fabricates the outer layer of the seminiferous tubules and set up direct connections with the basal surface of the Sertoli cells. PMC recruitment and deposition happen shortly after testis cord formation, and these are visible around 12 weeks of gestation in humans or 13.5 dpc in case of mice. The source of this layer is unknown in nature as mesonephric cells do not seem to contribute, and some intragonadal cell types appear to be responsible for the PMC. PMC differentiation depends on Sertoli cell factors, such as in the Desert hedgehog (DHH) (86,87). Knockout Dhh mice exhibited impaired PMC and Leydig differentiation, which leads to a malformed testis cord. (88). PMC results in the assembly of ECM proteins like laminin, fibronectin and collagen (89,90), which are important for cord delineation and basal surface formation. A similar condition of perturbed PMC and Leydig cell development was seen in the *Dax1* knockout mutant mouse (91), leading to the proposal that Leydig cells and PMCs may originate from a common intragonadal precursor cell population (92).

1.4.3 Formation of seminiferous tubules from testis cord by elongation

In order to accommodate the elongating testis cord, the horizontal axis of the testis increases in size, making the testis plumper in nature (80,82). This is the time where testis cords also fold themselves into "spaghetti"-like structures as observed in adult testis. It is interesting to note that the mature mouse testis has only a dozen of seminiferous tubules rather hundreds. It has been proposed that during late fetal development, the fetal Leydig cells are responsible for controlling testis cord expansion, not the Sertoli cells.

The lack of activin A, a TGF-β family member, particularly in fetal Leydig cells, affects the expansion and elongation of testis cord after 15.5 dpc, but not the formation of it (93).

1.5 CONCLUSION AND FUTURE DIRECTIONS

The organization and development of gonads into testis is a highly complex and, at the same time, well-organized process. The involvement of various genes, factors and regulators makes the story of gonad and testis development even more intriguing in nature. PGC migration in the mouse involves coverage of larger distance than other organisms. These underprivileged cells undergo extensive migration guidance along with a developmental makeover by external factors. These factors and chemicals work in supreme coordination to nurture PGC development. The entire process of PGC migration opens up crucial roles of many mechanisms and thus helps in the understanding of PGC development. Several studies have contributed substantially to the understanding of this process, but there is still a lot more to explore. The basic regulating factors of gonadal size and shape are elusive in nature. The lineage and source material of tunica albuginea and covering of the seminiferous tubule are poorly understood. Some components such as the PMC lineage and the tunica albuginea remain poorly characterized. The more we delve into the process, the more connections we find to explore. The understanding of testis building will push many investigations, which will, in turn, help us to uncover the mysteries associated with testicular diseases and disorders. The testicular organization is a long process starting right from the gastrulation stage, and no one has come across its end. Similarly, comprehension of how somatic cells and cord structures physically and molecularly cross talk to regulate proliferation, meiosis and maturation is likely to unearth the causes for infertility and germ cell cancers.

ACKNOWLEDGMENTS

The authors are thankful to the CSIR-CDRI for providing institutional infrastructure. Funding support of the ongoing project on PGC development by the SERB, DST is acknowledged.

REFERENCES

1. Chiquoine AD. The identification, origin, and migration of the primordial germ cells in the mouse embryo. *Anat Rec.* 1954 Feb;118(2):135–46.
2. Kobayashi T, Surani MA. On the origin of the human germline. *Development.* 2018 Jul 23;145(16).
3. Snow MH. Autonomous development of parts isolated from primitive-streak-stage mouse embryos. Is development clonal? *J Embryol Exp Morphol.* 1981 Oct;65(Suppl):269–87.
4. Copp AJ, Roberts HM, Polani PE. Chimaerism of primordial germ cells in the early postimplantation mouse embryo following microsurgical grafting of posterior primitive streak cells in vitro. *J Embryol Exp Morphol.* 1986 Jun;95:95–115.
5. Ginsburg M, Snow MH, McLaren A. Primordial germ cells in the mouse embryo during gastrulation. *Development.* 1990 Oct;110(2):521–8.
6. Downs KM, Inman KE, Jin DX, Enders AC. The Allantoic Core Domain: New insights into development of the murine allantois and its relation to the primitive streak. *Dev Dyn.* 2009 Mar;238(3):532–53.
7. Downs KM, Harmann C. Developmental potency of the murine allantois. *Development.* 1997 Jul;124(14):2769–80.
8. Saitou M, Barton SC, Surani MA. A molecular programme for the specification of germ cell fate in mice. *Nature.* 2002 Jul 18;418(6895):293–300.
9. Lawson KA, Dunn NR, Roelen BA, Zeinstra LM, Davis AM, Wright CV et al. Bmp4 is required for the generation of primordial germ cells in the mouse embryo. *Genes Dev.* 1999 Feb 15;13(4):424–36.
10. Ohinata Y, Payer B, O'Carroll D, Ancelin K, Ono Y, Sano M et al. Blimp1 is a critical determinant of the germ cell lineage in mice. *Nature.* 2005 Jul 14;436(7048):207–13.
11. Tam PP, Zhou SX. The allocation of epiblast cells to ectodermal and germ-line lineages is influenced by the position of the cells in the gastrulating mouse embryo. *Dev Biol.* 1996 Aug 25;178(1):124–32.
12. Chang DH, Cattoretti G, Calame KL. The dynamic expression pattern of B lymphocyte induced maturation protein-1 (Blimp-1) during mouse embryonic development. *Mech Dev.* 2002 Sep;117(1–2):305–9.
13. Hayashi K, de Sousa Lopes SM, Surani MA. Germ cell specification in mice. *Science.* 2007 Apr 20;316(5823):394–6.
14. Ohinata Y, Ohta H, Shigeta M, Yamanaka K, Wakayama T, Saitou M. A signaling principle for the specification of the germ cell lineage in mice. *Cell.* 2009 May 1;137(3):571–84.
15. Vincent SD, Dunn NR, Sciammas R, Shapiro-Shalef M, Davis MM, Calame K et al. The zinc finger transcriptional repressor Blimp1/Prdm1 is dispensable for early axis formation but is required for specification of primordial germ cells in the mouse. *Development.* 2005 Mar;132(6):1315–25.
16. Lawson KA, Hage WJ. Clonal analysis of the origin of primordial germ cells in the mouse. *Ciba Found Symp.* 1994;182:68–84; discussion 91.
17. Kurimoto K, Yabuta Y, Ohinata Y, Shigeta M, Yamanaka K, Saitou M. Complex genome-wide transcription dynamics orchestrated by Blimp1 for the specification of the germ cell lineage in mice. *Genes Dev.* 2008 Jun 15;22(12):1617–35.

18. Grabole N, Tischler J, Hackett JA, Kim S, Tang F, Leitch HG et al. Prdm14 promotes germline fate and naive pluripotency by repressing FGF signalling and DNA methylation. *EMBO Rep.* 2013 Jul;14(7):629–37.

19. Yamaji M, Seki Y, Kurimoto K, Yabuta Y, Yuasa M, Shigeta M et al. Critical function of Prdm14 for the establishment of the germ cell lineage in mice. *Nat Genet.* 2008 Aug;40(8):1016–22.

20. Magnusdottir E, Dietmann S, Murakami K, Gunesdogan U, Tang F, Bao S et al. A tripartite transcription factor network regulates primordial germ cell specification in mice. *Nat Cell Biol.* 2013 Aug;15(8):905–15.

21. Weber S, Eckert D, Nettersheim D, Gillis AJ, Schafer S, Kuckenberg P et al. Critical function of AP-2 gamma/TCFAP2C in mouse embryonic germ cell maintenance. *Biol Reprod.* 2010 Jan;82(1):214–23.

22. Magnusdottir E, Surani MA. How to make a primordial germ cell. *Development.* 2014 Jan;141(2):245–52.

23. Fuentealba LC, Eivers E, Ikeda A, Hurtado C, Kuroda H, Pera EM et al. Integrating patterning signals: Wnt/GSK3 regulates the duration of the BMP/Smad1 signal. *Cell.* 2007 Nov 30;131(5):980–93.

24. Moore H, Udayashankar R, Aflatoonian B. Stem cells for reproductive medicine. *Mol Cell Endocrinol.* 2008 Jun 25;288(1–2):104–10.

25. Yamaguchi YL, Tanaka SS, Kumagai M, Fujimoto Y, Terabayashi T, Matsui Y et al. Sall4 is essential for mouse primordial germ cell specification by suppressing somatic cell program genes. *Stem Cells.* 2015 Jan;33(1):289–300.

26. Tilgner K, Atkinson SP, Golebiewska A, Stojkovic M, Lako M, Armstrong L. Isolation of primordial germ cells from differentiating human embryonic stem cells. *Stem Cells.* 2008 Dec;26(12):3075–85.

27. Molyneaux KA, Stallock J, Schaible K, Wylie C. Time-lapse analysis of living mouse germ cell migration. *Dev Biol.* 2001 Dec 15;240(2):488–98.

28. McLaren A. Primordial germ cells in the mouse. *Dev Biol.* 2003 Oct 1;262(1):1–15.

29. Seki Y, Yamaji M, Yabuta Y, Sano M, Shigeta M, Matsui Y et al. Cellular dynamics associated with the genome-wide epigenetic reprogramming in migrating primordial germ cells in mice. *Development.* 2007 Jul;134(14):2627–38.

30. Laird DJ, Altshuler-Keylin S, Kissner MD, Zhou X, Anderson KV. Ror2 enhances polarity and directional migration of primordial germ cells. *PLOS Genet.* 2011 Dec;7(12):e1002428.

31. Tam PP, Snow MH. Proliferation and migration of primordial germ cells during compensatory growth in mouse embryos. *J Embryol Exp Morphol.* 1981 Aug;64:133–47.

32. Su TT, Campbell SD, O'Farrell PH. The cell cycle program in germ cells of the *Drosophila* embryo. *Dev Biol.* 1998 Apr 15;196(2):160–70.

33. Richardson BE, Lehmann R. Mechanisms guiding primordial germ cell migration: Strategies from different organisms. *Nat Rev Mol Cell Biol.* 2010 Jan;11(1):37–49.

34. De Melo Bernardo A, Sprenkels K, Rodrigues G, Noce T, Chuva De Sousa Lopes SM. Chicken primordial germ cells use the anterior vitelline veins to enter the embryonic circulation. *Biol Open.* 2012 Nov 15;1(11):1146–52.

35. Ewen KA, Koopman P. Mouse germ cell development: From specification to sex determination. *Mol Cell Endocrinol.* 2010 Jul 8;323(1):76–93.

36. Hara K, Kanai-Azuma M, Uemura M, Shitara H, Taya C, Yonekawa H et al. Evidence for crucial role of hindgut expansion in directing proper migration of primordial germ cells in mouse early embryogenesis. *Dev Biol.* 2009 Jun 15;330(2):427–39.

37. Ara T, Nakamura Y, Egawa T, Sugiyama T, Abe K, Kishimoto T et al. Impaired colonization of the gonads by primordial germ cells in mice lacking a chemokine, stromal cell-derived factor-1 (SDF-1). *Proc Natl Acad Sci USA.* 2003 Apr 29;100(9):5319–23.

38. Molyneaux KA, Zinszner H, Kunwar PS, Schaible K, Stebler J, Sunshine MJ et al. The chemokine SDF1/CXCL12 and its receptor CXCR4 regulate mouse germ cell migration and survival. *Development.* 2003 Sep;130(18):4279–86.

39. Gu Y, Runyan C, Shoemaker A, Surani A, Wylie C. Steel factor controls primordial germ cell survival and motility from the time of their specification in the allantois, and provides a continuous niche throughout their migration. *Development.* 2009 Apr;136(8):1295–303.

40. Cantu AV, Altshuler-Keylin S, Laird DJ. Discrete somatic niches coordinate proliferation and migration of primordial germ cells via Wnt signaling. *J Cell Biol.* 2016 Jul 18;214(2):215–29.

41. Di Carlo A, De Felici M. A role for E-cadherin in mouse primordial germ cell development. *Dev Biol.* 2000 Oct 15;226(2):209–19.

42. Bendel-Stenzel MR, Gomperts M, Anderson R, Heasman J, Wylie C. The role of cadherins during primordial germ cell migration and early gonad formation in the mouse. *Mech Dev.* 2000 Mar 1;91(1–2):143–52.

43. Anderson R, Fassler R, Georges-Labouesse E, Hynes RO, Bader BL, Kreidberg JA et al. Mouse primordial germ cells lacking β1 integrins enter the germline but fail to migrate normally to the gonads. *Development.* 1999 Apr;126(8):1655–64.

44. Jaglarz MK, Howard KR. The active migration of *Drosophila* primordial germ cells. *Development.* 1995 Nov;121(11):3495–503.

45. Lin Y, Page DC. Dazl deficiency leads to embryonic arrest of germ cell development in XY C57BL/6 mice. *Dev Biol.* 2005 Dec 15;288(2):309–16.

46. Ruggiu M, Speed R, Taggart M, McKay SJ, Kilanowski F, Saunders P et al. The mouse Dazla gene encodes a cytoplasmic protein essential for gametogenesis. *Nature.* 1997 Sep 4;389(6646):73–7.

47. Cooke HJ, Lee M, Kerr S, Ruggiu M. A murine homo-logue of the human DAZ gene is autosomal and expressed only in male and female gonads. *Hum Mol Genet*. 1996 Apr;5(4):513–6.

48. Tsui S, Dai T, Warren ST, Salido EC, Yen PH. Association of the mouse infertility factor DAZL1 with actively translating polyribosomes. *Biol Reprod*. 2000 Jun;62(6):1655–60.

49. Chen HH, Welling M, Bloch DB, Munoz J, Mientjes E, Chen X et al. DAZL limits pluripotency, differen-tiation, and apoptosis in developing primordial germ cells. *Stem Cell Reports*. 2014 Nov 11;3(5):892–904.

50. Van Doren M, Broihier HT, Moore LA, Lehmann R. HMG-CoA reductase guides migrating primordial germ cells. *Nature*. 1998 Dec 3;396(6710):466–9.

51. Reichman-Fried M, Minina S, Raz E. Autonomous modes of behavior in primordial germ cell migration. *Dev Cell*. 2004 Apr;6(4):589–96.

52. Merchant H. Rat gonadal and ovarian organogenesis with and without germ cells. An ultrastructural study. *Dev Biol*. 1975 May;44(1):1–21.

53. Hashimoto N, Kubokawa R, Yamazaki K, Noguchi M, Kato Y. Germ cell deficiency causes testis cord differ-entiation in reconstituted mouse fetal ovaries. *J Exp Zool*. 1990 Jan;253(1):61–70.

54. Pellas TC, Ramachandran B, Duncan M, Pan SS, Marone M, Chada K. Germ-cell deficient (gcd), an insertional mutation manifested as infertility in transgenic mice. *Proc Natl Acad Sci USA*. 1991 Oct 1;88(19):8787–91.

55. Buehr M, McLaren A, Bartley A, Darling S. Proliferation and migration of primordial germ cells in We/We mouse embryos. *Dev Dyn*. 1993 Nov;198(3):182–9.

56. Karl J, Capel B. Sertoli cells of the mouse testis origi-nate from the coelomic epithelium. *Dev Biol*. 1998 Nov 15;203(2):323–33.

57. Bullejos M, Koopman P. Spatially dynamic expres-sion of Sry in mouse genital ridges. *Dev Dyn*. 2001 Jun;221(2):201–5.

58. Schmahl J, Eicher EM, Washburn LL, Capel B. Sry induces cell proliferation in the mouse gonad. *Development*. 2000 Jan;127(1):65–73.

59. Gubbay J, Koopman P, Collignon J, Burgoyne P, Lovell-Badge R. Normal structure and expres-sion of Zfy genes in XY female mice mutant in Tdy. *Development*. 1990 Jul;109(3):647–53.

60. Koopman P, Munsterberg A, Capel B, Vivian N, Lovell-Badge R. Expression of a candidate sex-determining gene during mouse testis differentiation. *Nature*. 1990 Nov 29;348(6300):450–2.

61. Hacker A, Capel B, Goodfellow P, Lovell-Badge R. Expression of Sry, the mouse sex determining gene. *Development*. 1995 Jun;121(6):1603–14.

62. Albrecht KH, Eicher EM. Evidence that Sry is expressed in pre-Sertoli cells and Sertoli and granu-losa cells have a common precursor. *Dev Biol*. 2001 Dec 1;240(1):92–107.

63. Svingen T, Koopman P. Building the mammalian testis: Origins, differentiation, and assembly of the component cell populations. *Genes Dev*. 2013 Nov 15;27(22):2409–26.

64. Kent J, Wheatley SC, Andrews JE, Sinclair AH, Koopman P. A male-specific role for SOX9 in ver-tebrate sex determination. *Development*. 1996 Sep;122(9):2813–22.

65. Sekido R, Lovell-Badge R. Sex determination involves synergistic action of SRY and SF1 on a specific Sox9 enhancer. *Nature*. 2008 Jun 12;453(7197):930–4.

66. Kim Y, Kobayashi A, Sekido R, DiNapoli L, Brennan J, Chaboissier MC et al. Fgf9 and Wnt4 act as antago-nistic signals to regulate mammalian sex determina-tion. *PLOS Biol*. 2006 Jun;4(6):e187.

67. Moniot B, Declosmenil F, Barrionuevo F, Scherer G, Aritake K, Malki S et al. The PGD2 pathway, indepen-dently of FGF9, amplifies SOX9 activity in Sertoli cells during male sexual differentiation. *Development*. 2009 Jun;136(11):1813–21.

68. Eicher EM, Washburn LL, Whitney JB, 3rd, Morrow KE. Mus poschiavinus Y chromosome in the C57BL/6J murine genome causes sex reversal. *Science*. 1982 Aug 6;217(4559):535–7.

69. Wilhelm D, Washburn LL, Truong V, Fellous M, Eicher EM, Koopman P. Antagonism of the testis- and ovary-determining pathways during ovotestis devel-opment in mice. *Mech Dev*. 2009 May–Jun;126(5–6):324–36.

70. Hiramatsu R, Matoba S, Kanai-Azuma M, Tsunekawa N, Katoh-Fukui Y, Kurohmaru M et al. A critical time window of Sry action in gonadal sex determination in mice. *Development*. 2009 Jan;136(1):129–38.

71. Schmahl J, Capel B. Cell proliferation is necessary for the determination of male fate in the gonad. *Dev Biol*. 2003 Jun 15;258(2):264–76.

72. Katoh-Fukui Y, Miyabayashi K, Komatsu T, Owaki A, Baba T, Shima Y et al. Cbx2, a polycomb group gene, is required for Sry gene expression in mice. *Endocrinology*. 2012 Feb;153(2):913–24.

73. Griswold MD, Hogarth CA, Bowles J, Koopman P. Initiating meiosis: The case for retinoic acid. *Biol Reprod*. 2012 Feb;86(2):35.

74. Russo MA, Giustizieri ML, Favale A, Fantini MC, Campagnolo L, Konda D et al. Spatiotemporal pat-terns of expression of neurotrophins and neuro-trophin receptors in mice suggest functional roles in testicular and epididymal morphogenesis. *Biol Reprod*. 1999 Oct;61(4):1123–32.

75. Cupp AS, Kim GH, Skinner MK. Expression and action of neurotropin-3 and nerve growth factor in embry-onic and early postnatal rat testis development. *Biol Reprod*. 2000 Dec;63(6):1617–28.

76. Levine E, Cupp AS, Skinner MK. Role of neurotropins in rat embryonic testis morphogenesis (cord forma-tion). *Biol Reprod*. 2000 Jan;62(1):132–42.

77. Hiramatsu R, Harikae K, Tsunekawa N, Kurohmaru M, Matsuo I, Kanai Y. FGF signaling directs a center-to-pole expansion of tubulogenesis in mouse testis differentiation. *Development*. 2010 Jan;137(2):303–12.

78. McLaren A. Development of the mammalian gonad: The fate of the supporting cell lineage. *Bioessays*. 1991 Apr;13(4):151–6.

79. Coveney D, Cool J, Oliver T, Capel B. Four-dimensional analysis of vascularization during primary development of an organ, the gonad. *Proc Natl Acad Sci USA*. 2008 May 20;105(20):7212–7.

80. Combes AN, Wilhelm D, Davidson T, Dejana E, Harley V, Sinclair A et al. Endothelial cell migration directs testis cord formation. *Dev Biol*. 2009 Feb 1;326(1):112–20.

81. Cool J, DeFalco TJ, Capel B. Vascular-mesenchymal cross-talk through Vegf and Pdgf drives organ patterning. *Proc Natl Acad Sci U S A*. 2011 Jan 4;108(1):167–72.

82. Nel-Themaat L, Jang CW, Stewart MD, Akiyama H, Viger RS, Behringer RR. Sertoli cell behaviors in developing testis cords and postnatal seminiferous tubules of the mouse. *Biol Reprod*. 2011 Feb;84(2):342–50.

83. Vainio S, Heikkila M, Kispert A, Chin N, McMahon AP. Female development in mammals is regulated by Wnt-4 signalling. *Nature*. 1999 Feb 4;397(6718):405–9.

84. Yao HH, Aardema J, Holthusen K. Sexually dimorphic regulation of inhibin β B in establishing gonadal vasculature in mice. *Biol Reprod*. 2006 May;74(5):978–83.

85. Liu CF, Liu C, Yao HH. Building pathways for ovary organogenesis in the mouse embryo. *Curr Top Dev Biol*. 2010;90:263–90.

86. Clark AM, Garland KK, Russell LD. Desert hedgehog (Dhh) gene is required in the mouse testis for formation of adult-type Leydig cells and normal development of peritubular cells and seminiferous tubules. *Biol Reprod*. 2000 Dec;63(6):1825–38.

87. Yao HH, Capel B. Disruption of testis cords by cyclopamine or forskolin reveals independent cellular pathways in testis organogenesis. *Dev Biol*. 2002 Jun 15;246(2):356–65.

88. Pierucci-Alves F, Clark AM, Russell LD. A developmental study of the Desert hedgehog-null mouse testis. *Biol Reprod*. 2001 Nov;65(5):1392–402.

89. Hadley MA, Byers SW, Suarez-Quian CA, Kleinman HK, Dym M. Extracellular matrix regulates Sertoli cell differentiation, testicular cord formation, and germ cell development *in vitro*. *J Cell Biol*. 1985 Oct;101(4):1511–22.

90. Skinner MK, Tung PS, Fritz IB. Cooperativity between Sertoli cells and testicular peritubular cells in the production and deposition of extracellular matrix components. *J Cell Biol*. 1985 Jun;100(6):1941–7.

91. Meeks JJ, Crawford SE, Russell TA, Morohashi K, Weiss J, Jameson JL. Dax1 regulates testis cord organization during gonadal differentiation. *Development*. 2003 Mar;130(5):1029–36.

92. Wainwright EN, Wilhelm D. The game plan: Cellular and molecular mechanisms of mammalian testis development. *Curr Top Dev Biol*. 2010;90:231–62.

93. Archambeault DR, Yao HH. Activin A, a product of fetal Leydig cells, is a unique paracrine regulator of Sertoli cell proliferation and fetal testis cord expansion. *Proc Natl Acad Sci USA*. 2010 Jun 8;107(23):10526–31.

2

DNA methylation, imprinting and gene regulation in germ cells

SAUMYA SARKAR AND RAJENDER SINGH

HIGHLIGHTS

- At E6.5 (E6.25) day of embryonic development, a few cells are specified as the primordial germ cells (PGCs) and start their migration toward the developing gonad.
- At around E10.5–E11.5, the PGCs transform into gonocytes by undergoing extensive epigenetic reprogramming, via a genome-wide erasure and *de novo* rewriting of DNA methylation marks.
- DNA methylation erasure in the PGCs is completed in the gonadal stage and results in a globally hypomethylated state at E13.5, where the overall methylation level drops down to 10% in comparison to 70% for the entire embryo.
- At the onset of embryo sex determination at the E12.5 stage, new DNA methylation patterns are reestablished, reaching approximately 50% of the global methylation level in male PGCs by E16.5, while female PGCs retain the hypomethylated state from E13.5 to E16.5.

2.1 INTRODUCTION

DNA methylation is an elementary epigenetic modification in the mammalian genome that has a prevalent effect on the expression of genes. Regulation of gene expression is an important process in development and cell differentiation. At the E6.5 (E6.25) day of embryonic development, a few cells are specified as the primordial germ cells (PGCs) and start their migration toward the developing gonad. During germ-cell specification and maturation, epigenetic reprogramming occurs, and the DNA methylation landscape is profoundly remodeled. At around E10.5–E11.5, PGCs transform into gonocytes by undergoing extensive epigenetic reprogramming, via a genome-wide erasure and *de novo* rewriting of DNA methylation marks. Defects in this process can have major consequences on embryonic development and are associated with several genetic disorders.

DNA methylation marks established in the germline depict a key step toward genomic imprinting, epigenetic reprogramming and the establishment of the pluripotent state in early embryos.

2.2 DYNAMICS OF DNA METHYLATION DURING PGC DEVELOPMENT

Epigenetic marks are covalent modifications of the DNA or histone proteins that facilitate the regulation of genes by activating or inactivating them. Epigenetic marks are generally conserved in nature and thus are a key element for the maintenance of cellular identity. DNA methylation of promoter regions of genes is associated with transcriptional silencing. During development, the zygote is the only totipotent cell of the organism as it possesses every precursor cell of the embryo. Mammalian male and female gametes

11

have their own landscape of DNA methylation, and global DNA methylation levels differ significantly between them (1). The union of parental genomes at fertilization results in an embryo that has a heterogeneous composition of epigenetic marks. To establish germ cell specification and totipotency, these preexisting epigenetic marks reset themselves by a highly synchronized process termed *epigenetic reprogramming* (2). Reestablishment of DNA methylation marks is fundamentally important as any impairment in this process can lead to improper embryonic development and lethality. DNA methylation in sperm is mostly concentrated in repetitive and intergenic regions, whereas oocytes have significant methylation in CpG islands (CGIs) (1,3,4). Even after the passage of a few decades from the discovery of the importance of DNA methylation and DNA methylation machinery, why specific DNA sequences become epigenetically distinguished in germ cells is still only partially understood. Exceptional research has demonstrated the presence of global DNA methylation erasure and establishment in the embryonic stage. After the inception of the gastrulation stage, the founder germ cell precursors emerge from epiblast at E7.5 (<50 in number). These cells undergo proliferation and migration to colonize the developing genital ridge, the precursor of the gonad, at around E10.5–E11.5 (Figure 2.1). Since these PGCs originated from somatic embryonic cells, extensive remodeling of DNA methylation patterns for the development of a germ cell is essential (5–8). Current research has suggested that PGCs undergo two cycles of DNA methylation erasure during their development: the first one takes place during migration (E8.5), and the second cycle occurs during E10.5–E11.5 at the gonadal stage (9–12). DNA demethylation at the migration stage is more robust and global in nature as almost every genomic feature gets affected; however, certain regions escape this phase or rather show a very slow pace of demethylation. These regions include retrotransposons of the intracisternal

A-particle class (IAPs), imprinted control regions (ICRs), CGI promoters of germ cell–specific and meiosis-related genes and CGIs associated with inactive X chromosome (9,10,12). These protected regions attain demethylated status only after the second phase of the demethylation drive (13–15). DNA methylation erasure in PGCs is completed in the gonadal stage and results in a globally hypomethylated state at E13.5, where the overall methylation level drops down to 10% in comparison to 70% for the entire embryo (16–18) (Figure 2.1). As a result of this genome-wide global DNA methylation erasure, reestablishment by *de novo* DNA methylation takes place on a largely blank slate. At the onset of embryo sex determination at the E12.5 stage, new DNA methylation patterns are reestablished, reaching approximately 50% of the global methylation level in male PGCs by E16.5, while female PGCs retain the hypomethylated state from E13.5 to E16.5 (10), resulting in distinct methylation profiles of mature oocyte and sperm. *De novo* methylation in female germ cells takes place in postnatal growing oocytes arrested in meiotic prophase I to the characteristic methylation levels of about 40% (19,20). In the male germline, it initiates before birth in mitotically arrested prospermatogonia before the onset of meiosis; therefore, methylation reprogramming takes place during male germ cell development. Genome-wide methylation studies have discovered many oocyte- and sperm-specific CGIs, among which some are germline-specific differentially methylated regions of imprinted genes, which are responsible for parent-of-origin specific gene expression (4,21).

2.3 MECHANISM AND FACTORS OF DNA METHYLATION ERASURE

In the embryonic cells, the loss of DNA methylation is facilitated by the removal of Dnmt1 and Np95 from the nucleus (22). The erasure of DNA methylation is propagated through

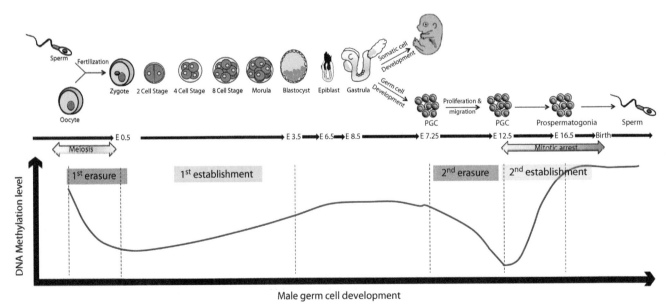

Figure 2.1 Early embryonic development showing the germ cell development and methylation events.

active and passive mechanisms of demethylation. The loss of methylation from the maternal genome is done through a passive mechanism, while in the paternal genome, it is via an active mechanism. Ten-eleven translocation (Tet) proteins involved in the first step of DNA demethylation pathway oxidize 5 mC to 5-hydroxymethylcytosine (5 hmC) and other intermediates. Tet3 plays a crucial role in active erasure in the zygote, in which oxidized intermediates get diminished gradually in their concentrations in the concomitant divisions, or provide substrate for enzymes of the base excision repair (BER) pathway (23–25). Evidence suggested that passive demethylation is responsible for global methylation erasure in the PGCs by gradual reduction of methylation levels with an increase in cell numbers along with the repression of Np95 and exclusion of Dnmt1 (9,10,26). Apart from the BER pathway, Aid- and Tdg-mediated DNA demethylation have also been implicated in PGCs (7,27). Tet1 and Tet2 proteins were also investigated for probable factors behind oxidative removal of 5 mC, but studies on Tet1 and Tet2 mutants in PGCs and ES-derived PGCs suggested these as dispensable for erasure of DNA methylation (10,28–30). It has also been suggested that the removal of 5 mC by oxidation could be a locus-specific activity, and global methylation erasure would occur in the early PGCs (E8.5–E10.5), mostly by a passive mechanism (29,30). Targeted demethylation of ICRs was suggested on the basis of the oxidative pathway, and the lack of Tet1 and Tet2 does not affect the process of global erasure in *in vitro* derived PGCs (31,32). These observations suggested that active and passive mechanisms work in synchrony for global erasure of DNA methylation marks.

2.4 MECHANISM AND FACTORS OF DNA METHYLATION ESTABLISHMENT

DNA methylation mark establishment is the next most crucial step for the proper development of the PGCs. The DNA methyltransferases 3 (Dnmt3) family of enzymes is responsible for *de novo* methylation in the PGCs. Dnmt3a and Dnmt3b are the enzymes, which act as the key players for methylation establishment along with Dnmt3L, which acts as their cofactor (33–35). These Dnmts show their expression in both female and male gonads but with differences in their involvement. In female PGCs, Dnmt3a and Dnmt3L showed their activity toward methylation of ICRs, gene CGIs and repetitive elements (4,36). In male PGCs, Dnmt3a, Dnmt3b and Dnmt3L play important roles in the establishment of the methylation pattern in ICRs and repetitive elements (37). Dnmt3a and Dnmt3b are reported to have their activity toward specific target sequences (38); however, the recruitment of Dnmt3L relaxes their specificity, thus expanding their sites of action (39). The methylation of CGIs is thought to have an influence from DNA sequences. Studies on the Dnmt3a-Dnmt3L complex have revealed the presence of two Dnmt3a catalytic sites with a distance corresponding to 8–10 bp of DNA, suggesting a prerequisite of CpG periodicity for their catalytic activity

(40). This particular type of gap was indeed found to be present in some genomic context with respect to imprinted DNA in female germ cells (40). However, this type of CpG sequence periodicity is not found in LINE elements whose methylation is also dependent on the Dnmt3a-Dnmt3L complex (41).

KRAB zing-finger proteins are transcriptional repressors in association with the KAP-1 co-repressor complex, recruiting factors responsible for DNA methylation and repressive chromatin state. A protein called ZFP57, a member of the KRAB zinc-finger protein family, has been implicated in facilitating establishment and maintenance of DNA methylation in the PGCs (42). The function of ZFP57 is varied in nature as it is required for *de novo* DNA methylation of imprinted gene Snrpn, but not for other imprinted genes like Nnat, Peg3 and Mest (42). ZFP57 is also required for maintenance methylation of several imprinted differentially methylated regions (DMRs) (42). A mutation in ZFP57 caused impaired DNA maintenance methylation and resulted in hypomethylation at several imprinted loci (43).

2.5 DNA METHYLATION AND HISTONE MODIFICATIONS

Interaction between specific domains of the DNMT3 proteins and histones is generally regulated by specific modifications on histones. *In vitro* studies have demonstrated that methylation at lysine residue 4 of histone 3 (H3K4) inhibits binding of both DNMT3A and DNMT3L, whereas DNMT3A binding is promoted by trimethylation at lysine 36 of histone 3 (H3K36me3) (44). Further, it has been postulated that KDM2A, a demethylase of H3K36me2, binds to the unmethylated CpG sites, resulting in site-specific depletion of H3K36me2 (45). During embryonic cell differentiation, DNA methylation leads to the loss of KDM2A and acquisition of H3K36me2 (45). Unmethylated CGIs are enriched in H3K4me3, which leads to the blockage of DNMT3 interaction with DNA, thus protecting the DNA from *de novo* methylation (46–48). Apart from protecting DNA from getting methylated, H3K4me3 also mediates the availability of DNA for *de novo* methylation in oocytes. Enrichment of H3K4me3 on unmethylated CGIs depends on CXXC1 (CXX finger complex 1), which interacts with the Setd1 complex, which is a H3K4 methyltransferase. The expression of Setd1 in oocytes keeps H3K4 in the methylated state so that DNA remains in unmethylated condition (4). This condition mediates the DNA methylation machinery and free access to their target CGIs. Further, the requirement of methylation in H3K4 is necessary for the setup of DNA methylation in PGCs, as supported by a genetic study (49). The study showed that oocytes lacking KDM1B, a H3K4 demethylase, exhibited impairment in DNA methylation (49). It is also observed that in male germ cells, maternal imprinted gene DMRs are enriched in H3K4me2, suggesting a possible rationale between this modification and their protection from DNA methylation during spermatogenesis (50).

2.6 CONCLUSION AND FUTURE DIRECTIONS

To establish the DNA methylation pattern, multiple factors work synergistically to result in proper PGC development. Experimental observations have suggested a complex and well-coordinated mechanism for the maintenance and removal of methylation. The erasure of DNA methylation involves active and passive processes, which are necessary to ensure error-free demethylation. DNA methylation establishment in imprinting and other CpG islands also relies on various factors like DNA sequences, DNA methylation machinery and histone marks. Despite significant progress in the understanding of crucial determinants of DNA methylation in the PGCs, many questions remain unanswered, in particular as to how the imprinted gDMRs and CGIs are specified during DNA methylation. The development of high-throughput next-generation sequencing technology has given an opportunity to profile genome-wide DNA methylation by using very small amounts of genomic DNA, providing an unparalleled chance to dissect the intricacies of *de novo* DNA methylation mechanisms in the germ cells. The interaction of the DNMT3 class of methyltransferases with nucleosomes is regulated by different histone modifications, which can be investigated by chromatin immunoprecipitation sequencing (ChIP-Seq) protocols to profile histone modifications in the field of epigenetic reprogramming. Germ-cell numbers will always pose a challenge, and the development of cell culture models that mimic imprinted gDMR DNA methylation establishment would be a breakthrough and provide new opportunities to identify the factors involved. In addition, genetic knock-out approaches available for the mouse will continue to be indispensable for studies of human epigenetic disorders to yield the way further.

ACKNOWLEDGMENTS

The authors are thankful to the CSIR-CDRI for providing institutional infrastructure. Funding support for the ongoing project on PGC development by the SERB, DST, Govt. of India (EMR/2017/003319) is acknowledged.

REFERENCES

1. Kobayashi H, Sakurai T, Imai M, Takahashi N, Fukuda A, Yayoi O et al. Contribution of intragenic DNA methylation in mouse gametic DNA methylomes to establish oocyte-specific heritable marks. *PLOS Genet.* 2012 Jan;8(1):e1002440.
2. Feng S, Jacobsen SE, Reik W. Epigenetic reprogramming in plant and animal development. *Science.* 2010 Oct 29;330(6004):622–7.
3. Borgel J, Guibert S, Li Y, Chiba H, Schubeler D, Sasaki H et al. Targets and dynamics of promoter DNA methylation during early mouse development. *Nat Genet.* 2010 Dec;42(12):1093–100.
4. Smallwood SA, Tomizawa S, Krueger F, Ruf N, Carli N, Segonds-Pichon A et al. Dynamic CpG island methylation landscape in oocytes and preimplantation embryos. *Nat Genet.* 2011 Jun 26;43(8):811–4.
5. Riddihough G, Zahn LM. Epigenetics. What is epigenetics? Introduction. *Science.* 2010 Oct 29;330(6004):611.
6. Hajkova P, Ancelin K, Waldmann T, Lacoste N, Lange UC, Cesari F et al. Chromatin dynamics during epigenetic reprogramming in the mouse germ line. *Nature.* 2008 Apr 17;452(7189):877–81.
7. Hajkova P, Jeffries SJ, Lee C, Miller N, Jackson SP, Surani MA. Genome-wide reprogramming in the mouse germ line entails the base excision repair pathway. *Science.* 2010 Jul 2;329(5987):78–82.
8. Bowles J, Koopman P. Sex determination in mammalian germ cells: Extrinsic versus intrinsic factors. *Reproduction.* 2010 Jun;139(6):943–58.
9. Guibert S, Forne T, Weber M. Global profiling of DNA methylation erasure in mouse primordial germ cells. *Genome Res.* 2012 Apr;22(4):633–41.
10. Seisenberger S, Andrews S, Krueger F, Arand J, Walter J, Santos F et al. The dynamics of genome-wide DNA methylation reprogramming in mouse primordial germ cells. *Mol Cell.* 2012 Dec 28;48(6):849–62.
11. Kagiwada S, Kurimoto K, Hirota T, Yamaji M, Saitou M. Replication-coupled passive DNA demethylation for the erasure of genome imprints in mice. *Embo J.* 2013 Feb 6;32(3):340–53.
12. Seki Y, Hayashi K, Itoh K, Mizugaki M, Saitou M, Matsui Y. Extensive and orderly reprogramming of genome-wide chromatin modifications associated with specification and early development of germ cells in mice. *Dev Biol.* 2005 Feb 15;278(2):440–58.
13. Hajkova P, Erhardt S, Lane N, Haaf T, El-Maarri O, Reik W et al. Epigenetic reprogramming in mouse primordial germ cells. *Mech Dev.* 2002 Sep;117(1–2):15–23.
14. Yamazaki Y, Low EW, Marikawa Y, Iwahashi K, Bartolomei MS, McCarrey JR et al. Adult mice cloned from migrating primordial germ cells. *Proc Natl Acad Sci USA.* 2005 Aug 9;102(32):11361–6.
15. Hackett JA, Reddington JP, Nestor CE, Dunican DS, Branco MR, Reichmann J et al. Promoter DNA methylation couples genome-defence mechanisms to epigenetic reprogramming in the mouse germline. *Development.* 2012 Oct;139(19):3623–32.
16. Seisenberger S, Peat JR, Hore TA, Santos F, Dean W, Reik W. Reprogramming DNA methylation in the mammalian life cycle: Building and breaking epigenetic barriers. *Philos Trans R Soc Lond B Biol Sci.* 2013 Jan 5;368(1609):20110330.
17. Anderson JS, Bauer G. Fighting HIV with stem cell therapy: One step closer to human trials? *Expert Rev Anti Infect Ther.* 2012 Oct;10(10):1071–3.
18. Popp C, Dean W, Feng S, Cokus SJ, Andrews S, Pellegrini M et al. Genome-wide erasure of DNA methylation in

mouse primordial germ cells is affected by AID deficiency. *Nature*. 2010 Feb 25;463(7284):1101–5.

19. Bourc'his D, Xu GL, Lin CS, Bollman B, Bestor TH. Dnmt3L and the establishment of maternal genomic imprints. *Science*. 2001 Dec 21;294(5551):2536–9.

20. Okano M, Bell DW, Haber DA, Li E. DNA methyltransferases Dnmt3a and Dnmt3b are essential for de novo methylation and mammalian development. *Cell*. 1999 Oct 29;99(3):247–57.

21. Ferguson-Smith AC. Genomic imprinting: The emergence of an epigenetic paradigm. *Nat Rev Genet*. 2011 Jul 18;12(8):565–75.

22. Howell CY, Bestor TH, Ding F, Latham KE, Mertineit C, Trasler JM et al. Genomic imprinting disrupted by a maternal effect mutation in the Dnmt1 gene. *Cell*. 2001 Mar 23;104(6):829–38.

23. Inoue A, Zhang Y. Replication-dependent loss of 5-hydroxymethylcytosine in mouse preimplantation embryos. *Science*. 2011 Oct 14;334(6053):194.

24. Inoue A, Shen L, Dai Q, He C, Zhang Y. Generation and replication-dependent dilution of 5fC and 5caC during mouse preimplantation development. *Cell Res*. 2011 Dec;21(12):1670–6.

25. He YF, Li BZ, Li Z, Liu P, Wang Y, Tang Q et al. Tet-mediated formation of 5-carboxylcytosine and its excision by TDG in mammalian DNA. *Science*. 2011 Sep 2;333(6047):1303–7.

26. Hackett JA, Sengupta R, Zylicz JJ, Murakami K, Lee C, Down TA et al. Germline DNA demethylation dynamics and imprint erasure through 5-hydroxymethylcytosine. *Science*. 2013 Jan 25;339(6118):448–52.

27. Cortellino S, Xu J, Sannai M, Moore R, Caretti E, Cigliano A et al. Thymine DNA glycosylase is essential for active DNA demethylation by linked deamination-base excision repair. *Cell*. 2011 Jul 8;146(1):67–79.

28. Yamaguchi S, Hong K, Liu R, Shen L, Inoue A, Diep D et al. Tet1 controls meiosis by regulating meiotic gene expression. *Nature*. 2012 Dec 20;492(7429):443–7.

29. Yamaguchi S, Hong K, Liu R, Inoue A, Shen L, Zhang K et al. Dynamics of 5-methylcytosine and 5-hydroxymethylcytosine during germ cell reprogramming. *Cell Res*. 2013 Mar;23(3):329–39.

30. Vincent JJ, Huang Y, Chen PY, Feng S, Calvopina JH, Nee K et al. Stage-specific roles for tet1 and tet2 in DNA demethylation in primordial germ cells. *Cell Stem Cell*. 2013 Apr 4;12(4):470–8.

31. Dawlaty MM, Breiling A, Le T, Raddatz G, Barrasa MI, Cheng AW et al. Combined deficiency of Tet1 and Tet2 causes epigenetic abnormalities but is compatible with postnatal development. *Dev Cell*. 2013 Feb 11;24(3):310–23.

32. Nakamura T, Arai Y, Umehara H, Masuhara M, Kimura T, Taniguchi H et al. PGC7/Stella protects against DNA demethylation in early embryogenesis. *Nat Cell Biol*. 2007 Jan;9(1):64–71.

33. Chedin F, Lieber MR, Hsieh CL. The DNA methyltransferase-like protein DNMT3L stimulates de novo methylation by Dnmt3a. *Proc Natl Acad Sci USA*. 2002 Dec 24;99(26):16916–21.

34. Hata K, Okano M, Lei H, Li E. Dnmt3L cooperates with the Dnmt3 family of de novo DNA methyltransferases to establish maternal imprints in mice. *Development*. 2002 Apr;129(8):1983–93.

35. Suetake I, Shinozaki F, Miyagawa J, Takeshima H, Tajima S. DNMT3L stimulates the DNA methylation activity of Dnmt3a and Dnmt3b through a direct interaction. *J Biol Chem*. 2004 Jun 25;279(26): 27816–23.

36. Kaneda M, Okano M, Hata K, Sado T, Tsujimoto N, Li E et al. Essential role for de novo DNA methyltransferase Dnmt3a in paternal and maternal imprinting. *Nature*. 2004 Jun 24;429(6994):900–3.

37. Kato Y, Kaneda M, Hata K, Kumaki K, Hisano M, Kohara Y et al. Role of the Dnmt3 family in de novo methylation of imprinted and repetitive sequences during male germ cell development in the mouse. *Hum Mol Genet*. 2007 Oct 1;16(19):2272–80.

38. Suetake I, Miyazaki J, Murakami C, Takeshima H, Tajima S. Distinct enzymatic properties of recombinant mouse DNA methyltransferases Dnmt3a and Dnmt3b. *J Biochem*. 2003 Jun;133(6):737–44.

39. Wienholz BL, Kareta MS, Moarefi AH, Gordon CA, Ginno PA, Chedin F. DNMT3L modulates significant and distinct flanking sequence preference for DNA methylation by DNMT3A and DNMT3B in vivo. *PLOS Genet*. 2010 Sep 9;6(9):e1001106.

40. Jia D, Jurkowska RZ, Zhang X, Jeltsch A, Cheng X. Structure of Dnmt3a bound to Dnmt3L suggests a model for de novo DNA methylation. *Nature*. 2007 Sep 13;449(7159):248–51.

41. Glass JL, Fazzari MJ, Ferguson-Smith AC, Greally JM. CG dinucleotide periodicities recognized by the Dnmt3a-Dnmt3L complex are distinctive at retroelements and imprinted domains. *Mamm Genome*. 2009 Sep–Oct;20(9–10):633–43.

42. Li X, Ito M, Zhou F, Youngson N, Zuo X, Leder P et al. A maternal-zygotic effect gene, Zfp57, maintains both maternal and paternal imprints. *Dev Cell*. 2008 Oct;15(4):547–57.

43. Mackay DJ, Callaway JL, Marks SM, White HE, Acerini CL, Boonen SE et al. Hypomethylation of multiple imprinted loci in individuals with transient neonatal diabetes is associated with mutations in ZFP57. *Nat Genet*. 2008 Aug;40(8):949–51.

44. Smallwood SA, Kelsey G. De novo DNA methylation: A germ cell perspective. *Trends Genet*. 2012 Jan;28(1):33–42.

45. Blackledge NP, Zhou JC, Tolstorukov MY, Farcas AM, Park PJ, Klose RJ. CpG islands recruit a histone H3 lysine 36 demethylase. *Mol Cell*. 2010 Apr 23;38(2):179–90.

46. Guenther MG, Levine SS, Boyer LA, Jaenisch R, Young RA. A chromatin landmark and transcription initiation at most promoters in human cells. *Cell*. 2007 Jul 13;130(1):77–88.

47. Barski A, Cuddapah S, Cui K, Roh TY, Schones DE, Wang Z et al. High-resolution profiling of histone methylations in the human genome. *Cell.* 2007 May 18;129(4):823–37.

48. Thomson JP, Skene PJ, Selfridge J, Clouaire T, Guy J, Webb S et al. CpG islands influence chromatin structure via the CpG-binding protein Cfp1. *Nature.* 2010 Apr 15;464(7291):1082–6.

49. Ciccone DN, Su H, Hevi S, Gay F, Lei H, Bajko J et al. KDM1B is a histone H3K4 demethylase required to establish maternal genomic imprints. *Nature.* 2009 Sep 17;461(7262):415–8.

50. Delaval K, Govin J, Cerqueira F, Rousseaux S, Khochbin S, Feil R. Differential histone modifications mark mouse imprinting control regions during spermatogenesis. *Embo J.* 2007 Feb 7;26(3):720–9.

Testicular stem cells, spermatogenesis and infertility

DEEPA BHARTIYA, SANDHYA ANAND, HIREN PATEL, ANKITA KAUSHIK, AND SREEPOORNA PRAMODH

HIGHLIGHTS

- Mammalian testes are understood to harbor spermatogonial stem cells (SSCs) that undergo self-renewal and expansion prior to differentiation to maintain the production of large numbers of sperm every day. These SSCs are established at puberty; however, their ontogeny largely remains unknown.
- Various models explaining SSC biology have been proposed including the A$_s$, fragmentation and hierarchical model. The "A$_s$ model" for spermatogonial multiplication and stem cell renewal in mice suggests that A$_s$ are SSCs (reserve, rarely divide) that give rise to A$_{pr}$ and A$_{al}$ spermatogonial cells. In human testes, A$_{dark}$ and A$_{pale}$ SSCs exist, wherein A$_{pale}$ cells divide regularly and are historically defined as the "active" stem cell pool. There is lack of clarity on the two new models including the "fragmentation" and the "hierarchical" model, since the stem cells identified in these models are located far away from the basal lamina (natural niche for testicular stem cells) of the seminiferous tubules.
- Work done by our group over a decade has focused on a novel population of more primitive, pluripotent stem cells (PSCs) that exist in addition to SSCs in the mammalian testes. These PSCs are developmentally equivalent to the primordial germ cells (PGCs) that rather than getting converted into gonocytes and ceasing to exist during early development, survive in few numbers throughout life. These PSCs are spherical in shape, small in size, have high nucleo-cytoplasmic ratio and are termed very small embryonic-like stem cells (VSELs). They have been reported in both human and mouse testes.
- VSELs are quiescent in nature, survive oncotherapy and are reported in chemoablated mouse testes and also in azoospermic human testes of cancer survivors who survived various kinds of cancers during childhood. This stem cell population has been overlooked by reproductive biologists, possibly due to their small size and rare occurrence.

- VSELs express embryonic markers including nuclear OCT-4A, undergo asymmetrical cell divisions whereby they self-renew and give rise to slightly bigger "progenitors"—SSCs that express cytoplasmic OCT-4B. The SSCs undergo symmetric cell division and clonal expansion to form chains before entering meiosis and differentiation. Thus, mammalian testes harbor two populations of stem cells, i.e., VSELs and SSCs, of which VSELs are the quiescent "true" stem cells, whereas SSCs are the actively dividing "progenitors." This understanding calls for a paradigm shift of our understanding of basic testicular stem cells biology.
- Any alteration in VSELs biology, such as exposure to endocrine disruptors, leads to disturbed tissue homeostasis. Excessive self-renewal at the expense of differentiation of the stem cells (whose function is regulated by the factors secreted by the niche) can initiate testicular tumors, whereas compromised differentiation (spermatogenesis) could lead to reduced sperm count and infertility.

3.1 INTRODUCTION

Every tissue in the body is expected to harbor two populations of stem cells, namely, a quiescent population and an actively dividing population (1,2). However, there is still ambiguity on the presence of a quiescent stem cell population in the testis (3). The testis harbors spermatogonial stem cells (SSCs), which are one of the best-studied adult stem cells besides hematopoietic stem cells (HSCs) in the bone marrow. How to define different adult stem cells was recently elaborated by Clevers (4). Basically, stem cells are expected to be quiescent in nature, should be able to self-renew and give rise to tissue-specific progenitors by undergoing asymmetrical cell division (ACD) and exhibit plasticity. The progenitors, in turn, undergo symmetrical cell divisions and clonal expansion to form chains followed by further differentiation.

Understanding testicular stem cells biology is of utmost importance, since it regulates the daily production of sperm by a process termed *spermatogenesis*. In this chapter, we describe the journey of sperm production that begins early on during development with the migration of primordial germ cells (PGCs). With recent advances in technologies available, like lineage tracing, germ cell transplantation, germ cell ablation, etc., reproductive biologists are now well equipped to unfold the mysteries behind the true nature and biology of testicular stem cells. Any adverse effect on spermatogenesis would result in reduced sperm count, infertility and sometimes could even lead to cancer. This basic understanding of testicular stem cells is also required to comprehend the deleterious effects of oncotherapy on the testes and whether the non-functional testis could be coaxed to enter a regeneration pathway to produce sperm that will help improve the quality of life of cancer survivors.

Our group has been studying testicular stem cell biology for more than a decade now, and the results suggest the existence of a sub-population of more primitive pluripotent stem cells (PSCs) among SSCs (5,6). The PSCs have been detected by a few other groups as well, but detailed characterization has been done by our group. Lim et al. (7), while studying the expansion of spermatogonial cells *in vitro* from obstructive and non-obstructive azoospermia patients, observed that GFRa (SSC marker) and SSEA-4 (pluripotent marker) do not co-localize but were expressed on different cells, implying that different types of cells (ES-like and SSCs) coexist. Izadyar et al. (8) demonstrated the presence of SSEA-4 positive cells co-expressing OCT-4 and NANOG close to the basement membrane. Sorting and transplantation of SSEA-4$^+$ cells in nude busulphan-treated mice showed that these cells colonized the recipient testis, and about one-third of the repopulating cells co-expressed SSEA-4 with NANOG/OCT-4. These results also indicated the presence of a population in adult human testis with pluripotent characteristics. Our group has studied these "pluripotent" stem cells extensively and published on various aspects of their biology using adult mouse testes as a study model. These PSCs termed very small embryonic-like stem cells (VSELs) have remained undetected over decades due to their relatively small size and their presence in very few numbers. VSELs are indeed developmentally equivalent to PGCs that rather than ceasing to exist during early development, survive throughout life in various adult tissues including the testis. Thus, the testis harbors VSELs/SSCs similar to VSELs/HSCs in the bone marrow and VSELs/ovarian stem cells (OSCs) in the ovary, and this basic insight is set to bring about a paradigm shift in our understanding of the testicular biology. Keeping in mind that a wider acceptance of the presence of VSELs in adult testes is yet to happen, we have also provided simple protocols to confirm their presence in testicular tissue.

3.2 DEVELOPMENT OF MALE GERMLINE CELLS

Life begins with the fertilization of the egg with a sperm leading to the formation of a totipotent zygote that develops into a blastocyst-stage embryo with pluripotent cells comprising the inner cell mass. It further develops into an epiblast-stage embryo, where a few cells arise in the yolk sac and are destined to become PGCs, which are precursors to the functional gametes and provide the link between generations and deliver genetic/epigenetic information to develop a new organism. These PGCs migrate along the dorsal mesentery to reach the genital ridge; during migration, PGCs undergo active proliferation but do not differentiate, express core pluripotency genes (Oct-4, Sox2 and Nanog) and undergo unique genome-wide modifications, including imprinting erasure, which enables them to initiate gametogenesis. Upon arrival at the gonadal ridge and in response to the somatic microenvironment, PGCs undergo a global change in gene expression. A set of genes is turned on that enables them to undergo gametogenesis, and the pluripotency program is shut down leading to the formation of gametogenesis-committed cells by a process termed *germ cell licensing*. For more detailed information on these aspects, one could refer to detailed reviews in the field (9–13).

PGCs continue to proliferate by mitosis after entering the gonadal ridge and maintain bipotentiality for about a week. Upon sex determination in males, the germ cells continue to expand over time, termed *gonocytes*, and form the foundation for life-long spermatogenesis. Then, germ cells in the male gonad become enclosed in the seminiferous cords and differentiate into the spermatogonial lineage, which does not enter meiosis until the onset of puberty. Prevention of entry into meiosis is a specific effect of male somatic Sertoli cells. Retinoic acid produced by the mesonephros acts as a meiosis inducer; however, Sertoli cells express CYP26B1, an enzyme that catabolizes retinoic acid, thus behaving as a meiosis-preventing factor (14,15).

The testes are divided into tubules termed as *seminiferous tubules* (about 200 μm diameter), which have a simple structural framework composed of Sertoli and peritubular myoid cells, the two somatic cell types that cover the inside and outside of the basement membrane. Each mouse testis contains about 20 tubules that are highly convoluted and tightly packed inside the testicular capsule (tunica albuginea). Their total length is up to 2 m, and spermatogenesis occurs evenly throughout the seminiferous epithelium.

Leydig cells (the main producers of testosterone) are somatic cells located outside the tubules. Blood vessels nourish the tubules but do not penetrate them and exist in the inter-tubular interstitial space to form a network. Sertoli cells are somatic testicular cells derived from the coelomic epithelium. They form a typical epithelium that provides the main structural component of the seminiferous tubules, create the blood-testis barrier (BTB) and perform multiple functions facilitating the transformation of SSCs into haploid sperm. They are the "nurse" cells that support germ cell development, phagocytose degraded germ cells and debris and assist in the release of sperm. The Sertoli cells secrete an anti-Müllerian hormone (AMH), whereas the Leydig cells secrete androgens that are essential for fetal sex differentiation.

The two distinct compartments, the basal compartment and the adluminal compartment, constitute the seminiferous tubule. The tight junctions between the Sertoli cells are the anatomical basis of the blood-testis barrier, which separates the tubules into the two compartments. The basal compartment is occupied with spermatogonial cells that contain stem cells and their differentiating progeny. Then, germ cells translocate to the adluminal compartment when entering meiosis, through the tight junction. While entering meiosis subsequently, the post-meiotic round and elongating spermatids are pushed up toward the lumen, which results in the beautifully arranged organization of the seminiferous epithelium. The mature sperm are released into the lumen and ejaculated outside via the rete testes, epididymis and vas deferens. The BTB limits access to nutrients, hormones and other substances to the adluminal compartment of the seminiferous tubule and physically protects the post-meiotic germ cells from the immune system. During infancy and childhood, the Sertoli cells remain immature both morphologically and functionally and secrete high levels of AMH. The significant increase in testicular volume, the changes in hormone secretion and the activation of full spermatogenesis that occur during pubertal development are due to the reactivation of pituitary gonadotropin secretion. Luteinizing hormone (LH) drives Leydig cell maturation resulting in active steroidogenesis and the elevation of intra-testicular androgen concentration. Testosterone induces morphological and functional maturation of the Sertoli cells, resulting in down-regulation of AMH expression, and germ cells undergo meiosis and attain sperm production—the hallmark of adult spermatogenesis.

The entire process of spermatogenesis including the massive entry of germ cells into meiosis is established on attaining puberty. The first round of spermatogenesis bypasses the stage of self-renewing stem cells and originates directly from the gonocytes. SSCs are also thought to be established at puberty; however, their ontogeny largely remains unknown (16,17).

Spermatogenesis comprises three main phases (mitosis, meiosis and post-meiosis spermiogenesis). Spermatogonia are present as undifferentiated type A spermatogonia (A_{single}, A_{paired}, $A_{aligned}$), which retain stem cell properties; differentiated type A spermatogonia (A1, A2, A3, A4); intermediate spermatogonia; and type B spermatogonia. Type B spermatogonia divide by mitosis to form preleptotene, leptotene and zygotene spermatocytes, which subsequently undergo meiosis I to form secondary spermatocytes and meiosis II to form haploid round spermatids. Spermiogenesis is the post-meiotic process that transforms spherical, haploid spermatids into elongated spermatids and mature sperm that are released into the lumen of the seminiferous tubules (18). Various molecular controls of spermatogenesis are well described (19).

3.3 TESTICULAR STEM CELLS

SSCs are the adult stem cells in the testes that balance self-renewal divisions and differentiation to maintain sperm production throughout the adult life of men. SSCs are rare cells located at the basement membrane of the seminiferous tubules. These stem cells give rise to undifferentiated progenitor spermatogonia that undergo several transit-amplifying mitotic divisions, followed by two meiotic divisions and morphological differentiation to produce sperm. Spermatogenesis produces approximately 40 million sperm per gram of tissue per day in mice and 5.5 million sperm per gram of tissue per day in men. The difference in sperm production in mice and men can be explained in part by differences in the number of transit-amplifying mitotic divisions that precede meiosis (20).

Which germ cell population acts as the SSCs? How do they behave in the testis to achieve stem cell functions? In humans, the SSCs pool is composed of A_{dark} and A_{pale} spermatogonia. A_{dark} are relatively quiescent, while A_{pale} are mitotically active and undergo one to two transit-amplifying divisions before giving rise to differentiating type B spermatogonia and then primary spermatocytes, which enter meiosis and migrate off the basement membrane of the seminiferous tubule (21–23).

In mice, SSCs are the "undifferentiated spermatogonia," the most primitive set of spermatogonia, comprising A_{single} (isolated spermatogonia, also known as A_s), A_{paired} (interconnected pairs of spermatogonia A_{pr}) and $A_{aligned}$ (chains of 4, 8, 16, or occasionally 32 spermatogonia; A_{al}). Undifferentiated SSCs constitute the smallest population that has been shown to have the stem cell function on the basis of transplantation and regeneration experiments. It has long been proposed and widely believed that A_{single} spermatogonia represent the stem cells, although this still warrants experimental evaluation. Their progeny remains interconnected by intercellular bridges due to incomplete cytokinesis, forming chains.

A_{undiff} spermatogonial cells persist throughout the cycle and give rise to A1 differentiating spermatogonia once every cycle. A1 spermatogonia subsequently go through six mitoses (each forming A2, A3, A4 and B spermatogonia, and pre-leptotene primary spermatocytes) and two meiotic divisions before forming haploid spermatids, in a highly synchronous manner within a particular seminiferous tubule segment; therefore, A_{undiff} act as the stem cell population in the basal compartment. A_{undiff} is often found to survive after any kind of stress like chemicals, radiation, or high temperature. However, A_{undiff} is a heterogeneous population, and it is unlikely that all A_{undiff} act equivalently as the stem cells. The A_s model is currently the most widely accepted model in mice. This model proposes that A_s is the only cell type that can act as stem cells, whereas the interconnected population of A_{undiff} (A_{pr} and A_{al}) cells are devoid of stem cell capacity. De Rooij (24–26) has elegantly summarized recent evolving concepts of SSCs. Other reviews are also available describing these recent advances in the understanding of testicular stem cell biology (27). Various models describing testicular stem cells biology are discussed later.

3.3.1 A_s model for spermatogonial multiplication and stem cell renewal

The A_s model, where A_s spermatogonia are the SSCs, was put forth by Huckins (28) and has been in use for almost four decades. A_s divides and gives rise to A_{pr} and A_{al} spermatogonia (Figure 3.1). Among these undifferentiated spermatogonia lies a population of SSCs, which can both self-renew and differentiate to give rise to a large number of spermatogonial cells that support daily production of a large number of sperm throughout life. In the last decade, however, two alternative models have been proposed based on studies done using emerging technologies like live cell imaging and more specific markers for SSCs.

3.3.2 Fragmentation model

Based on live-cell imaging studies to follow spermatogonial cells proliferation kinetics, on the basal lamina of the seminiferous tubules over 3 days, Yoshida's group has suggested that all A_s, A_{pr}, A_{al} spermatogonial cells have stem cells properties, and stem cell renewal is achieved by fragmentation of pairs and chains of these spermatogonia (29,30) (Figure 3.1). They studied SSC markers neurogenin 3 (Ngn3: which marks spermatogonia that could have taken a first step toward differentiation) and GDNF family receptor-α1 (Gfra1: which marks early spermatogonia that have not yet initiated differentiation). It was found that A_s spermatogonia divided into A_{pr} spermatogonia, and that the pairs and chains of spermatogonia fragmented into singles and pairs. These findings led the authors to propose that stem cell renewal primarily takes place by fragmentation of clones of two to eight A_{pr} and A_{al} spermatogonia into singles and pairs. They also observed that Ngn3 expressing spermatogonial cells could revert to acquire stem cell properties. In the live-cell imaging experiments, it was found that A_s, A_{pr} and A_{al} spermatogonia proliferate slowly, only once per 10, 12 and 13 days, respectively (29). Such a low proliferative activity is incompatible with normal steady-state kinetics of the seminiferous epithelium (26). Thus, the "fragmentation model" could not fully explain the general behavior of A_s, A_{pr} and A_{al} spermatogonia in the mouse seminiferous epithelium. It is possible that the live cell imaging did not faithfully reflect the true *in vivo* situation. The conditions during the live-imaging experiments might be damaging to spermatogonia, possibly because of phototoxic damage to the cells. This may inhibit the proliferative activity of A_s, A_{pr} and A_{al} spermatogonia and/or disrupt intercellular bridges, causing a subsequent fragmentation of spermatogonial clones. Second, and perhaps more likely, the areas with A_s, A_{pr} and A_{al} spermatogonia selected for live imaging might not be representative of the entire population of A_s, A_{pr} and A_{al} spermatogonia. In the live-cell imaging setup used, only those seminiferous tubules that run directly under the testicular tunica albuginea can be observed (29,31). Stretches of interstitial tissue with its blood vessels, which is thought to be the spermatogonial niche, could not be studied by a live-cell imaging system, as it only allows one to see cells on the basal lamina, not germ cells covered by the interstitial cells or arterioles and venules. Also, most of the niche area was in a plane perpendicular to that followed in the live-cell imaging setup. Thus, live cell imaging probably gathered evidence of spermatogonial cells poised to differentiate rather than the primitive stem cells that initiate spermatogenesis (26).

3.3.3 Hierarchical model

This model seems more probable and suggests that A_s spermatogonia are heterogeneous with respect to their capacity for self-renewal, and there exists a hierarchy among SSCs. This model is based on studies undertaken on the

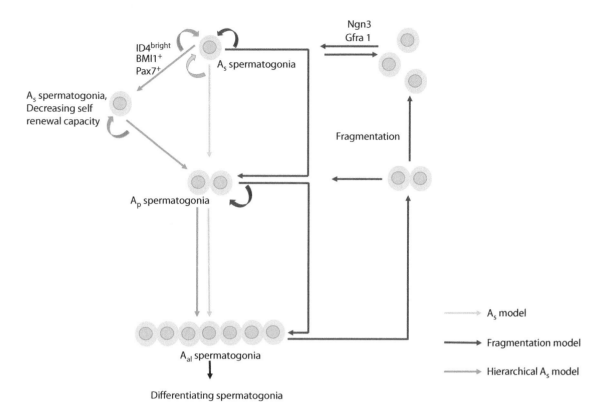

Figure 3.1 Three available models for spermatogonial stem cells (SSCs) divisions and clonal expansion prior to spermato-genesis. According to the oldest hypothesis, A_s SSCs divide into A_{pr} and A_{al} spermatogonia by undergoing transit amplifica-tion. Based on recent advances and live cell imaging studies, the Yoshida group has proposed the fragmentation model and identifying ID4+, Bmi1+ and Pax7+ subpopulation of SSCs led to the hierarchical model put forth by the Oatley group. (From Hara K et al. *Cell Stem Cell.* 2014;14:658–72; Helsel AR et al. *Development.* 2017;144:624–34.)

expression of inhibitor of differentiation 4 (ID4) as a marker for SSCs (Figure 3.1). ID4 is almost exclusively expressed in A_s spermatogonia and in a few A_{pr} (required for proper self-renewal of cultured SSCs) (32). Upon transplantation, only ID4+ cells can form repopulating spermatogenic colonies demonstrating their stem cell capacity (33). The Oatley group reported that about 20% of A_s spermatogonia are ID4 Bright, 40% are ID4 Dim and 40% have an intermediate level of staining with the ID4 bright population having the greatest capacity of self-renewal (34). Another marker for SSCs undergoing self-renewal is paired box 7 (PAX7) (35). Pax7 is expressed in A_s spermatogonia, and in lineage-tracing experiments, Pax7+ cells were found to be able to form long-term spermatogenic patches and repopulating colonies after transplantation. These cells also co-express ID4 and are actively proliferating, although they are even more rare than ID4+ cells, as there are only about 400 of these cells per mouse testis. This group has given the term "ultimate" SSCs to cells marked by bright Id4 and Bmi1 and "transitory" SSCs to A_s spermatogonia with lower ID4-eGFP signal that exhibit lower self-renewal capacity (34). De Rooij (26) further discussed whether these cells represent true SSCs. According to him, if only ID4+/BMI1+ cells are able to self-renew, one-fifth of the A_s population would have to carry out all self-renewing divisions, which would be an unrealistic number of divisions for these cells. Helsel and

Oatley (36) have discussed that ID4− A_s spermatogonia may have the ability of self-renewal and an enhanced chance of differentiation. This begs the question of which cells should be called SSCs, and which ones should be termed as the progenitor cells?

Generally, tissue stem cells are localized in a specific area, a niche, in which they preferentially self-renew, whereas daughter cells that move out of the niche differentiate. Only about 6,000 of the approximately 35,000 A_s spermatogonia in mouse testis express ID4 and surprisingly are not localized in the conventional spermatogonial niche. The "ultimate" SSCs have been found to only be localized outside the conventional niche (37). This implies that there may be a separate niche for "ultimate" SSCs in areas of the basal lamina of seminiferous tubules opposing other tubules. The idea that emerges then is that "ultimate" SSCs self-renew and form "transitory" SSCs, which move to the A_s, A_{pr} and A_{al} spermatogonial niche; there the transitory SSCs both self-renew and form A_{pr} spermatogonia that enter the differentiation pathway forming chains of A_{al} spermatogonia. However, further studies are clearly needed to determine if this is indeed the case. It is also not yet clear which cell types might constitute the "ultimate" and "transitory" SSC niches.

It seems logical that Sertoli cells play an important role as they produce a number of growth factors, such as GDNF, FGF2, CXCL12 and WNT5A, which influence spermatogonial behavior. However, as yet, no morphological differences have been observed between Sertoli cells inside and outside of the A_s, A_{pr} and A_{al} spermatogonial niche. Besides Sertoli cells, a number of other cell types contribute to the establishment of the niche. Peritubular myoid cells, for instance, produce colony stimulating factor 1 (CSF1) and GDNF, both of which have a role in the regulation of SSC behavior. Peritubular macrophages also are important in the A_s, A_{pr} and A_{al} spermatogonial niche, producing CSF1 and expressing enzymes involved in the biosynthesis of retinoic acid, which regulates spermatogonial differentiation (38–41). However, although Sertoli cells, peritubular myoid cells and peritubular macrophages together can regulate spermatogenesis, they have not yet been reported to form recognizable associations/structures that could correspond to two distinct niches—one for the ultimate SSCs and one for the transitory SSCs/A_s, A_{pr} and A_{al} spermatogonia.

Factors like ID4, PAX7 and BMI1 are the marker proteins for "ultimate" SSCs but are not crucial for their function and/or behavior since the effects of the deficiency of these proteins remain surprisingly small. Mice deficient in ID4 have spermatogenic problems, but fertility is only significantly decreased after 8 months of age; the epididymal sperm concentration in these mice is still at 20% of the normal concentration (32). No effect on spermatogenesis is observed in mice in which PAX7 is specifically knocked out in the germ cells (35). Mice deficient in BMI1, epithelial stages are disturbed in only 1% of tubule cross-sections. This could be due to a redundancy of these genes, i.e., other genes may take over. Kumar (42) discussed that PAX7 is a bona fide marker expressed uniquely in a rare subset of SSCs in mouse testes, but germline-specific deletion of *Pax7* indicates that it is dispensable for spermatogenesis.

Thus, to conclude, it seems that the seminiferous epithelium harbors few "ultimate" SSCs and a great many "transitory" stem cells. Ultimate SSCs produce transitory SSCs, which have a higher chance of differentiation, to the extent that they are not completely capable of maintaining themselves. The "ultimate" SSCs are more resistant to irradiation and cytotoxic agents than the transitory SSCs (35,43). The number of PAX7+ cells increases after administration of busulphan or cyclophosphamide and also after irradiation. In contrast, the number of FOXO1+ cells that mark all A_s, A_{pr} and A_{al} spermatogonia decreases quickly (35). The number of ultimate versus transitory SSCs per mouse testis is also not yet clear. There are 5,000–6,000 ID4+ and IBM1+ cells per testis, but the number of ultimate SSCs is much lower. What composes the niche of "ultimate" stem cells? What is the trigger for the daughter cells of ultimate stem cells to become transitory stem cells? What makes ultimate SSCs resistant to the cytotoxic drug busulphan and irradiation? These are questions that largely remain unanswered.

3.4 OUR VIEWS

3.4.1 Pluripotent very small embryonic-like stem cells (VSELs) are the most primitive stem cells in adult mammalian testis

We propose that the testicular stem cells that undergo self-renewal by undergoing asymmetrical cell divisions have not yet been identified. This quest for the most primitive stem cells that undergo self-renewal and give rise to SSCs comes to an end with the discovery of VSELs. This is similar to the hematopoietic system where specific markers to purify HSCs remain unknown, and rather than transplanting HSCs, mononuclear cells purified in the "buffy coat" by density gradient centrifugation (supposedly enriched for HSCs) get transplanted during bone marrow transplantation (BMT). According to our studies, rather than ceasing to exist during early development, PGCs survive in adult testes as well as in the ovaries as pluripotent VSELs. These stem cells were first reported by the Ratajczak group (44) and have been recently reviewed (5,45,46). Here we focus only on the testis and describe our contribution toward the understanding of testicular stem cell biology.

Our group reported two populations of OCT-4+ stem cells in both human testicular tissue smears and sections (5). Smaller cells were spherical in shape, expressed nuclear OCT-4A and were the pluripotent VSELs, whereas slightly bigger cells with cytoplasmic OCT-4 were the SSCs. We used three different antibodies for immunolocalization, Western blotting and specific primers/probes for OCT-4 A and B for *in situ* hybridization and quantitative reverse transcriptase polymerase chain reaction (qRT-PCR) studies. The cells with cytoplasmic OCT-4B were in higher abundance and also existed as chains with cytoplasmic connectivity in testicular sections. VSELs are located along the basement membrane of the seminiferous tubules in human testis (5) and are clearly visualized in mouse testis after chemoablation (8). These stem cells have escaped the attention of reproductive biologists until today because of their small size and presence in very few numbers. Zuba-Surma et al. (47) described a strategy to study VSELs in mouse bone marrow with a surface phenotype of LIN−/CD45−/SCA-1+ and also were the first to detect them as OCT-4+ and SCA-1+ cells in various adult mouse tissues including testes by Image stream analysis. However, these stem cells get unknowingly discarded while processing tissues (48) and are still struggling to get acknowledged and widely accepted by the scientific community (49).

Anand et al. (50,51) have reported that these stem cells survive chemotherapy in mouse testes and rather increase in numbers on D15 after busulphan treatment. Flow cytometry studies on small-sized, viable cells with a surface phenotype of LIN− CD45− SCA-1+ show that almost 0.03% cells in the normal testis are VSELs, and their numbers increase after chemoablation to about 0.06%, where percentage denotes the total events studied by flow cytometry. In this study, the number of VSELs on

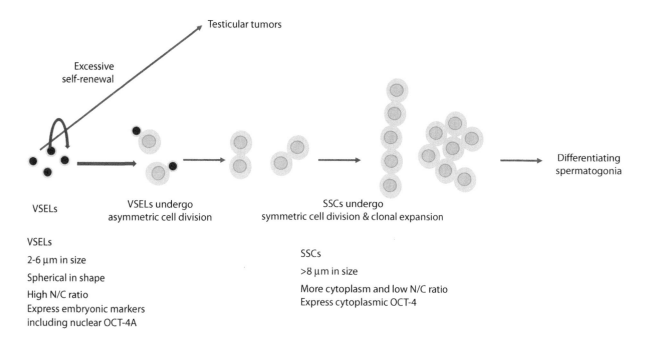

VSELs

VSELs undergo
asymmetric cell division

SSCs undergo
symmetric cell division & clonal expansion

Differentiating
spermatogonia

VSELs

2-6 μm in size

Spherical in shape

High N/C ratio

Express embryonic markers
including nuclear OCT-4A

SSCs

>8 μm in size

More cytoplasm and low N/C ratio

Express cytoplasmic OCT-4

Figure 3.2 Our model to explain testicular stem cell biology. We reported the presence of a sub-population of small-sized, pluripotent, very small embryonic-like stem cells (VSELs) among the spermatogonial stem cells (SSCs). These stem cells undergo asymmetrical cell division to give rise to SSCs that in turn undergo symmetrical cell division and clonal expansion prior to initiating differentiation (spermatogenesis). This basic stem cell biology is common in rodents, non-human primates and human testes. Being pluripotent, VSELs have abundant euchromatin and thus have dark-stained nuclei in all the species. (A_{dark} spermatogonial cells are not limited to only human testes.) Excessive self-renewal of VSELs possibly leads to testicular cancer.

different days after chemotherapy was monitored and found to initially increase on D15 after busulphan treatment and then to return to basal numbers. The total percentage of VSELs was back-calculated in the total cell count obtained per animal to obtain absolute numbers of LIN⁻ CD45⁻ SCA-1⁺ VSELs per animal. Normal adult mouse testis harbors $3,856 \pm 1,968.78$ VSELs, which increase to $23,396.67 \pm 8,830.570$ on D15 and later return to basal numbers $5,880 \pm 4,129.504$ on D30 after busulphan treatment. Small-sized stem cells were also studied for their ability to efflux the vital dye Hoechst using ABC transporter proteins in the side population (SP). The percentage of SP cells in normal testis within the total testicular cell population was $0.166 \pm 0.07\%$, and a similar SP was also observed in chemoablated testis and composed of $0.2 \pm 0.07\%$ of the total population. This indicates that the verapamil-sensitive SP remains unaffected by busulphan treatment. Further, approximately $5 \pm 0.02\%$ of SP cells were SCA-1⁺ in normal testes and $8.6 \pm 2.02\%$ of cells in the SP were SCA-1⁺ in chemoablated testes. The results confirmed that SCA-1⁺ cells in the SP resist chemotherapy and increase in numbers in response to busulphan treatment.

Similar PSCs have been reported in azoospermic human testicular biopsies in infertile men (52,53). Kurkure et al. (54) have reported VSELs in azoospermic testicular biopsies of adult survivors of childhood cancer. VSELs survive oncotherapy due to their quiescent nature. Studies done exclusively on mouse bone marrow show that being equivalent to PGCs, VSELs show biallelic open expression of imprinted genes including high expression of H19 and minimal IGF2 (55,56), whereas the HSCs show proper genetic imprinting

and express IGF2. It is for this reason that VSELs remain quiescent and survive oncotherapy, whereas the HSCs get destroyed (57). However, similar studies are yet to be performed on testicular VSELs.

Thus, we propose that VSELs are the most primitive stem cells in the testis. They undergo ACD to self-renew and give rise to the SSCs that undergo SCD and further clonal expansion prior to initiating spermatogenesis (Figure 3.2). Excessive self-renewal of VSELs in the testes could lead to testicular cancer (58) (discussed ahead).

3.4.2 Protocols to detect VSELs in testicular tissue

VSELs of small size (3–5 μm), spherical shape and high N/C ratio can be studied by flow cytometry with a surface phenotype of LIN⁻/CD45⁻/SCA-1⁺ in mouse and LIN⁻/CD45⁻/CD133⁺ in human testis. These stem cells express nuclear OCT-4 along with SSEA-1 in mice and SSEA-4 in human testes. They can also be enriched by FACS/MACS, and we have successfully isolated them from mouse testis using MACS. Care should be taken to always centrifuge cell suspension during processing at 3000 rpm, as these stem cells get unknowingly discarded when cells are spun at 1200 rpm (5,49). It is best to first isolate them from chemoablated mouse testis, where they get enriched due to the loss of actively dividing spermatogonial cells and haploid sperm. Subject chemoablated testes to enzymatic digestion (after detunication, incubate the tubules in 1 mg/mL collagenase type IV for 15 minutes at 37°C with intermittent shaking, wash twice with phosphate buffer saline for 5 minutes each, add 1 mL of 0.25% trypsin EDTA; incubate for another 7 minutes at 37°C, stop the reaction by adding 20% fetal bovine serum (FBS) and filter the cells through 70 and 40 μm filters to remove undigested pieces/debris. Then spin the cells at 1,000 rpm (250 g) when most of the cells settle down. VSELs remain suspended in the supernatant at this stage and can be obtained by spinning at 3,000 rpm (1,000 g) (8,49). This is a very simple method to obtain an enriched (not pure) population of VSELs. Hematoxylin and Eosin (H&E) staining of cell smears pelleted at 1,200 and 3,000 rpm reveal that while cells at 1,200 rpm have pale stained nuclei and abundant pink cytoplasm, cells at 3,000 rpm are spherical in shape, are 3–5 μm in diameter, have a high N/C ratio, stain dark blue with hematoxylin and have minimal pink cytoplasm (51) (Figure 3.3). They can also be visualized in 15 days old mouse testis and also after pregnant mare serum gonadotropin/follicle-stimulating hormone (PMSG/FSH) treatment by studying OCT-4/PCNA expression (59) and can be separated by using the immuno-magnetic separation method (5).

3.4.3 Pluripotent VSELs in adult testes undergo asymmetrical cell divisions

VSELs being developmentally equivalent to the PGCs, besides expressing embryonic markers, also express receptors for sex and gonadotropin hormones in various tissues, including the hematopoietic system, ovary, testis and uterus. FSHR

expression was first shown for ovarian stem/progenitor cells, and FSH treatment was found to stimulate them *in vitro* to form germ cell nests (60). Ratajczak et al. recently discussed and provided an explanation as to why the HSCs are so "sexy" (61). We also showed that stem cells expressing FSHR are activated by FSH treatment by up-regulating alternately spliced growth factor type 1 receptor isoform Fshr3 that acts via MAPK and not via the canonical G protein-coupled receptor FSHR1 that acts via cAMP. Alternately, spliced FSHR isoforms have been reported in the past (62). Recently, all four FSHR isoforms were detected in uterine tissue (63). We reported FSHR expression on testicular stem/progenitor cells and that FSH treatment increased the number of VSELs in the chemoablated mouse testis ($0.045 \pm 0.008\%$ in the chemoablated testis to $0.1 \pm 0.03\%$ of total cells after FSH treatment). We discussed the ubiquitous expression of FSHR in various adult organs (64).

Evidence has accumulated suggesting that VSELs both *in vitro* and *in vivo* undergo asymmetrical cell divisions in various adult tissues including bone marrow, ovary, testis, uterus and pancreas (65) to self-renew and give rise to slightly bigger tissue-specific progenitors including SSCs in the testes (59). PCNA expression in testicular sections from chemoablated mouse testis after FSH treatment provided evidence for ACDs occurring *in vivo* (Figures 3.3 and 3.4). Cells isolated from the seminiferous tubules of chemoablated mouse testis clearly showed that small-sized VSELs undergo ACD to give rise to slightly bigger SSCs that in turn undergo SCD and clonal expansion, associated with

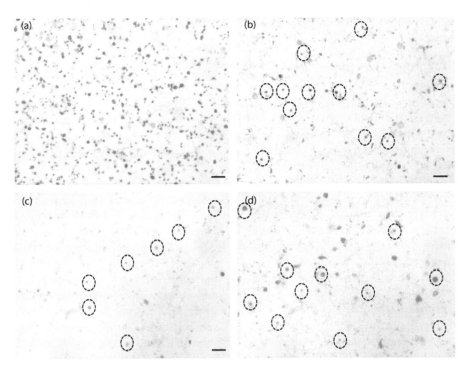

Figure 3.3 Detection of VSELs in adult mouse testicular cells suspension. The testis is subjected to enzymatic digestion (please refer to the main text for further details). **(a)** Spinning the cells suspension at 1200 rpm (250 g) results in large numbers of cells of bigger and variable sizes in the H&E stained smears. **(b)** Small-sized spherical cells are clearly visualized when the supernatant was spun at 3000 rpm (1000 g). **(c)** VSELs can be further enriched by overnight filtration through a 5 μm filter. **(d)** Higher magnification of cells observed in (b).

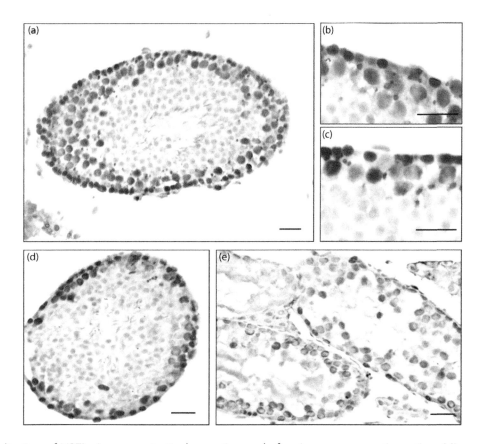

Figure 3.4 Visualization of VSELs in mouse testicular section and after immuno-magnetic sorting. Mice were treated with PMSG (10 IU) for 24 hours and then testicular sections were studied for PCNA expression using standard methods. Small-sized cells are clearly visualized, and the division of these cells was observed at higher magnification. A distinct gradient of PCNA expression from dark brown nuclear to cytoplasmic expression in different-sized spermatogonial cells was observed. (From Patel H, Bhartiya D. Testicular stem cells express follicle-stimulating hormone receptors and are directly modulated by FSH. *Reprod Sci*. 2016;23(11):1493–508.)

selective up-regulation of Fshr3. Interestingly, being developmentally equivalent to PGCs, which are natural precursors of gametes, the testicular VSELs *in vitro* spontaneously differentiate into sperm (66). Even VSELs enriched from adult mouse bone marrow and cultured on a Sertoli cell bed, differentiate into Gfra and Dazl expressing germ cells (67). Testicular VSELs have better potential to differentiate into sperm compared to ES/iPS cells, since they are epigenetically more mature (derived from epiblast stage embryo compared to inner cell mass from which ES cells are derived) (68,69).

To conclude, rather than Pax7, which is currently considered the ideal marker for SSCs, nuclear OCT-4 positive, small-sized VSELs are the bona fide and most primitive stem cells in the testis. They largely remain quiescent, undergo rare ACD to give rise to slightly bigger SSCs (that express Id4, Pax7, Ngn3 and other markers), which in turn undergo SCD and clonal expansion (rapid proliferation with incomplete cytokinesis) prior to meiosis, followed by further differentiation into sperm. Pax7 and Id4 are also expressed by the spermatogonial cells undergoing rapid proliferation, SCD and also clonal expansion. Compared to about 3,856 + 1,968.78 VSELs in normal testis, the number of ID4+ cells are 5,000–6,000 and PAX7+ cells are about 500. In comparison to the quiescent VSELs, ID4+ and PAX7+

stem cells are actively dividing and undergo symmetric cell divisions. ID4 and PAX7 are expressed on A_{single} spermatogonia, but all A_{single} cells are not SSCs. VSELs are located in the basal lamina of the tubules unlike the Pax7+ and Id4+ cells that are located outside the conventional niche (37). It is possible that Pax7+ cells appear to be resistant to oncotherapy, possibly because the quiescent VSELs increase in number after busulphan treatment and undergo ACD to give rise to Pax7+ SSCs in an attempt to restore homeostasis. Thus, Pax7 cells do not survive but rather increase in number by ACD of VSELs in response to chemotherapy-induced stress.

3.4.4 Pluripotent VSELs provide an alternate premise to explain testicular germ cell tumors

Excessive self-renewal at the expense of differentiation of the stem cells (whose function is regulated by the factors secreted by the niche) can cause tumorigenesis, including tumors in the testes (also develop in extra-gonadal sites along the midline of the body and the brain), whereas compromised differentiation (spermatogenesis) could lead to reduced sperm count and infertility. Recently, the incidences of testicular tumors and infertility have increased along with a reduction in sperm count possibly due to perinatal exposure to endocrine disruptors. Factors within the niche regulate a balance between stem cell self-renewal and differentiation. A recent review has elegantly summarized various aspects of testicular tumors (70). It is intriguing to note that testicular tumors express embryonic markers, and OCT-4 is reported to be a sensitive and specific marker for testicular tumors (71). This observation intrigued scientists since embryonic markers are limited to early fetal development. It has been proposed that fetal cells survive in individuals who are prone to form testicular tumors later in life (as pre-carcinoma *in situ* CIS, now termed pre–germ cell neoplasia *in situ* pre-GCNIS). However, tumors occur due to excessive self-renewal of pluripotent VSELs, which express embryonic markers including OCT-4. We recently discussed this concept and explained possible mechanisms that could lead to the initiation of different types of testicular cancers (72). It is likely that endocrine disruptors affect normal tissue homeostasis by affecting the epigenetic status of VSELs that in turn leads to various pathologies.

A possible role of VSELs in cancers was first proposed by Ratajczak et al. (73). During the nineteenth and early twentieth centuries, "embryonic rest hypothesis of cancer origin" was proposed by Virchow in 1855 and Cohnheim in 1875. According to this hypothesis, adult tissues contain embryonic remnants that normally lie dormant but can be "activated" to become malignant. VSELs residing in various adult tissues could possibly be the embryonic remnants that initiate various cancers (74,75). Recently, Virant-Klun et al. (76) showed that VSELs may be possible stem cells that initiate ovarian cancers.

3.5 DISCUSSION AND FUTURE DIRECTIONS

A wider consensus needs to be arrived at regarding the presence of VSELs in adult testes. In fact, it is not only the testes, but it has been proposed that the PGCs migrate to all developing organs and survive throughout life as VSELs. They are the quiescent PSCs that serve as a back-up pool to give rise to tissue-specific "progenitor" cells by undergoing asymmetric cell divisions (65).

A better understanding of the VSELs/SSCs in the testes will be of great use in the field of oncofertility. VSELs resist oncotherapy and survive in azoospermic mouse (50,51,59) and human (52–54) testes. Rather their number increases after chemotherapy, but they are unable to restore spermatogenesis since oncotherapy adversely affects the niche (51). Thus, we could successfully restore spermatogenesis in azoospermic testes by transplanting the niche cells (Sertoli or bone marrow–derived mesenchymal cells). This strategy to restore spermatogenesis embodies the concept of "seed and soil" (77) and is beyond the scope of this chapter.

It is also intriguing to note that testicular VSELs/SSCs express FSHR, and FSH exerts a direct action on them via alternately spliced growth factor type 1 Fshr3 isoform (59). This observation calls for a paradigm shift, since the current understanding is that only Sertoli cells express FSHR, and FSH exerts an indirect action on testicular stem cells.

Being equivalent to PGCs which are natural precursors of gametes, we have reported that testicular VSELs that survive chemotherapy can spontaneously differentiate into sperm when cultured on a Sertoli cell bed and exposed to Sertoli cell conditioned medium (66). We have also shown that bone marrow VSELs also have the ability to differentiate into germ cells when cultured on a Sertoli cell bed (67). To conclude, our studies on testicular VSELs open a venue for further research and have huge translational potential.

ACKNOWLEDGMENTS

The authors acknowledge all the fellow colleagues' contributions whose work may be relevant but may not have been quoted. Also, we acknowledge ICMR for financial support. NIRRH Accession Number: OTH/694/11-2018.

REFERENCES

1. Li L, Clevers H. Coexistence of quiescent and active adult stem cells in mammals. *Science.* 2010;327(5965):542–45.
2. De Rosa L, De Luca M. Cell biology: Dormant and restless skin stem cells. *Nature.* 2012;489:215–7.
3. Clevers H, Watt FM. Defining adult stem cells by function, not by phenotype. *Annu Rev Biochem.* 2018;87:1015–27.
4. Clevers H. Stem cells. What is an adult stem cell? *Science.* 2015;350(6266):1319–20.
5. Bhartiya D, Shaikh A, Anand S, Patel H, Kapoor S, Sriraman K, Parte S, Unni S. Endogenous, very small embryonic-like stem cells: Critical review, therapeutic potential and a look ahead. *Hum Reprod Update* 2016;23(1):41–476.
6. Bhartiya D, Kasiviswanathan S, Unni SK, Pethe P, Dhabalia JV, Patwardhan S, Tongaonkar HB. Newer insights into premeiotic development of germ cells in adult human testis using Oct-4 as a stem cell marker. *J Histochem Cytochem.* 2010;58(12):1093–106.
7. Lim JJ, Sung SY, Kim HJ, Song SH, Hong JY, Yoon TK, Kim JK, Kim KS, Lee DR. Long-term proliferation and characterization of human spermatogonial stem cells obtained from obstructive and non-obstructive azoospermia under exogenous feeder-free culture conditions. *Cell Prolif.* 2010;43:405–17.
8. Izadyar F, Wong J, Maki C, Pacchiarotti J, Ramos T, Howerton K, Yuen C et al. Identification and characterization of repopulating spermatogonial stem cells from the adult human testis. *Hum Reprod.* 2011;26:1296–306.
9. Gill ME, Hu YC, Lin Y, Page DC. Licensing of gametogenesis, dependent on RNA binding protein DAZL, as a gateway to sexual differentiation of fetal germ cells. *Proc Natl Acad Sci USA.* 2011;108:7443–8.

10. Hu YC, Nicholls PK, Soh YQ, Daniele JR, Junker JP, van Oudenaarden A, Page DC. Licensing of primordial germ cells for gametogenesis depends on genital ridge signaling. *PLOS Genet.* 2015;11(3):e1005019.

11. Tan H, Tee WW. Committing the primordial germ cell: An updated molecular perspective. *Wiley Interdiscip Rev Syst Biol Med.* 2018;17:e1436.

12. Hen G, Sela-Donenfeld D. "A narrow bridge home": The dorsal mesentery in primordial germ cell migration. *Semin Cell Dev Biol.* 2019;92:97–104.

13. Lebedeva LA, Yakovlev KV, Kozlov EN, Schedl P, Deshpande G, Shidlovskii YV. Transcriptional quiescence in primordial germ cells. *Crit Rev Biochem Mol Biol.* 2018;3:1–17.

14. Bowles J, Knight D, Smith C, Wilhelm D, Richman J, Mamiya S, Yashiro K et al. Retinoid signaling determines germ cell fate in mice. *Science.* 2006;312:596–600.

15. Koubova J, Menke DB, Zhou Q, Capel B, Griswold MD, Page DC. Retinoic acid regulates sex-specific timing of meiotic initiation in mice. *Proc Natl Acad Sci USA.* 2006;103(8):2474–9.

16. Yoshida S. From cyst to tubule: Innovations in vertebrate spermatogenesis. *Wiley Interdiscip Rev Dev Biol.* 2016;5(1):119–31.

17. Spradling A, Fuller MT, Braun RE, Yoshida S. Germline stem cells. *Cold Spring Harb Perspect Biol.* 2011;3(11):a002642.

18. Ehmcke J, Schlatt S. A revised model for spermatogonial expansion in man: Lessons from non-human primates. *Reproduction.* 2006;132(5):673–80.

19. Jan SZ, Hamer G, Repping S, de Rooij DG, van Pelt AM, Vormer TL. Molecular control of rodent spermatogenesis. *Biochim Biophys Acta.* 2012;1822(12):1838–50.

20. Valli H, Phillips BT, Shetty G, Byrne JA, Clark AT, Meistrich ML, Orwig KE. Germline stem cells: Toward the regeneration of spermatogenesis. *Fertil Steril.* 2014;101(1):3–13.

21. Fayomi AP, Orwig KE. Spermatogonial stem cells and spermatogenesis in mice, monkeys and men. *Stem Cell Res.* 2018;29:207–14.

22. Hermann BP, Sukhwani M, Hansel MC, Orwig KE. Spermatogonial stem cells in higher primates: Are there differences from those in rodents? *Reproduction.* 2010;139(3):479–93.

23. Hermann BP, Sukhwani M, Simorangkir DR, Chu T, Plant TM, Orwig KE. Molecular dissection of the male germ cell lineage identifies putative spermatogonial stem cells in rhesus macaques. *Hum Reprod.* 2009;24(7):1704–16.

24. de Rooij DG, Griswold MD. Questions about spermatogonia posed and answered since 2000. *J Androl.* 2012;33(6):1085–95.

25. de Rooij DG, Russell LD. All you wanted to know about spermatogonia but were afraid to ask. *J Androl.* 2000;21(6):776–98.

26. de Rooij DG. The nature and dynamics of spermatogonial stem cells. *Development.* 2017;144(17):3022–30.

27. Lord T, Oatley JM. A revised single model to explain stem cell dynamics in the mouse male germline. *Reproduction.* 2017;154(2):R55–64.

28. Huckins C. The spermatogonial stem cell population in adult rats. I. Their morphology, proliferation and maturation. *Anat. Rec.* 1971;169:533–57.

29. Hara K, Nakagawa T, Enomoto H, Suzuki M, Yamamoto M, Simons BD, Yoshida S. Mouse spermatogenic stem cells continually interconvert between equipotent singly isolated and syncytial states. *Cell Stem Cell.* 2014;14:658–72.

30. Nakagawa T, Sharma M, Nabeshima Y, Braun RE, Yoshida S. Functional hierarchy and reversibility within the murine spermatogenic stem cell compartment. *Science.* 2010;328:62–7.

31. Klein AM, Nakagawa T, Ichikawa R, Yoshida S, Simons BD. Mouse germ line stem cells undergo rapid and stochastic turnover. *Cell Stem Cell.* 2010;7(2):214–24.

32. Oatley MJ, Kaucher AV, Racicot KE, Oatley JM. Inhibitor of DNA binding 4 is expressed selectively by single spermatogonia in the male germline and regulates the self-renewal of spermatogonial stem cells in mice. *Biol Reprod.* 2011;85:347–356.

33. Sun F, Xu Q, Zhao D, Degui Chen C. Id4 marks spermatogonial stem cells in the mouse testis. *Sci Rep.* 2015;5:17594.

34. Helsel AR, Yang QE, Oatley MJ, Lord T, Sablitzky F, Oatley JM. ID4 levels dictate the stem cell state in mouse spermatogonia. *Development.* 2017;144:624–34.

35. Aloisio GM, Nakada Y, Saatcioglu HD, Peña CG, Baker MD, Tarnawa ED, Mukherjee J et al. PAX7 expression defines germline stem cells in the adult testis. *J. Clin. Invest.* 2014;124:3929–44.

36. Helsel AR, Oatley JM. Transplantation as a quantitative assay to study mammalian male germline stem cells. *Methods Mol Biol.* 2017;1463:155–72.

37. Chan F, Oatley MJ, Kaucher AV, Yang QE, Bieberich CJ, Shashikant CS, Oatley JM. Functional and molecular features of the Id4+ germline stem cell population in mouse testes. *Genes Dev.* 2014;28(12):1351–62.

38. Meistrich ML, Shetty G. The new director of "the spermatogonial niche": Introducing the peritubular macrophage. *Cell Rep.* 2015;12(7):1069–70.

39. Potter SJ, DeFalco T. Role of the testis interstitial compartment in spermatogonial stem cell function. *Reproduction.* 2017;153(4):R151–62.

40. DeFalco T, Potter SJ, Williams AV, Waller B, Kan MJ, Capel B. Macrophages contribute to the spermatogonial niche in the adult testis. *Cell Rep.* 2015;12(7):1107–19.

41. Chen Y, Ma L, Hogarth C, Wei G, Griswold MD, Tong MH. Retinoid signaling controls spermatogonial differentiation by regulating expression of replication-dependent core histone genes. *Development.* 2016;143(9):1502–11.

42. Kumar TR. The quest for male germline stem cell markers: PAX7 gets ID'd. *J Clin Invest.* 2014;124(10):4219–22.

43. Komai Y, Tanaka T, Tokuyama Y, Yanai H, Ohe S, Omachi T, Atsumi N et al. Bmi1 expression in long-term germ stem cells. *Sci Rep.* 2014;4:6175.

44. Kucia M, Reca R, Campbell FR, Zuba-Surma E, Majka M, Ratajczak J, Ratajczak MZ. A population of very small embryonic-like (VSEL) CXCR4+ SSEA-1+ Oct-4+ stem cells identified in adult bone marrow. *Leukemia.* 2006;20(5):857–69.

45. Ratajczak MZ, Ratajczak J, Suszynska M, Miller DM, Kucia M, Shin DM. A novel view of the adult stem cell compartment from the perspective of a quiescent population of very small embryonic-like stem cells. *Circ Res.* 2017;120(1):166–78.

46. Bhartiya D, Patel H. Ovarian stem cells—Resolving controversies. *J Assist Reprod Genet.* 2018;35(3):393–8.

47. Zuba-Surma EK, Kucia M, Wu W, Klich I, Lillard JW Jr, Ratajczak J, Ratajczak MZ. Very small embryonic-like stem cells are present in adult murine organs: Image Stream-based morphological analysis and distribution studies. *Cytometry A.* 2008;73(12):1116–27.

48. Bhartiya D, Shaikh A, Nagvenkar P, Kasiviswanathan S, Pethe P, Pawani H, Mohanty S, Rao SG, Zaveri K, Hinduja I. Very small embryonic-like stem cells with maximum regenerative potential get discarded during cord blood banking and bone marrow processing for autologous stem cell therapy. *Stem Cells Dev.* 2012;21(1):1–6.

49. Bhartiya D. Pluripotent stem cells in adult tissues: Struggling to be acknowledged over two decades. *Stem Cell Rev.* 2017;13(6):713–24.

50. Anand S, Bhartiya D, Sriraman K, Patel H, Manjramkar DD. Very small embryonic-like stem cells survive and restore spermatogenesis after busulphan treatment in mouse testis. *J Stem Cell Res Ther.* 2014;4:216.

51. Anand S, Bhartiya D, Sriraman K, Mallick A. Underlying mechanisms that restore spermatogenesis on transplanting healthy niche cells in busulphan treated mouse testis. *Stem Cell Rev.* 2016;12(6):682–97.

52. Stimpfel M, Skutella T, Kubista M, Malicev E, Conrad S, Virant-Klun I. Potential stemness of frozen-thawed testicular biopsies without sperm in infertile men included into the in vitro fertilization programme. *J Biomed Biotechnol.* 2012. doi: 10.1155/2012/291038.

53. Virant-Klun I, Stimpfel M, Cvjeticanin B, Vrtacnik-Bokal E, Skutella T. Small SSEA-4-positive cells from human ovarian cell cultures: Related to embryonic stem cells and germinal lineage? *J Ovarian Res.* 2013;6:24.

54. Kurkure P, Prasad M, Dhamankar V, Bakshi G. Very small embryonic-like stem cells (VSELs) detected in azoospermic testicular biopsies of adult survivors of childhood cancer. *Rep Biol Endocrinol.* 2015. doi: 10.1186/s12958-015-0121-1.

55. Shin DM, Zuba-Surma EK, Wu W, Ratajczak J, Wysoczynski M, Ratajczak MZ, Kucia M. Novel epigenetic mechanisms that control pluripotency and quiescence of adult bone marrow-derived Oct4+ very small embryonic-like stem cells. *Leukemia.* 2009;23(11):2042–51.

56. Ratajczak MZ. Igf2-H19, an imprinted tandem gene, is an important regulator of embryonic development, a guardian of proliferation of adult pluripotent stem cells, a regulator of longevity, and a 'passkey' to cancerogenesis. *Folia Histochem Cytobiol.* 2012;50(2):171–9.

57. Ratajczak J, Wysoczynski M, Zuba-Surma E, Wan W, Kucia M, Yoder MC, Ratajczak MZ. Adult murine bone marrow-derived very small embryonic-like stem cells differentiate into the hematopoietic lineage after coculture over OP9 stromal cells. *Exp Hematol.* 2011;39(2):225–37.

58. Kaushik A, Bhartiya D. Pluripotent very small embryonic-like stem cells in adult testes—An alternate premise to explain testicular germ cell tumors. *Stem Cell Rev.* 2018;14(6):793–800.

59. Patel H, Bhartiya D. Testicular stem cells express follicle-stimulating hormone receptors and are directly modulated by FSH. *Reprod Sci.* 2016;23(11):1493–508.

60. Patel H, Bhartiya D, Parte S, Gunjal P, Yedurkar S, Bhatt M. Follicle stimulating hormone modulates ovarian stem cells through alternately spliced receptor variant FSH-R3. *J Ovarian Res.* 2013;6:52.

61. Ratajczak MZ. Why are hematopoietic stem cells so 'sexy'? on a search for developmental explanation. *Leukemia.* 2017;31(8):1671–7.

62. Sairam MR, Babu PS. The tale of follitropin receptor diversity: A recipe for fine tuning gonadal responses? *Mol Cell Endocrinol.* 2007;260–262:163–171.

63. James K, Bhartiya D, Ganguly R, Kaushik A, Gala K, Singh P, Metkari SM. Gonadotropin and steroid hormones regulate pluripotent very small embryonic-like stem cells in adult mouse uterine endometrium. *J Ovarian Res.* 2018;11(1):83.

64. Bhartiya D. Ubiquitous expression of FSH/LH/hCG receptors, OCT-4 and CD133 in adult organs and cancers reflects novel VSELs biology. *J Rep Health and Medicine.* 2016;2(1):33–36.

65. Bhartiya D, Patel H, Ganguly R, Shaikh A, Shukla Y, Sharma D, Singh P. Novel insights into adult and cancer stem cell biology. *Stem Cells Dev.* 2018;27(22):1527–1539.

66. Anand S, Patel H, Bhartiya D. Chemoablated mouse seminiferous tubular cells enriched for very small embryonic-like stem cells undergo spontaneous spermatogenesis in vitro. *Reprod Biol Endocrinol.* 2015;13:33.

67. Shaikh A, Anand S, Kapoor S, Ganguly R, Bhartiya D. Mouse bone marrow VSELs exhibit differentiation into three embryonic germ lineages and germ and hematopoietic cells in culture. *Stem Cell Rev.* 2017;13(2):202–16.

68. Bhartiya D, Anand S, Patel H, Parte S. Making gametes from alternate sources of stem cells: Past, present and future. *Reprod Biol Endocrinol.* 2017.

69. Bhartiya D. Shifting gears from embryonic to very small embryonic-like stem cells for regenerative medicine. *Indian J Med Res*. 2017;146(1):15–21.

70. Cheng L, Albers P, Berney DM, Feldman DR, Daugaard G, Gilligan T, Looijenga LHJ. Testicular cancer. *Nat Rev Dis Primers*. 2018;4(1):29.

71. Jones TD, Ulbright TM, Eble JN, Baldridge LA, Cheng L. OCT4 staining in testicular tumors: A sensitive and specific marker for seminoma and embryonal carcinoma. *Am J Surg Pathol*. 2004;28(7):935–40.

72. Ratajczak MZ, Shin DM, Liu R, Marlicz W, Tarnowski M, Ratajczak J, Kucia M. Epiblast/germ line hypothesis of cancer development revisited: Lesson from the presence of Oct-4+ cells in adult tissues. *Stem Cell Rev*. 2010;6(2):307–16.

73. Ratajczak MZ, Bujko K, Mack A, Kucia M, Ratajczak J. Cancer from the perspective of stem cells and misappropriated tissue regeneration mechanisms. *Leukemia*. 2018. doi: 10.1038/s41375-018-0294-7.

74. Ratajczak MZ, Marycz K, Poniewierska-Baran A, Fiedorowicz K, Zbucka-Kretowska M, Moniuszko M. Very small embryonic-like stem cells as a novel developmental concept and the hierarchy of the stem cell compartment. *Adv Med Sci*. 2014;59(2):273–80.

75. Virant-Klun I, Stimpfel M. Novel population of small tumour-initiating stem cells in the ovaries of women with borderline ovarian cancer. *Sci Rep*. 2016;6:34730.

76. Virant-Klun I, Kenda-Suster N, Smrkolj S. Small putative NANOG, SOX2, and SSEA-4-positive stem cells resembling very small embryonic-like stem cells in sections of ovarian tissue in patients with ovarian cancer. *J Ovarian Res*. 2016;9:12.

77. Bhartiya D, Anand S. Effects of oncotherapy on testicular stem cells and niche. *Mol Hum Reprod*. 2017;23(9):654–5.

4

Testicular germ cell apoptosis and spermatogenesis

BINETA SINGH AND GOPAL GUPTA

HIGHLIGHTS

- Male fertility relies on successful and incessant production of sperm.
- Spermatogenesis is a complex process of mitotic and meiotic proliferation of germ cells, which takes place inside the seminiferous tubules.
- About 25%–75% of germ cells undergo spontaneous apoptosis to remove surplus germ cells as well as those with defects.
- Germ cells develop an intricate contact with fixed population of somatic Sertoli cells for nutrition, anchorage and paracrine support.
- Spontaneous apoptosis maintains the germ cell homeostasis by eliminating superfluous and defective cells produced by continual cell proliferation and thus preventing space, paracrine and nutrition crisis.
- Apoptosis of germ cells is significantly augmented under stress conditions of hormonal imbalance, radiation, increased temperature and treatment with testicular toxicants.
- Fas/FasL, extrinsic, intrinsic and p53-mediated pathways are involved in germ cell apoptosis along with cytochrome c, caspases 9,8,3 and Bcl-2 family proteins.
- Premeiotic (spermatogonia), meiotic (spermatocytes) and postmeiotic (spermatids) undergo spontaneous apoptosis; however, the stage of spermatogenesis and germ cell type affected depend on the kind of stimulus.

4.1 INTRODUCTION

4.1.1 Proliferative phase of spermatogonia

Successful completion of spermatogenesis ensures the production of a highly differentiated cell, the spermatozoon, which functions as a delivery vehicle for the paternal DNA to the oocyte. Production of a single spermatozoon is a very complex but well-organized process, which takes place in the testis and can broadly be divided into three phases. The first phase is the proliferative phase, during which spermatogonial stem cells undergo mitotic divisions to maintain the stem cell population and to produce spermatogonia cells ready to proceed for spermatogenesis (1,2). Thus, the proliferative phase is strongly committed to a cyclic and continual expansion of spermatogonia (3,4). The first division of spermatogenesis is known as spermatocytogenesis, and its function is to maintain a pool of stem cells and to produce spermatogonia for further proliferation and differentiation (5,6). Three types of spermatogonia have been described, which are type-A spermatogonia, intermediate-type and type-B spermatogonia (7–9). Type-A spermatogonia are primitive spermatogonia due to the absence of heterochromatin, while the intermediate spermatogonia have a lower amount of heterochromatin. Type-B spermatogonia possess a higher amount of heterochromatin and are highly differentiated. Type-A spermatogonia can be subdivided into A-single, A-paired and A-aligned spermatogonia, which differ only in their topographical arrangement on the basement membrane of the seminiferous tubule. Type-B spermatogonia enter into the meiosis phase by giving rise to primary spermatocyte after the mitotic division (8–10).

4.1.2 Entry of spermatogenic cells into meiosis

The transition of spermatogenesis from mitosis to meiosis is a highly coordinated and regulated process (11,12). During meiosis, the genetic material exchange takes place through recombination, and chromosome numbers are halved to form haploid gametes. Type-B spermatogonia entering meiotic prophase result in the formation of primary spermatocytes that passes through various stages like the preleptotene, leptotene, zygotene and pachytene stages. Active DNA synthesis and recombination of maternal and paternal DNA characterize this stage, resulting in the formation of 4n (tetraploid DNA content, diploid chromosome number) cells that have a genetic endowment different from their parent spermatogonia (13). These cells divide into two 2n (diploid DNA content, haploid chromosome number) secondary spermatocytes that further divide to produce two 1n (haploid DNA content, haploid chromosome number) haploid spermatids each (14,15).

4.1.3 Spermiogenesis and attainment of the motility appendage

Spermiogenesis is morphological differentiation of spermatids after completion of successful meiotic division to form the most physically and functionally differentiated haploid cells, called the spermatozoa (7–9). Round spermatids undergo a series of changes for their transition into spermatozoa. The process of spermiogenesis includes several steps, which could broadly be divided into (a) formation of acrosome by modification of lysosome, (b) changes in nucleus through condensation of genetic material and its movement toward the periphery of the cell, (c) reorganization of cellular contents and the cytoplasm,

and (d) development of a flagella or tail as a filamentous structure emanating from one pair of centrioles (14,15). In rats, spermiogenesis has been recognized as a nineteen-step metamorphosis of round spermatid to form a fully differentiated, flagellated sperm (16).

4.1.4 Spermatogenic wave

Spermatogenesis progresses in seminiferous tubules in the form of waves. A spermatogenic wave is usually described as the spatial arrangement or association of germ-cells along the tubule (17). A large number of spermatozoa are produced inside the seminiferous tubule in a form of wave known as a spermatogenic wave (18). The spermatogenic wave ensures the continual release of spermatozoa, which reduces the competition for space, hormone and metabolites at any specific stage (7).

4.2 GERM CELL APOPTOSIS

Apoptosis of the germ cell is necessary for the maintenance of a proper germ cell to Sertoli cell ratio, as well as for the elimination of abnormal germ cells formed by errors during mitotic and meiotic cell divisions. Normally, about 25%–75% of spermatogenic germ cells undergo apoptosis (19). Thus, a large number of germ cells are removed by apoptosis to ensure germ cell homeostasis (20,21). Apoptosis is either spontaneous for removal of surplus germ cells or takes place under stress caused by hormonal imbalance, temperature, radiation or toxicants. Rodents, like the rat, have been studied extensively for germ cell apoptosis during spermatogenesis (22). The spermatogenesis in rats is distinctly classified into 14 stages (stages I–XIV) and spermiogenesis with 19-step maturation (steps 1–19) of round spermatids into mature sperm. During spontaneous apoptosis, the pre-meiotic spermatogonia undergo apoptosis at their mitotic peaks, mostly at stages XII and XIV (23,24) in large numbers to maintain the germ cell homeostasis. An imbalance in germ cell to Sertoli cell ratio is known to cause severe male infertility (25). Spermatogonia seem to die during the G2 phase when the cell prepares itself for mitosis, and the depolymerization of the cytoskeletal elements takes place (26). Several reports have suggested that programmed cell death (PCD) or apoptosis is the sole path of germ cell death, which is distinct from necrosis and is necessary for the normal process of spermatogenesis (23,27). Gross membrane damage during necrosis causes inflammation and affects neighboring cells, while apoptosis is genetically encoded cell death that does not cause inflammation and is seen in scattered single cells without affecting the neighboring cells (23). When spermatogonia divide mitotically to differentiate into sperm, the progeny cells remain connected by cytoplasmic intercellular bridges through all the subsequent mitotic and meiotic divisions to form large clones of spermatogenic cells that develop synchronously (28,29). However, the apoptosis of a single cell induced spontaneously or by radiation does not affect the neighboring cells of the clone (30). Spermatocytes undergo apoptosis during preleptotene, leptotene, zygotene, pachytene and metaphase I, and spermatids at all steps of their maturation (23). Preleptotene, leptotene and zygotene spermatocytes have been considered as most sensitive to apoptosis at stages VII and VIII due to their active DNA synthesis for meiosis, chromosomal pairing and movement from basal to the adluminal compartment. Any error in DNA synthesis, chromosomal pairing or surplus number of cells crossing the blood-testis barrier results in cells receiving signals for apoptosis for maintaining the optimum germ cell to Sertoli cell ratio (23). Apoptotic pachytene spermatocytes have been seen at almost all the stages of spermatogenesis in rodents including stages I, II, VII–IX, XII and XIV (23), and stages VII and VIII (31), since these cells are committed to meiosis and need to maintain the integrity of genetic information. Postmeiotic spermatids are haploid cells that carry the paternal genetic information for transmission to the female gamete; hence, apoptosis is crucial at this stage to maintain the genetic integrity of spermatozoa. Apoptosis has been recorded in spermatids at steps 1, 2, 4, 5 (23) and at 10, 11, 19 during chromatin condensation (32).

Spontaneous death of testicular germ cells by apoptosis during normal spermatogenesis has also been studied in humans, and apoptosis has been reported in spermatogonia, spermatocytes and spermatids. The incidence was found to be higher in Chinese men than in Caucasian men though the differences were statistically nonsignificant (33,34). Since testosterone-sensitive stages of spermatogenesis were also involved in apoptosis, the study indirectly supported the greater efficacy of hormonal contraception in Chinese men than Caucasian men (33). Also, the rates of spermatocyte and spermatid apoptosis were higher in humans than

in rats (35) resulting in lower sperm output of the former (36). Spermatogonial cell apoptosis is also seen in normal, prepubertal human testis (37).

4.2.1 Pathways of apoptosis in testis

Apoptosis entails two major pathways; the first one is described as an extrinsic pathway and the second one as the intrinsic pathway. The extrinsic pathway is normally carried out by the extracellular ligand, FasL, which binds with the death receptor Fas that ultimately culminates in cell death. On the other side, the intrinsic pathway involves a signaling mechanism carried out by the mitochondria (Figure 4.1). Cytochrome c, an important protein released from mitochondria, is the main initiator of apoptosis leading to the activation of caspase-9 that results in the activation of a series of caspases including caspase-3, which leads to germ cell death (38,39). The apoptotic machinery includes a complex network of different proteins including the Bcl-2 family proteins, the caspases, cytochrome c, which along with the mitochondria constitute the intracellular system of apoptosis (40).

4.2.2 Fas/FasL system: Central regulator of testicular germ cell population

The throttle mechanism of germ cell loss occurs during different stages, and approximately 25%–75% apoptotic germ cell death occurs during the course of spermatogenesis (41). The Fas/FasL signal transduction system is the key pathway for germ cell apoptosis in the testis (42,43). Sertoli cells generally have full control over the apoptosis of developing germ cell population through the activation of the Fas/FasL system. Fas (APO-1, CD95) is a member of the tumor

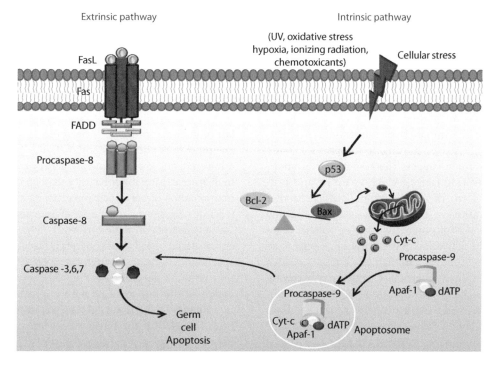

Figure 4.1 The extrinsic and intrinsic pathways of testicular germ cell apoptosis.

necrosis factor (TNF) family, which possesses a "death domain" close to the carboxy-terminal region (44,45). It is a transmembrane protein with two to six cysteine-rich extracellular domains that carry the signal when bound to FasL. FasL (Fas ligand, CD95L) is a 40KD transmembrane protein belonging to the TNF family that binds with Fas and initiates its trimerization (46). In rats, spermatocytes and few spermatogonia show high expression levels of Fas associated with activation of caspases 8, 9, 3, 6 and 2, predisposing them to apoptosis by extrinsic or intrinsic pathways (47,48). The Fas ligand is expressed on the surface of Sertoli cells, and Fas receptors are present on spermatogenic cells (49). During the process of "shedding," the Fas ligand/CD95L undergoes processing for activation and becomes accessible to its receptor (50,51). Sertoli cells expressing FasL initiate apoptosis of germ cells expressing Fas (42) when Fas-FasL get in line with each other, thereafter recruiting the Fas-associated death domain (FADD). FADD comes up with a dimerized form of procaspase-8 leading to the formation of a death-inducing signaling complex (DISC). Caspase-8 endows its proteolytic action on its downstream effector caspases 3 and 7 in their mature forms and comes with its autoactivation. The effector caspases cause transition to cell death by apoptosis, and key takeaways of apoptosis characterized by DNA fragmentation, condensation of cytoplasm, etc., are observed. The resulting debris are taken up by the cell and degraded inside the phagosomes.

4.2.3 Activation of caspase-9 via the intrinsic pathway

This pathway serves to remove germ cells in response to external and internal stimuli, leading to mitochondrial permeabilization, which causes leakage of cytochrome c and activation of caspase-9. Mitochondria are armed with both proapoptotic and antiapoptotic machinery, which governs the cell fate (52). Cytochrome c is the most prominent among these (45) that get transported into the intermembranous space of mitochondria. The permeability of the mitochondria allows the cytochrome c to cross the outer mitochondrial membrane into the cytosol. This is a critical event for the initiation of mitochondria-dependent activation of caspases leading to apoptosis (53,54). Cytosolic cytochrome c triggers the association of apoptotic protease activating factor (APAF-1), dATP and procaspase-9 (55) to form the "apoptosome," which further triggers the activation of the caspase cascade entailing cell death (56,57). Apoptosome, an adapter protein complex, carries out the activation of the initiator caspase (caspase-9) (58). Apoptosome is a multimeric complex, which includes Apaf-1 (apoptotic protease activating factor-1), procaspase-9, cytochrome c and dATP/ATP. The binding of cytochrome c and the hydrolysis of dATP induce a conformational change in Apaf-1 to unmask the caspase activation domain recruitment domain (CARD) at the C-terminal. The N-terminal CARD of Apaf-1 is proposed to function via interaction with the prodomain of

procaspase-9, resulting in its activation (59). The activated caspase-9 gets detached from its complex, cleaves and activates its downstream executioner caspases 3, 6 and 7. The male germ cells respond to extracellular stimuli through changes in the internal environment, which decide the fate of the cell. In the course of the first wave of spermatogenesis, Bax is shown to be necessary for normal spermatogenesis, and its expression is increased on those cells, which are destined to undergo apoptosis. Studies have revealed that the Bax knockout mice possess a high number of spermatogonia and preleptotene spermatocytes due to failure of apoptosis during the first wave of spermatogenesis, and their spermatogenesis is unable to proceed normally (60). Insulin-like growth factor binding protein-3 (IGFBP-3) and Bax interaction activates germ cell apoptosis by the mitochondrial pathway (61). Another study has shown that phosphorylation of BCL2 at serine residue and activation of the MAPK14-mediated mitochondria-dependent pathway regulate male germ cell death in monkeys (61). The Bcl-2 family includes both proapoptotic (Bax, Bak, Bcl-$_{xs}$ and Bad) and antiapoptotic (Bcl-2, Bcl-$_{XL}$, Mcl and M1) proteins, which are important for germ cell apoptosis (62). The ratio of pro- and antiapoptotic proteins decides whether a cell would survive or undergo apoptotic cell death (63,64). A high Bcl-2/Bax ratio results in cell survival, and on the contrary, a high Bax/Bcl-2 ratio leads to cell death (65). A dynamic change in Bcl-2 family proteins is continuous during the first cycle of spermatogenesis. The competitive action of proapoptotic and antiapoptotic Bcl-2 family proteins controls the activation of caspases and apoptosis (66).

In humans, Bcl-2 and Bak are preferentially expressed in spermatocytes and differentiating spermatids, Bcl-x is expressed in spermatogonia, while Bax is seen in nuclei of round spermatids, which indicates a specific role of these proteins in spermatogenesis (67) through spontaneous apoptosis and germ cell homeostasis.

4.2.4 P53 and spermatogenic cell apoptosis

The tumor suppressor protein p53 plays an important role in mammalian spermatogenesis and acts as a guardian of genome integrity. It has been shown that p53 plays an important role in testicular germ cell apoptosis. With a lowered rate of spontaneous germ cell apoptosis, p53$^{-/-}$ male mice exhibit lower fertility than p53$^{+/+}$ (68), indicating maintenance of germ cell integrity by spontaneous apoptosis during spermatogenesis. Overexpression of p53 may cause infertility in male cattle-yak (69). Testicular atrophy encountered in p53 knockout rats is plausibly due to elevated spermatocyte death, though the spermatogonial proliferation remains normal (70). But p53 gene polymorphism in codon 72 did not correlate with idiopathic male infertility in humans (71,72). In rats, strong p53 immunoreactivity has been reported in the nuclei of several spermatogonia and premeiotic spermatocytes, and almost all spermatids, which has been correlated with their susceptibility to spontaneous apoptosis for quality control (72).

4.3 EXECUTIONER CASPASES

Caspases are the initiators and executioners of apoptosis. They are synthesized in the form of procaspases, which get activated during the apoptotic process (73). These procaspases contain three domains: an NH_2 domain and the p20 and p10 domains. Caspases are cysteine proteases that cleave their substrate protein after the aspartic acid residue that leads to cell death (45). The executioner caspases exist in the cytosol in the form of inactive dimers, and their activation is carried out by the initiator caspases through proteolytic cleavage of its catalytic domain to an active scaffold. The proteolytic cleavage allows the rearrangement of its mobile loop conferring it the catalytic activity (74,75). In the cytosol, caspase-3 and caspase-7 exist in their dimeric forms, and activation is through the cleavage within their respective linker segments (76). In human testis biopsies, effector caspase-7 seemed to be absent from normal human testes, whereas procaspase-3 and procaspase-6 were detected in germ cells. Increased germ cell apoptosis in patients with the spermatogenic arrest was associated with increased levels of active caspase-3, which indicates that caspase-3 is the major executioner of apoptosis in human infertility (77).

Similarly, in rodents also caspase-3 appears to be the major executioner of apoptosis (78,79).

4.4 APOPTOSIS OF GERM CELLS CAUSED BY HORMONAL, TEMPERATURE AND CHEMICAL INSULT

Spontaneous apoptosis of male germ cells under normal conditions maintains the required germ cell to Sertoli cell ratio and also maintains the quality of spermatozoa by removing surplus/defective cells. However, the apoptotic process is augmented during a variety of stress conditions, e.g., hormonal variations, heat stress and/or treatment with antispermatogenic chemicals. A brief account of testicular germ cell apoptosis under different stress conditions is discussed with emphasis on the susceptible spermatogenic cell type and the mechanism of action (Figure 4.2).

4.4.1 Hormonal variations

Gonadotrophins act as survival factors for spermatogonia by regulating the intrinsic pathway, though they do not promote cellular proliferation in normal men (80). Testicular germ

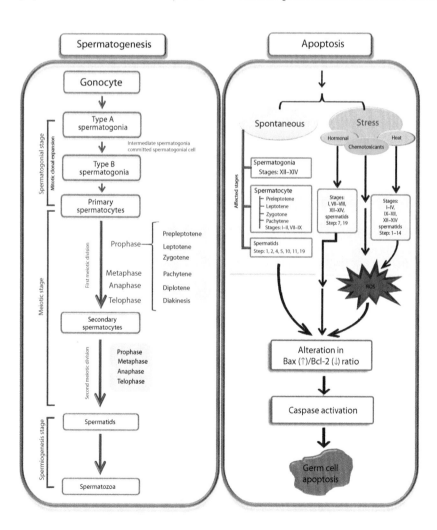

Figure 4.2 Spermatogenic phases and their susceptibility to spontaneous and stress apoptosis.

cell apoptosis caused by immunization against gonadotrophin-releasing hormone (GnRH) in boars (81) caused significant reduction in LH and testosterone levels, with a twofold increase in apoptosis of spermatogonia (except type-A spermatogonia) and pachytene spermatocytes (82). Similarly, treatment with GnRH antagonist in rats (83) caused apoptosis of spermatocytes mainly at stages I and XII-XIV compared with stage VIII (84) that could be corrected largely by the administration of exogenous estradiol and testosterone (83). Another study detected apoptosis at preleptotene and pachytene spermatocytes, and step 7 and 19 spermatids at stages VII and VIII (85,86). However, maximum inhibition of spermatogenesis was achieved by coadministration of an antiandrogen (flutamide) with a long-acting GnRH antagonist, with significant germ cell apoptosis at stages VII–VIII accompanied by reduced preleptotene and pachytene spermatocytes, as well as round spermatids (87). GnRH agonist buserelin caused apoptosis of testicular germ cells in rats (88). Spermatogonial apoptosis is induced by suppressing FSH, and the pathway of cell death is predominantly via the intrinsic pathway accompanied with lowered BCL2 (89) and increased caspase activity (90). Suppression of endogenous testosterone production by exogenous testosterone and progestin administration causes inhibition of spermatogenesis with mass germ cell apoptosis and has shown the potential of male contraception. Apoptosis was seen in all the germ cell types with the level of apoptosis being in spermatid > spermatocyte > spermatogonia (91). Progestin induces germ cell apoptosis at stages I–IV and XII–XIV, while testosterone stimulates apoptosis at stages VII–VIII (92). The mechanism of programmed cell death was through both extrinsic and intrinsic pathways of apoptosis with upregulation of caspases 8, 9 and 3, accompanied with increased levels of Fas/FasL and Bax proteins (93).

4.4.2 Heat stress

The germ cell apoptotic index in normal rats is augmented several-folds by mild hyperthermia within 24–48 hours with apoptosis, which is seen predominantly at stages I–IV and XII–XIV, while stages V–VI and VII–VIII are reported to be relatively resistant to heat stress. Pachytene spermatocytes (at stages I–IV and IX–XII), diplotene spermatocytes (at stages XIII–XIV), and round spermatids (steps 1–4) were the most susceptible cell types to heat (94). Apoptosis was initiated by movement of Bax from the cytoplasmic to the perinuclear region after heating, with Bcl-2 being redistributed to the cytoplasmic and nuclear compartments in heat-susceptible cells (95). Both constitutive and inducible heat shock proteins HSP70/70i were unable to protect spermatocytes and spermatids from apoptosis caused by heat stress (96). Fibroblast growth factor-4 and lactate were shown to act as antiapoptotic agents for germ cells under heat stress (97). Lactate is known to protect testicular germ cells from apoptosis in humans via the Fas/FasL pathway (98), and heat stress is known to increase lactate production by Sertoli cells (62).

4.5 TESTICULAR TOXICANTS AND GERM CELL APOPTOSIS

Germ cell apoptosis is massively upregulated in the testis by the influence of a variety of testicular toxicants, which include chemicals and radiations. The Fas/FasL system of germ cell apoptosis has been shown to be upregulated in the testis after treatment with a testicular toxicant. Fas was overexpressed in germ cells after exposure to radiation, and both Fas and FasL were upregulated in germ cells and Sertoli cells, respectively, after treatment with mono-(2-ethylhexyl) phthalate and 2,5-hexanedione (99). Mono(2-ethylhexyl) phthalate (MEHP) targets germ cells indirectly through Sertoli cells. An initial inhibition of germ cell apoptosis after MEHP treatment is followed by significantly enhanced apoptosis, which is caused by the detachment of germ cells from Sertoli cells. The initial drop in apoptosis could be due to disconnection from the Fas/FasL system controlled by Sertoli cells, which is followed by massive apoptosis of germ cells by autocrine mechanisms (100), perhaps involving the intrinsic pathway. Translocation of Fas from the cytosolic to the membrane fraction of the testis has been seen after MEHP treatment (100). Methoxyacetic acid causes a significant increase in apoptosis of germ cells, mainly at the pachytene spermatocyte stage of mice (101), rats and humans (102). Endocrine disruptors like bBisphenol-A and nonylphenol that are ubiquitously distributed in plastic products used by humans, induce testicular germ cell apoptosis at spermatocyte and spermatogonial stages, respectively, and reduce sperm output (103). Most of the testicular toxicants including cadmium, bisphenol A, perfluorooctanesulfonate, phthalates, glycerol and some male contraceptive candidates like adjudin and gamendazole, induce testicular germ cell apoptosis partly by disrupting Sertoli cell–germ cell and/or Sertoli cell–Sertoli cell junctions (104).

4.6 CONCLUSION

Spontaneous germ cell apoptosis in the normal testis is a critical process to limit the germ cell clones to a number that can be supported by the fixed population of Sertoli cells and also to eliminate germ cells with defective DNA integrity or chromosomal pairing. This is a very critical step in normal spermatogenesis, and its inhibition results in disruption of spermatogenesis and male fertility. The Sertoli cell number determines the spermatogenic output, as these cells remain intimately associated with the spermatogenic cells and support sperm production by providing metabolic, nutritional, physical and paracrine support. The Fas/FasL pathway is a major regulator of germ cell apoptosis and is under the control of Sertoli cells, which express FasL that binds to Fas expressed on germ cells, and initiates cell death. Both the extrinsic and intrinsic pathways of cell apoptosis regulate the spermatogenic cell number mainly with the help of initiator and executioner caspases. During the course of this pursuit, both the effector and initiator caspases share a common feature of their catalytic activation, but they achieve this activation by different mechanistic pathways. Initiator caspases require their activation by means of apoptosome, which is an adapter protein complex, while effector caspases are activated via interchain cleavage. Mitochondria play an essential role in cell death by the intrinsic pathway, with the release of cytochrome c and translocation of Bcl-2 family proteins. The antiapoptotic Bcl-2 family proteins like Bcl-$_{XL}$ prevent leakage of cytochrome c into the cytosol, while the proapoptotic proteins like Bax facilitate the process to maintain the optimal Sertoli cell to germ cell ratio and eliminate superfluous spermatogenic cells or cells with a genetic defect. These mechanisms are upregulated to enhance the apoptosis of germ cells under stressful conditions of hormonal imbalance, increased temperature and treatment with testicular toxicants. However, the germ cell type and the stages of spermatogenesis are differentially susceptible to various kinds of antispermatogenic stimuli.

REFERENCES

1. Print CG, Loveland KL, Gibson L, Meehan T, Stylianou A, Wreford N et al. Apoptosis regulator bcl-w is essential for spermatogenesis but appears otherwise redundant. *Proc Natl Acad Sci USA*. 1998 Oct 13;95(21):12424–31.
2. Wistuba J, Stukenborg JB, Luetjens C. Mammalian spermatogenesis. *Funct Dev Embryol*. 2007;1:99–117.
3. Amann RP. The cycle of the seminiferous review epithelium in humans: A need to revisit? *J Androl*. 2008 Sep–Oct;29(5):469–87.
4. O'Donnell L, Robertson KM, Jones ME, Simpson ER. Estrogen and spermatogenesis. *Endocrine Rev*. 2001 Jun;22(3):289–318.
5. AtiaTarek AM. Review: Genetics of spermatogenesis. *Scholars J Appl Med Sci (SJAMS)*. 2014;2:1171–81.
6. D'Cruz SC, Vaithinathan S, Jubendradass R, Mathur PP. Effects of plants and plant products on the testis. *Asian J Androl*. 2010;12(4):468–79.
7. Johnson L. Efficiency of spermatogenesis. *Microsc Res Tech*. 1995 Dec 1;32(5):385–422.
8. O'Donnell L, Stanton P, de Kretser DM. Endocrinology of the male reproductive system and spermatogenesis. In: McLachlan R (ed.), *Endocrinology of the Male Reproductive System*. South Dartmouth, MA: Endotext; 2013, pp. 1–57.
9. Rato L, Alves MG, Socorro S, Duarte AI, Cavaco JE, Oliveira PF. Metabolic regulation is important for spermatogenesis. Nature review. *Urology*. 2012 May 1;9(6):330–8.
10. Phillips BT, Gassei K, Orwig KE. Spermatogonial stem cell regulation and spermatogenesis. *Philos Trans the R Soc Lond B, Biol Sci*. 2010 May 27;365(1546):1663–78.
11. Chu DS, Shakes DC. Spermatogenesis. *Adv Exp Med Biol*. 2013 June;757:171–203.
12. Griswold MD (ed.). The initiation of spermatogenesis and the cycle of the seminiferous epithelium. *Sertoli Cell Biol*. 2015 December; 2nd Edition, 233–45. Elsevier Inc, Amsterdam, Netherlands.
13. Chocu S, Calvel P, Rolland AD, Pineau C. Spermatogenesis in mammals: Proteomic insights. *Syst Biol Reprod Med*. 2012 Aug;58(4):179–90.
14. DeKretser DM, Loveland KL, Meinhardt A, Simorangkir D, Wreford N. Spermatogenesis. *Human Reprod*. 1998 Apr 1;13(suppl_1):1–8.
15. Amann RP. A critical review of methods for evaluation of spermatogenesis from seminal characteristics. *J Androl*. 1981 Feb;2:37–58.
16. Leblond CP, Clermont Y. Definition of the stages of the cycle of the seminiferous epithelium in the rat. *Ann NY Acad Sci*. 1952 Nov 20;55(4):548–73.
17. Staub C, Hue D, Nicolle JC, Perrard-Sapori MH, Segretain D, Durand P. The whole meiotic process can occur in vitro in untransformed rat spermatogenic cells. *Exp Cell Res*. 2000 Oct 10;260(1):85–95.
18. Hai Y, Hou J, Liu Y, Liu Y, Yang H, Li Z, He Z. The roles and regulation of Sertoli cells in fate determinations of spermatogonial stem cells and spermatogenesis. *Semin Cell Dev Biol*. 2014 May;29:66–75.
19. Shaha C, Tripathi R, Mishra DP. Male germ cell apoptosis: Regulation and biology. *Phil Trans R Soc Lond B Biol Sci*. 2010 May 27;365(1546):1501–15.
20. Alves MG, Rato L, Carvalho RA, Moreira PI, Socorro S, Oliveira PF. Hormonal control of Sertoli cell metabolism regulates spermatogenesis. *Cell Mol Life Sci*. 2013 Mar;70(5):777–93.
21. Feng L, Yang Y. Origin and Quantitative Control of Sertoli Cells. 2017 June. https://arxiv.org/ftp/arxiv/papers/1706/1706.00721.pdf
22. Francavilla S, D'Abrizio P, Cordeschi G, Pelliccione F, Necozione S, Ulisse S, Properzi G, Francavilla F. Fas expression correlates with human germ cell degeneration in meiotic and post meiotic arrest of spermatogenesis. *Mol Hum Reprod*. 2002 Mar;8(3):213–20.
23. Blanco-Rodríguez J, Martínez-García C. Spontaneous germ cell death in the testis of the adult rat takes the form of apoptosis: Re-evaluation of cell types that exhibit the ability to die during spermatogenesis. *Cell Prolif*. 1996 Jan;29(1):13–31.
24. Hentrich A, Wolter M, Szardening-Kirchner C, Lüers GH, Bergmann M, Kliesch S, Konrad L. Reduced numbers of Sertoli, germ, and spermatogonial stem cells in impaired spermatogenesis. *Modern Pathol*. 2011 Oct;24(10):1380–9.
25. Aitken RJ, Baker MA. Causes and consequences of apoptosis in spermatozoa; contributions to infertility and impacts on development. *Int J Dev Biol*. 2013;57(2–4):265–72.
26. Huckins C. The morphology and kinetics of spermatogonial degeneration in normal adult rats: An analysis using a simplified classification of the germinal epithelium. *Anat Rec*. 1978 Apr;190(4):905–26.
27. Xiong W, Wang H, Wu H, Chen Y, Han D. Apoptotic spermatogenic cells can be energy sources for Sertoli cells. *Reproduction*. 2009 Mar;137(3):469–79.

28. Shimizu S, Konishi A, Kodama T, Tsujimoto Y. BH4 domain of antiapoptotic Bcl-2 family members closes voltage-dependent anion channel and inhibits apoptotic mitochondrial changes and cell death. *Proc Natl Acad Sci USA.* 2000 Mar 28;97(7):3100–5.

29. Shiratsuchi A, Umeda M, Ohba Y, Nakanishi Y. Recognition of phosphatidylserine on the surface of apoptotic spermatogenic cells and subsequent phagocytosis by Sertoli cells of the rat. *J Biol Chem.* 1997 Jan 24;272(4):2354–8.

30. Hamer G, Roepers-Gajadien HL, Gademan IS, Kal HB, De Rooij DG. Intercellular bridges and apoptosis in clones of male germ cells. *Int J Androl.* 2003 Dec;26(6):348–53.

31. Kerr JB. Spontaneous degeneration of germ cells in normal rat testis: Assessment of cell types and frequency during the spermatogenic cycle. *J Reprod Fertil.* 1992 Aug;95(3):825–30.

32. Russell LD, Malone JP, Karpas SL. Morphological pattern elicited by agents affecting spermatogenesis by disruption of its hormonal stimulation. *Tissue Cell.* 1981 Jan 1;13(2):369–80.

33. Hikim AP, Wang C, Lue Y, Johnson L, Wang XH, Swerdloff RS. Spontaneous germ cell apoptosis in humans: Evidence for ethnic differences in the susceptibility of germ cells to programmed cell death. *J Clin Endocrinol Metab.* 1998 Jan;83(1):152–6.

34. Svingen T, Koopman P. Building the mammalian testis: Origins, differentiation, and assembly of the component cell populations. *Gene Dev.* 2013 Nov 15;27(22):2409–26.

35. SinhaHikim AP, Wang C, Lue YH, Johnson L, Wang XH, Swerdloff RS. Spontaneous germ cell apoptosis in human evidence for ethnic differences in the susceptibility of germ cells to programmed cell death. *J Clin Endocrinol Metab.* 1998 Jan;83(1):152–6

36. Johnson L, Petty CS, Neaves WB. A comparative study of daily sperm production and testicular composition in humans and rats. *Biol Reprod.* 1980 Jun;22(5):1233–43.

37. Heiskanen P, Billig H, Toppari J, Kaleva M, Arsalo A, Rapola J, Dunkel L. Apoptotic cell death in the normal and cryptorchid human testis: The effect of human chorionic gonadotropin on testicular cell survival. *Pediatr Res.* 1996 Aug;40(2):351.

38. Bejarano I, Rodríguez AB, Pariente JA. Apoptosis is a demanding selective tool during the development of fetal male germ cells. *Front Cell Dev Biol.* 2018 Jun 28;6:65.

39. Czabotar PE, Lessene G, Strasser A, Adams JM. Control of apoptosis by the BCL-2 protein family: Implications for physiology and therapy. *Nat Rev: Mol Cell Biol.* 2014 Jan;15(1):49–63.

40. Antonsson B, Montessuit S, Lauper S, Eskes R, Martinou JC. Bax oligomerization is required for channel-forming activity in liposomes and to trigger cytochrome c release from mitochondria. *Biochem J.* 2000 Jan 15;345(Pt 2):271–8.

41. Koji T. Male germ cell death in mouse testes: Possible involvement of Fas and Fas ligand. *Med Electron Microsc.* 2001 Dec;34(4):213–22.

42. Lee J, Richburg JH, Younkin SC, Boekelheide K. The Fas system is a key regulator of germ cell apoptosis in the testis. *Endocrinology.* 1997 May 1;138(5):2081–8.

43. Kiess W, Gallaher B. Hormonal control of programmed cell death/apoptosis. *Eur J Endocrinol.* 1998 May;138(5):482–91.

44. Vaishnaw AK, Orlinick JR, Chu JL, Krammer PH, Chao MV, Elkon KB. The molecular basis for apoptotic defects in patients with CD95 (Fas/Apo-1) mutations. *J Clin Investig.* 1999 Feb 1;103(3):355–63.

45. Hengartner MO. The biochemistry of apoptosis. *Nature.* 2000 June 12;407:770–6.

46. Schneider P, Bodmer JL, Holler N, Mattmann C, Scuderi P, Terskikh A, Peitsch MC, Tschopp J. Characterization of Fas (Apo-1, CD95)-Fas ligand interaction. *J Biol Chem.* 1997 Jul 25;272(30):18827–33.

47. Lizama C, Alfaro I, Reyes JG, Moreno RD. Up-regulation of CD95 (Apo-1/Fas) is associated with spermatocyte apoptosis during the first round of spermatogenesis in the rat. *Apoptosis.* 2007 Mar;12(3):499–512.

48. Orlinick JR, Elkon KB, Chao MV. Separate domains of the human Fas ligand dictate self-association and receptor binding. *J Biol Chem.* 1997 Dec 19;272(51):32221–9.

49. Rojas J, Lizbeth, Fahiel C, Socorro RM. Stress and cell death in testicular cells. *Androl (Los Angel).* 2017 Jun 10;6:183.

50. Kierszenbaum AL. Apoptosis during spermatogenesis: The thrill of being alive. *Molecular Reprod Dev.* 2001 Jan;58(1):1–3.

51. Wang M, Su P. The role of the Fas/FasL signaling pathway in environmental toxicant-induced testicular cell apoptosis: An update. *Syst Biol Reprod Med.* 2018 Apr;64(2):93–102.

52. Green DR. Apoptotic pathways: Paper wraps stone blunts scissors. *Cell.* 2000 Jul 7;102(1):1–4.

53. Vander Heiden MG, Thompson CB. Bcl-2 proteins: Regulators of apoptosis or of mitochondrial homeostasis? *Nat Cell Biol.* 1999 Dec;1(8):E209–16.

54. Kumar S. Mechanisms mediating caspase activation in cell death. *Cell Death Differ.* 1999 Nov;6(11):1060–6.

55. McDonnell MA, Wang D, Khan SM, Vander Heiden MG, Kelekar A. Caspase-9 is activated in a cytochrome c-independent manner early during TNFα-induced apoptosis in murine cells. *Cell Death Differ.* 2003 Sep;10(9):1005.

56. Joza N, Susin SA, Daugas E, Stanford WL, Cho SK, Li CY et al. Essential role of the mitochondrial apoptosis-inducing factor in programmed cell death. *Nature.* 2001 Mar 29;410(6828):549–54.

57. Thornberry NA, Lazebnik Y. Caspases: Enemies within. *Science.* 1998 Aug 28;281(5381):1312–6.

58. Bao Q, Shi Y. Apoptosome: A platform for the activation of initiator caspases. *Cell Death Differ.* 2007 Jan;14(1):56–65.

59. Budihardjo I, Oliver H, Lutter M, Luo X, Wang X. Biochemical pathways of caspase activation during apoptosis. *Annu Rev Cell Dev Biol.* 1999;15:269–90.

60. Print CG, Loveland KL. Germ cell suicide: New insights into apoptosis during spermatogenesis. *Bioessays: News Rev Mol, Cell Dev Biol.* 2000 May;22(5):423–30.

61. Jia Y, Lee KW, Swerdloff R, Hwang D, Cobb LJ, SinhaHikim A, Lue YH, Cohen P, Wang C. Interaction of insulin-like growth factor-binding protein-3 and BAX in mitochondria promotes male germ cell apoptosis. *J Biol Chem.* 2010 Jan 15;285(3):1726–32.

62. Tsujimoto Y, Shimizu S. Bcl-2 family: Life-or-death switch. *Federation Eur Biochem Soc.* 2000 Jan 21;466(1):6–10.

63. SinhaHikim AP, Swerdloff RS. Hormonal and genetic control of germ cell apoptosis in the testis. *Rev Reprod.* 1999 Jan;4(1):38–47.

64. Vaithinathan S, D'Cruz SC, Mathur PP. Apoptosis and male infertility. In: Parekattil SJ and Agarwal A (eds.), *Male Infertility: Contemporary Clinical Approaches, Androl, ART & Antioxidants.* New York, NY: Springer, 2012; pp. 329–36.

65. Xu YR, Dong HS, Yang WX. Regulators in the apoptotic pathway during spermatogenesis: Killers or guards? *Gene.* 2016 May 15;582(2):97–111.

66. Yan W, Samson M, Jégou B, Toppari J. Bcl-w forms complexes with Bax and Bak, and elevated ratios of Bax/Bcl-w and Bak/Bcl-w correspond to spermatogonial and spermatocyte apoptosis in the testis. *Mol Endocrinol.* 2000 May;14(5):682–99.

67. Oldereid NB, Angelis PD, Wiger R, Clausen OP. Expression of Bcl-2 family proteins and spontaneous apoptosis in normal human testis. *Mol Hum Reprod.* 2001 May;7(5):403–8.

68. Yin Y, Stahl BC, DeWolf WC, Morgentaler A. p53-mediated germ cell quality control in spermatogenesis. *Dev Biol.* 1998 Dec 1;204(1):165–71.

69. Liu P, Yu S, Cui Y, He J, Zhang Q, Sun J et al. Regulation by Hsp27/P53 in testis development and sperm apoptosis of male cattle (cattle-yak and yak). *J Cell Physiol.* 2018 Jan;234(1):650–60.

70. Dai MS, Hall SJ, VantangoliPolicelli MM, Boekelheide K, Spade DJ. Spontaneous testicular atrophy occurs despite normal spermatogonial proliferation in a Tp53 knockout rat. *Andrology.* 2017 Nov;5(6):1141–52.

71. Luciano RP, Wajchenberg M, Almeida SS, Amorim CE, Rodrigues LM, Araujo RC, Puertas EB, Faloppa F. Genetic ACE I/D and ACTN3 R577X polymorphisms and adolescent idiopathic scoliosis. *Genet Mol Res.* 2016 Nov 3;15(4).

72. Stephan H, Polzar B, Rauch F, Zanotti S, Ulke C, Mannherz HG. Distribution of deoxyribonuclease-I (DNase I) and p53 in rat testis and their correlation with apoptosis. *Histochem Cell Biol.* 1996 Oct;106(4):383–93.

73. Jiang X, Wang X. Cytochrome c promotes caspase-9 activation by inducing nucleotide binding to Apaf-1. *J Biol Chem.* 2000 Oct 6;275(40):31199–203.

74. Pop C, Salvesen GS. Human caspases: Activation, specificity, and regulation. *J Biol Chem.* 2009 Aug 14;284(33):21777–81.

75. Parone PA, James D, Martinou JC. Mitochondria: Regulating the inevitable. *Biochimie.* 2002 Feb–Mar;84(2–3):105–11.

76. Boatright KM, Salvesen GS. Mechanisms of caspase activation. *Curr Opin Cell Biol.* 2003 Dec;15(6):725–31.

77. Bozec A, Amara S, Guarmit B, Selva J, Albert M, Rollet J et al. Status of the executioner step of apoptosis in human with normal spermatogenesis and azoospermia. *Fertil Steril.* 2008 Nov;90(5):1723–31.

78. Xiong Q, Xie P, Li H, Hao L, Li G, Qiu T, Liu Y. Involvement of Fas/FasL system in apoptotic signaling in testicular germ cells of male Wistar rats injected i.v. with microcystins. *Toxicon.* 2009 Jul;54(1):1–7.

79. Juárez-Rojas AL, García-Lorenzana M, Aragón-Martínez A, Gómez-Quiroz LE, Retana-Márquez Mdel S. Intrinsic and extrinsic apoptotic pathways are involved in rat testis by cold water immersion-induced acute and chronic stress. *Syst Biol Reprod Med.* 2015;61(4):211–21.

80. Ruwanpura SM, McLachlan RI, Matthiesson KL, Meachem SJ. Gonadotrophins regulate germ cell survival, not proliferation, in normal adult men. *Human Reprod.* 2008(a) Feb;23(2):403–11.

81. Wagner A, Messe N, Bergmann M, Lekhkota O, Claus R. Effects of estradiol infusion in GnRH immunized boars on spermatogenesis. *J Androl.* 2006 Nov–Dec;27(6):880–9.

82. Wagner A, Claus R. Involvement of glucocorticoids in testicular involution after active immunization of boars against GnRH. *J Androl.* 2004 Feb;127(2):275–83.

83. Walczak-Jedrzejowska R, Kula K, Oszukowska E, Marchlewska K, Kula W, Slowikowska-Hilczer J. Testosterone and oestradiol in concert protect seminiferous tubule maturation against inhibition by GnRH-antagonist. *Int J Androl.* 2011 Oct;34(5 Pt 2):e378–85.

84. Billig H, Furuta I, Rivier C, Tapanainen J, Parvinen M, Hsueh AJ. Apoptosis in testis germ cells: Developmental changes in gonadotropin dependence and localization to selective tubule stages. *Endocrinology.* 1995 Jan;136(1):5–12.

85. Hikim AP, Wang C, Leung A, Swerdloff RS. Involvement of apoptosis in the induction of germ cell degeneration in adult rats after gonadotropin-releasing hormone antagonist treatment. *Endocrinology.* 1995 Jun;136(6):2770–5.

86. Sasagawa I, Yazawa H, Suzuki Y, Nakada T. Stress and testicular germ cell apoptosis. *Archives of Androl.* 2001 Nov–Dec;47(3):211–6.

87. Hikim AP, Vera Y, Elhag RI, Lue Y, Cui YG, Pope V, Leung A, Atienza V, Wang C, Swerdloff RS. Mouse model of male germ cell apoptosis in response to a lack of hormonal stimulation. *Indian J Exp Biol.* 2005 Nov;43(11):1048–57.

88. Peirouvi T, Salami S. GnRH agonist induces apoptosis in seminiferous tubules of immature rats: Direct gonadal action. *Andrologia.* 2010 Aug;42(4):231–5.

89. Ruwanpura SM, McLachlan RI, Stanton PG, Meachem SJ. Follicle-stimulating hormone affects spermatogonial survival by regulating the intrinsic apoptotic pathway in adult rats. *Biol Reprod.* 2008(b) Apr;78(4):705–13.

90. Ruwanpura SM, McLachlan RI, Stanton PG, Loveland KL, Meachem SJ. Pathways involved in testicular germ cell apoptosis in immature rats after FSH suppression. *J Endocrinol.* 2008(c) Apr;197(1):35–43.

91. Ilyas S, Lestari SW, Moeloek N, Asmarinah, Siregar NC. Induction of rat germ cell apoptosis by testosterone undecanoate and depot medroxyprogesterone acetate and correlation of apoptotic cells with sperm concentration. *Acta Medica Indonesiana.* 2013 Jan;45(1):32–7.

92. Lue Y, Wang C, Lydon JP, Leung A, Li J, Swerdloff RS. Functional role of progestin and the progesterone receptor in the suppression of spermatogenesis in rodents. *Andrology.* 2013 Mar;1(2):308–17.

93. Meena R, Misro MM, Ghosh D. Complete sperm suppression in rats with dienogest plus testosterone undecanoate is facilitated through apoptosis in testicular cells. *Reprod Sci.* 2013 Jul;20(7):771–80.

94. Lue YH, Hikim AP, Swerdloff RS, Im P, Taing KS, Bui T, Leung A, Wang C. Single exposure to heat induces stage-specific germ cell apoptosis in rats: Role of intra testicular testosterone on stage specificity. *Endocrinology.* 1999 Apr;140(4):1709–17.

95. Yamamoto CM, SinhaHikim AP, Huynh PN, Shapiro B, Lue Y, Salameh WA, Wang C, Swerdloff RS. Redistribution of Bax is an early step in an apoptotic pathway leading to germ cell death in rats, triggered by mild testicular hyperthermia. *Biol Reprod.* 2000 Dec;63(6):1683–90.

96. Widlak W, Winiarski B, Krawczyk A, Vydra N, Malusecka E, Krawczyk Z. Inducible 70 kDa heat shock protein does not protect spermatogenic cells from damage induced by cryptorchidism. *Int J Androl.* 2007 Apr;30(2):80–7.

97. Hirai K, Sasaki H, Yamamoto H, Sakamoto H, Kubota Y, Kakizoe T, Terada M, Ochiya T. HST-1/FGF-4 protects male germ cells from apoptosis under heat-stress condition. *Exp Cell Res.* 2004 Mar 10;294(1):77–85.

98. Erkkilä K, Aito H, Aalto K, Pentikäinen V, Dunkel L. Lactate inhibits germ cell apoptosis in the human testis. *Mol Hum Reprod.* 2002 Feb;8(2):109–17.

99. Lee J, Richburg JH, Shipp EB, Meistrich ML, Boekelheide K. The Fas system, a regulator of testicular germ cell apoptosis, is differentially up-regulated in Sertoli cell versus germ cell injury of the testis. *Endocrinology.* 1999 Feb;140(2):852–8.

100. Richburg JH. The relevance of spontaneous and chemically induced alterations in testicular germ cell apoptosis to toxicology. *Toxicol Lett.* 2000 Mar 15;112–113:79–86.

101. Krishnamurthy H, Weinbauer GF, Aslam H, Yeung CH, Nieschlag E. Quantification of apoptotic testicular germ cells in normal and methoxyacetic acid-treated mice as determined by flow cytometry. *J Androl.* 1998 Nov–Dec;19(6):710–7.

102. Li LH, Wine RN, Chapin RE. 2-Methoxyacetic acid (MAA)-induced spermatocyte apoptosis in human and rat testes: An in vitro comparison. *J Androl.* 1996 Sep–Oct;17(5):538–49.

103. Urriola-Muñoz P, Lagos-Cabré R, Moreno RD. A mechanism of male germ cell apoptosis induced by bisphenol-A and nonylphenol involving ADAM17 and p38 MAPK activation. *PLOS ONE.* 2014;9(12):e113793.

104. Cheng CY. (2015) Toxicants target cell junctions in the testis: Insights from the indazole-carboxylic acid model. *Spermatogenesis.* 21;4(2):e981485.

5

Hormonal regulation of spermatogenesis

PALLAV SENGUPTA, MOHAMED ARAFA, AND HAITHAM ELBARDISI

HIGHLIGHTS

- The hypothalo-pituitary-gonadal (HPG) axis holds prime control over the process of spermatogenesis.
- The hypothalamus secretes gonadotropin-releasing hormone (GnRH) in a pulsatile manner and stimulates the release of gonadotrophins from the pituitary, i.e., follicle-stimulating hormone (FSH) and luteinizing hormone (LH).
- FSH triggers androgen binding protein (ABP) production and also aids in forming the blood-testis barrier (BTB).
- LH stimulates testosterone production from the Leydig cells.
- Testosterone is vital to support and maintain spermatogenesis and the BTB.
- The testicular cells maintain their local interactions via their own paracrine secretion as well as via the influence of gonadotropins.

5.1 INTRODUCTION

Spermatogenesis, the process to produce spermatozoa, occurs within the seminiferous tubule of the testis under strict endocrine regulation. It commences at the pubertal phase of a man's life, as the seminiferous tubules remain quiescent in the childhood phase. The onset of spermatogenesis is induced by elevated levels of gonadotropins and testosterone and persists throughout life, slightly declining in old age. It takes about 65–70 days to produce mature spermatozoa from the very first stage of spermatogonia (1). Since spermatogenic cells have to undergo numerous developmental stages during a particular time frame, these developmental stages are together called the spermatogenic cycle (1).

The hypothalo-pituitary-gonadal (HPG) axis holds prime control over the process of spermatogenesis. The hypothalamus induces gonatropin secretion from the anterior pituitary by the pulsatile release of gonadotropin-releasing hormone (GnRH) (2,3). Uninterrupted proper spermatogenesis is maintained through steady high intratesticular testosterone. Testosterone production is induced by the gonadotropin, luteinizing hormone (LH)–stimulated Leydig cells. Testosterone crosses the tubular basement membrane and diffuses into the Sertoli cells to bind with androgen binding protein (ABP) (4,5). Sertoli cells also possess receptors for follicle-stimulating hormone (FSH) that are probably required for the initiation of spermatogenesis (6,7). Sertoli cells also produce glycoprotein hormones such as inhibins, activins and follistatin that mediate feedback regulations of the principal hormones. Apart from the classical hormones, there are several metabolic hormones, growth factors as well as paracrine factors that influence spermatogenesis either via their direct effect on the testicular cells or by affecting the hormonal cross-talks (8). This chapter presents an easy understanding of the complex hormonal regulations of spermatogenesis.

5.2 SPERMATOGENESIS: AN OVERVIEW

Spermatogenesis is the process by which germ cells present in the seminiferous tubules of the testis develop into haploid spermatozoa. The process begins with stem cells (a diploid spermatogonium) adjacent to the tubular basement membrane undergoing mitotic division producing type A and type B cells (1,9). Type A cells restore the stem cell milieu, while type B cells differentiate into diploid intermediate primary spermatocytes (9). The primary spermatocyte travels to the adluminal compartment of the seminiferous tubules and duplicates its DNA undergoing meiosis I to yield two haploid secondary spermatocytes, each of which via meiosis II gives rise to two equal haploid spermatids (9). Therefore, each primary spermatocyte ultimately produces four spermatids. Henceforth, an individual spermatid is transformed functionally and morphologically into spermatozoa (sperm) by the process of spermiogenesis. While they are transferred through the male reproductive tract and during their transduction through female tracts, they attain their fully matured state. Each cell division starting from each spermatogonium to a haploid spermatid remains incomplete; the cells stay attached to one another by cytoplasmic bridges allowing synchronous development. Moreover, not all spermatogonia divide to yield spermatocytes to avoid insufficiency of spermatogonia, while spermatogonial stem cells undergo mitosis to replicate themselves, ensuring constancy and adequacy of spermatogonia to keep fueling spermatogenesis (10). Spermatogenesis is highly dependent on optimal physiological conditions and strict neuroendocrine regulation for its precision and continuity (4).

In order to distinctly discuss the process of spermatogenesis, three phases can be identified, namely, stem cell renewal, the proliferation of germ cells, and spermiogenesis (9). The stem cell renewal mechanism is to ensure an adequate consistent supply of stem cells to continue the subsequent phases of spermatogenesis. Out of the two types of stem cell populations, dark type A (Ad) and pale type A (Ap) spermatogonia, the former rarely divide to maintain the number of undifferentiated stem cells and are termed as renewing stem cells (10). The pale type Ap cells divide to yield to daughter cells that again divide such that half of them replicate themselves and half define the first generation of differentiated spermatogonia (type B1). Formation of type B spermatogonia marks the commencement of the proliferative phase of spermatogenesis (4).

5.3 GERM CELL REGENERATION AND DEATH

Like most other tissues, cell numbers in the seminiferous tubules maintain a dynamic balance between their regeneration and death (11). The first wave of spermatogenesis thereby follows stem cell differentiation, in a unique hormonal microenvironment. Excess cells produced during this period die by apoptosis, which is mainly mediated via Bcl-xL and Bax (12,13). As the gonocytes differentiate to form spermatogonia, the stage of elevated apoptosis or the first wave of spermatogenesis commences involving caspases 2, 3, 8 and 9, suggesting an association of both extrinsic and intrinsic pathways of apoptosis (12). Spontaneous as well as induced cell death (inadequacy of intratesticular testosterone and/or gonadotrophins, toxicants from the Sertoli cell, chemotherapeutic drug, etc.) occur via apoptosis (12). Thus, the germinal epithelium undergoes species-specific sets of cellular changes referred to as stages of the seminiferous epithelial cycle (12). Apoptosis is a normal spermatogenic component to ascertain a modest yet regulated number of productions of testicular spermatozoa from undifferentiated spermatogonia (4,12).

It is also required for subsequent waves of spermatogenesis, via synchronizing the Sertoli cell–germ cell ratio. From observations using rodents and nonhuman primates, it may be suggested that, besides the Sertoli cells, the number of type Ap spermatogonia contributes in determining the maximum spermatogenic capacity, referred to as the "ceiling of the testis" (4). From the endocrine perspectives, it is to be stated that FSH, LH, testosterone and human chorionic gonadotropin all reportedly participate in regulation of germ cell survival and apoptosis (14). It is postulated that Fas/FasL expression in the human testis is developmentally monitored via gonadotropin regulations (15). Either deprivation of these hormones or excess exposure can induce testicular cell apoptosis (16). Sertoli cells bear both FSH and testosterone receptors, and these two hormones are the direct hormonal regulators of spermatogenesis. During seminiferous tubule maturation, synergistic effects of testosterone and FSH along with estradiol aid germ cell survival (12,16,17). However, estradiol alone imposes an inhibitory or proapoptotic effect on germ cells. FSH functions mostly to aid in germ cell survival and, to less of an extent, in proliferation, in the window period between 14 and 18 days of testicular maturation, and this phase coincides with the termination of proliferation of Sertoli cells as well as the onset of meiosis among the germ cells marking the first wave of spermatogenesis (17). Testicular germ cells may undergo apoptosis via both extrinsic and intrinsic apoptotic death pathways when there is diminished FSH and testosterone levels, stimulates caspase activity and produces DNA fragmentation in both Sertoli cells and germ cells (17,18). An excess of these hormones may trigger the expressions of Fas/FasL in testis. Thus, FSH and testosterone levels are the key regulators of spermatogenic homeostasis (17).

5.4 HYPOTHALAMIC-PITUITARY-GONADAL AXIS

Spermatogenesis comprises complex yet precisely disciplined cellular events orchestrated by numerous paracrine, endocrine and intracrine factors. The hypothalamic-pituitary-testicular axis operates in both positive and negative feedback loops, in accordance with internal and external cues, thereby precisely regulating the reproductive events. The hypothalamus secretes GnRH in pulsatile fashion stimulating gonadotropins from the pituitary, namely, lutropin or LH, and follitropin or FSH. The gonadotrophins regulate testicular spermatogenesis and steroidogenesis. LH acts through their receptors on the interstitially placed Leydig cells to induce testosterone synthesis (19,20). Testosterone, in turn, exerts extragonadal sexual (libido) and anabolic (muscle strength, bone density) functions as well as intratesticular paracrine function to maintain spermatogenesis, which again occurs via stimulating Sertoli cells. FSH stimulates spermatogenesis by acting on the Sertoli cells in the seminiferous tubular compartment, through their specific receptor cells. Testosterone and Sertoli cell secretions, such as inhibins (inhibitory) and activins (stimulatory) along with several other paracrine factors mediate the qualitative and quantitative regulation of spermatogenesis (Figure 5.1a). This regulation is processed by feedback mechanisms influencing the secretion of both hypothalamic GnRH and subsequent gonadotropins from the anterior pituitary (19,20).

The evolving era in male reproductive physiology has surfaced several other male reproductive regulatory factors. These include groups of small RF-amide peptides with Arg-Phe-NH2 motif at C-terminus, namely, gonadotropin-inhibiting hormone (GnIH) and related peptides (19). Another important regulatory peptide is a 54–amino acid containing kisspeptin, which is encoded by the KiSS-1 gene. It seems to operate through the G protein–coupled receptor (GPR54) in the hypothalamus to bring about the onset of puberty and also is responsible for male precocious puberty (21).

5.5 ENDOCRINE REGULATION OF SPERMATOGENESIS

5.5.1 Follicle-stimulating hormone

FSH is an anterior pituitary gonadotropin, induced by low-frequency GnRH pulses from the hypothalamus. The synergistic actions of FSH with testosterone in stimulating all the steps of spermatogenesis are well documented, but the individual exact role of FSH is still elusive. It is suggested to be essential in determining the Sertoli cell numbers besides maintaining robust sperm production (7).

The effects of FSH on the spermatogonial cells are mediated via their actions on the Sertoli cells expressing the FSH receptor (FSH-R). The activation of the receptor is attained through dissociation of its α-subunit–linked Gs protein that activates adenylyl cyclase yielding cyclic adenosine monophosphate (cAMP) (4). The latter releases the catalytic subunit of protein kinase (PKA) in order to phosphorylate several intracellular proteins, such as the transcription factors, cAMP response element binding protein,

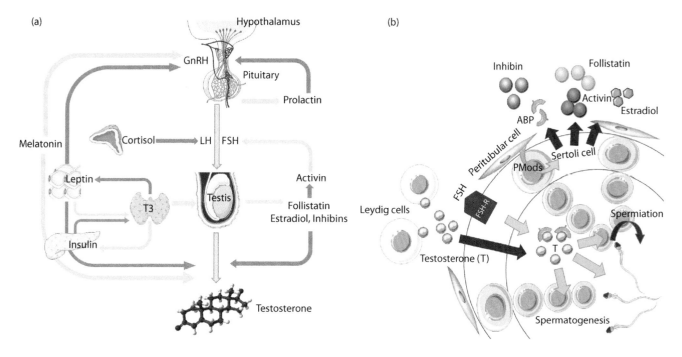

Figure 5.1 The hormonal cross talks **(a)** and endocrine, paracrine interactions among testicular cells in mediating spermatogenesis **(b)**.

etc. In other proposed mechanisms FSH signal transduction does prevail, but they are relatively elusive in an *in vivo* scenario (22).

FSH triggers the production of ABP by Sertoli cells and also aids the formation of the blood-testis barrier. ABP is required to sequester and concentrate testosterone in levels that are adequately high (even 50–200 times higher than that in the blood) to stimulate and maintain spermatogenesis (23). After FSH has initiated spermatogenesis via providing a signal to set the rate of sperm production above the basal level, it has been suggested that testosterone alone is sufficient in maintaining and continuing the process. However, with an increase in the FSH level, spermatozoa production also has been shown to elevate via the prevention of apoptosis of type A spermatogonia (24).

Although FSH secretion depends on the pulsatile GnRH stimulation, it is shown to be not highly sensitive to frequency modulation of the hypothalamic signal. FSH secretion is selectively regulated by the negative feedback loop mediated by the Sertoli cell protein, inhibin B, probably via antagonizing the activin drive to stimulate FSH β gene expression (4).

5.5.2 Luteinizing hormone

Luteinizing hormone (LH, also known as lutropin and sometimes lutrophin [25]) is a hormone produced by gonadotropic cells in the anterior pituitary gland (26). In males, where LH had also been called interstitial cell-stimulating hormone (ICSH), it stimulates Leydig cell production of testosterone. It acts synergistically with FSH (26).

LH mediates its action, mostly steroidogenesis to produce testosterone, through its receptors on the plasma membrane of the Leydig cells, which amounts to almost 15,000 in number (27). The occupancy of LH receptors of less than 5% of total receptors reportedly is sufficient for robust steroidogenesis (28). Leydig cells thereby produce testosterone via the LH-dictated pathway. An LH receptor is a single 93 kDa glycoprotein with three functional domains, namely, a glycosylated extracellular LH binding domain, a seven-segmented transmembrane spanning domain and an intracellular message conveying domain (27). These receptors are G-protein-coupled receptors that activate adenylyl cyclase to produce cAMP, which, in turn, leads to the activation of PKA. LH-mediated activated PKA may phosphorylate cholesterol esterase to release cholesterol from the intracellular stores, and/or activate CYP11A1, in order to stimulate steroidogenesis. LH also determines 17β-hydroxysteroid dehydrogenase expression that converts testicular androstenedione to testosterone (29).

LH secretion from the anterior pituitary is induced by high-frequency GnRH pulses from the hypothalamus. During a decrease in T levels, GnRH from the hypothalamus induces pituitary LH secretion, while during increased levels of T, it inhibits GnRH and LH release via negative feedback mechanisms. T may also inhibit LH by itself getting aromatized to estradiol (E2) that decreases the GnRH pulse amplitude and responsiveness of the anterior pituitary to GnRH (30).

5.5.3 Prolactin

Prolactin (PRL) or luteotropin, is a protein hormone secreted from the anterior pituitary. Prolactin self-regulates its release by a short feedback loop that operates by the activation of specific autoreceptors placed on the hypothalamic tuberoinfundibular dopaminergic neurons. These neurons, once stimulated, release dopamine (DA) that is transported via the long portal vessels reaching the adenohypophysis. Dopamine then acts on the lactotrophs via its cognate D2 dopaminergic receptors and thereby inhibits further prolactin release (31). Testicular steroids also affect prolactin release, such as a high estrogen level reportedly modulates the dopaminergic neurons and renders them refractory toward prolactin autofeedback (32). The association of prolactin with male reproductive functions is beyond the cross-talks with gonadal hormones for regulation of prolactin release and action. Prolactin has also been reported to play a role in testosterone synthesis by stimulating the LH receptors on Leydig cells and thus may account for the upregulation of spermatogenesis (33,34).

5.5.4 Inhibin, activin and follistatin

Sertoli cells produce several glycoprotein hormones to regulate the secretion of FSH from the anterior pituitary. These proteins are inhibins, activins and follistatins. Inhibin is a protein having two known forms, inhibin A and inhibin B (35). Both forms of inhibin have been documented to inhibit FSH secretion from the anterior pituitary without influencing the LH secretion (35). The complexity of regulation of FSH further increased with the isolation of proteins named as activins, which showed stimulatory effects over the HPG axis to increase FSH secretion (Figure 5.1a). These comprise mainly three forms, activin A, activin B and activin AB (36). They are disulfide-linked dimers of inhibin b-subunits and also reportedly are members of the protein superfamily of transforming growth factor-beta (TGF-β) (36). The third most important operator of the feedback loop to assure precise hormonal regulation of spermatogenesis is follistatin. The conventional function of follistatin in spermatogenesis attributes to its capability to potentially bind to activins with a strong affinity to neutralize the FSH stimulatory effects of the latter (37).

5.5.5 Sex steroids

5.5.5.1 TESTOSTERONE

Besides FSH, androgenic sex steroids are the most important hormones regulating spermatogenesis, their production being stimulated mainly by LH. Androgens regulate their own production by Leydig cells by modulating LH levels through feedback mechanisms. Biologically, most active androgens are testosterone and its 5α-reduced derivative dihydrotestosterone (DHT).

As discussed earlier, testosterone is a Leydig cell product that is produced via LH stimulation. It acts as a paracrine hormone diffusing into the seminiferous compartments to act via its receptors in the Sertoli cells. The effects of T are mediated through 110 KD androgen receptors (AR or NR3C4), which are located in the nucleus and cytoplasm and invoke functional responses needed to support spermatogenesis. It is noteworthy that the germ cells themselves do not possess any functional AR, while besides Sertoli cells, they are found in other testicular cells such as the Leydig cells, peritubular myoid cells, arteriole smooth muscle as well as the vascular endothelial cells. The classical pathway of testosterone involves its binding to the AR in the cytoplasm followed by its translocation to the nucleus and binding on specific gene promoter regions, thereby regulating gene transcription (38). The nonclassical T pathway involves its binding to AR and recruiting of Src kinase, which induces the epidermal growth factor receptor (EGFR) to activate MAPK cascade kinases (RAF, MAPK kinase [MEK] and ERK), followed by downstream kinase-dependent steps terminating in transcriptional regulation (6,39).

Testosterone levels are maintained at relatively constant high levels in the testis, while AR expressions in Leydig and peritubular cells are also almost constant, conveying a constitutively activated testosterone signal in these cells. AR expression in Sertoli cells undergoes cyclical alterations in accordance with the subsequent stages of the seminiferous epithelial cycle, with the highest being in stage 3 of the six stages (39). About two-thirds of testicular T is bioavailable, which is either free or weakly bound to albumen, while one-third remains tightly associated with ABP or the sex hormone binding globulin (SHBG). Bioavailable testosterone exceeds the level required for saturating the expressed AR.

Testosterone is vital to support and maintain the consistency of spermatogenesis, mainly by regulating four critical processes. First, it contributes to maintaining the dynamic blood-testis barrier (BTB) by aiding reassembly of its machinery on the basal side of the spermatocyte after the old BTB has been dismantled (18). Second, it has been reported that without testosterone signaling, spermatogenesis halts during the stage of meiosis, letting only very few spermatogonia develop up to the stage of haploid spermatid, and elongated spermatid production is inhibited. The interruption or halt in spermatogenesis may be explained by loss of testosterone signaling leading to cellular stresses associated with unfolded protein response, generation of reactive oxygen and nitrogen species and oxidative damage, DNA damage and alterations of regulatory proteins vital for RNA splicing, post-translational modifications, DNA repair and other functions for meiotic divisions. Third, the inadequacy of testosterone signaling leads to the premature release of round spermatid from the Sertoli cells, as the attachment between the Sertoli cell with elongated spermatid cannot be maintained without proper testosterone signaling via activated AR. Finally, even if the matured sperm are released

normally during stage VIII, owing to a lack of testosterone, they are retained followed by phagocytosis by the Sertoli cells (18). Src, which is related to the proteins at the ectoplasmic specialization, mediates activation of the release of sperm. Src phosphorylates and activates the N-cadherin and β-catenin proteins in Sertoli cells, aiding the building of ectoplasmic specialization adhesion sites with maturing elongated spermatids. β-catenin and N-cadherin, on getting activated, diffuse away from each other, breaking the cell linkage and thereby releasing the mature sperm. Suppression of testosterone and FSH in rats has displayed an expression of genes by Sertoli cells that are associated with adhesion of sperm with ectoplasmic specialization (18).

5.5.5.2 ESTROGEN

Estrogen has a substantial influence on male reproductive functions, interfering both in the hormonal cross talks and directly on testicular components. Evidence presents that male reproductive tissues mediate estrogen biosynthesis by aromatase and also express its receptors. Testes produce estrogen right from the fetal period and continuing throughout adulthood (40). Estrogen receptors (ERa and ERb) have been found to be present in juvenile, young as well as old-aged testis (40). Some cells, such as the Leydig cells, possess both ERa and ERb, while the seminiferous epithelial cells express only the ERb (40,41). It has been suggested that estrogen can modulate spermatogenesis acting at multiple levels of regulation. The most prominent function of estrogen is its participation in the negative feedback regulation of testosterone by acting on the pituitary gonadotropin secretion. Therefore, absence or inadequate exposure to estrogen results in disrupted hypothalamo-pituitary-testis axis balance. In view of the fact that this axis is a major determinant of the spermatogenic potential of the testis, its impairment via estrogen is likely to impose deleterious effects on spermatogenesis.

It has also been shown that estrogen possesses a functional role in male germ cells, as the latter contain ERs as well as the enzyme, aromatase. Thus, estrogen may take up an intracrine mode of action in the germ cells regulating their viability/apoptosis and possibly also play a role in acrosome biogenesis. Moreover, the nongenomic mechanism of action of estrogen in regulating various sperm functions has also been claimed (40).

5.5.5.3 PROGESTERONE

Progesterone, a natural progestin, is produced from cholesterol. It has long been established that progesterone acts as an antagonist to testosterone and displays strong negative feedback action upon hypothalamus and pituitary secretions (42). Hence, such a feedback loop reduces the plasma levels of LH and testosterone, which may justify the inhibitory action of progesterone on the process of spermatogenesis. Deleterious effects of progesterone on male reproductive functions may also be presumed from the study that showed that a potent derivative of progesterone, namely, cyproterone acetate, results in atrophy of the male accessory sex glands (43).

5.5.6 Metabolic hormones and growth factors

Metabolic hormones can affect spermatogenesis either via interfering in the HPG axis or acting directly on the testicular cells. The physiological mechanisms regulating energy balance and reproduction are intrinsically related. The neural apparatus to modulate metabolic rate and energy balance is referred to as the body "metabolic sensor," which converts specific signals provided by the circulating hormones into neuronal signals, thereby ultimately regulating the hypothalamic GnRH pulse generator to control spermatogenesis and other reproductive functions (44). In the realm of reproductive biology, metabolic syndrome and related disorders have garnered considerable attention because of the connection that exists between diabetes mellitus (DM), hyperleptinemia and infertility. Metabolic indicator hormones, such as insulin, leptin, growth hormone (GH) and insulin-like growth factor-I (IGF-I), suggestively provide signals of nutritional status to the hypothalamus and links to the HPG axis affecting spermatogenesis (44,45).

Leptin is best known as a regulator of food intake and energy expenditure via hypothalamic-mediated effects. An increasing body of data suggests that leptin also acts as a metabolic and neuroendocrine hormone. It is involved in glucose metabolism as well as in normal sexual maturation and reproduction. Three leptin receptor isoforms have been reported to be present in gonadal tissue, suggesting that leptin could exert a direct endocrine action on the gonads. The crucial roles of leptin on reproduction have been demonstrated by the observation of the ob/ob mouse, which lacks a functional leptin gene; these mice have impaired gonadotropin secretion and are infertile, but treatment with exogenous leptin restored fertility (46). Leptin may increase hypothalamic GnRH secretion and pituitary LH secretion, although these effects are still controversial (47). Chronic administration of antileptin antibody to rats was shown to inhibit LH release. Humans deficient in leptin exhibit effects similar to those observed in animal models. The importance of leptin during the process of spermatogenesis was demonstrated by the observation that a leptin deficiency in mice was associated with impaired spermatogenesis, increased germ cell apoptosis and upregulated expression of proapoptotic genes within the testes (48). This resulted in a reduction in germ cell numbers and the absence of mature spermatozoa in the seminiferous tubules. This finding adds further support to the importance of physiological leptin levels in the normal production of male gametes. Conversely, leptin has also been reported to have an inhibitory effect on the testis, reducing steroidogenesis and testosterone and estradiol levels in the serum. This, in turn, imposes inhibitory effects on spermatogenesis (49).

5.5.7 Other hormones

There are numerous other hormones that influence spermatogenesis by meddling with its main hormonal regulations, or also by acting on testicular cells under certain conditions. This chapter would be incomplete if some of such important hormones are not covered.

Melatonin (MLT) (tryptophan-derived hormone) is secreted from the pineal gland and stimulates gonadotropin as well as testosterone secretion. Thus, this pineal hormone may upregulate spermatogenesis (50,51). Anti-Müllerian hormone (AMH) (dimeric glycoprotein hormone) is produced by Sertoli cells in the fetus and has a structural resemblance to inhibin. It has been reported to account for Müllerian duct regression during the initial 8 weeks of embryogenesis. It reflects the functions of the Sertoli cell and is negatively regulated by testosterone and LH (2,52,54). Other vital hormones regulating male reproductive functions are the thyroid hormones. Association of the hypothalamo-pituitary-thyroid axis with the HPG axis potentially modulates testicular development (3,55). Actions of the thyroid hormones (T_4 and T_3) on GnRH and gonadotropin secretion remain controversial. However, thyroid hormones evidently stimulate steroidogenesis and hence may positively influence spermatogenesis (3,56,57). In addition, the hypothalamic-pituitary-adrenal (HPA) axis activation mainly owing to stress and an increase in glucocorticoid concentrations in plasma may be detrimental to male reproductive functions, including that upon spermatogenesis. Cortisol may disrupt GnRH, LH and FSH secretions (58). Several studies have also reported a significant decline in testosterone level with a rise in serum cortisol levels. These reports suggest that cortisol downregulates the hormones essential for normal spermatogenesis, thus adversely affecting the process (59–62).

5.6 SERTOLI CELL INTERACTION WITH LEYDIG AND PERITUBULAR MYOID CELLS

Testis, being an endocrine-responsive tissue, needs pristine cell-cell interactions to regulate cellular growth and differentiation. Sertoli cells in the seminiferous tubules confer cytoarchitectural support and a proper microenvironment for sperm to develop. Peritubular myoid cells encase the seminiferous tubule. Networks of extracellular matrix separate them from the basal surface of the Sertoli cells. Leydig cells are present in the interstitium of the testis and are involved in androgen synthesis. Testicular cell-cell interactions primarily showcase the interactions among the Sertoli, Leydig, peritubular and germinal cells. However, there are other cell types that contribute to the proper reproductive functioning, including steroidogenesis and spermatogenesis. Cells such as the lymphatic endothelial, stromal cells, testicular macrophages, lymphocytes, etc., are involved in local cell-cell interactions, but their associations are yet to be elaborately revealed (8).

The interactions between Leydig and Sertoli cells are bidirectional. Sertoli cells produce estradiol and cannot produce testosterone. But Sertoli cells bear testosterone receptors along with FSH-dependent aromatase. On the contrary, Leydig cells produce testosterone and cannot produce estradiol. But these cells possess estradiol receptors so that estradiol from Sertoli cells can act on it to suppress Leydig cell responses toward LH. Testosterone, produced by the Leydig cells, diffuses through the basement membrane of seminiferous tubule and binds to ABP in the Sertoli cell. Testosterone is obligatory in maintaining robust spermatogenesis and is vital to ensure the appropriate functioning of Sertoli cells (Figure 5.1b). Testosterone is also a precursor for estradiol production in the Sertoli cells (27,63).

The Sertoli cells produce several paracrine factors that may act on the germinal cells to regulate their differentiation. These factors include insulin-like growth factor-I (IGF-I), transforming growth factor-alpha (TGF-α), growth inhibitor transforming growth factor-beta (TGF-β), interleukin-1 (IL-I), etc. The potential paracrine interactions between the Sertoli and spermatogenic cells are supposedly influenced by endocrine factors. FSH, via its receptors on Sertoli cells, regulates cellular differentiation and function (64).

Peritubular cells, besides maintaining the structural integrity of the tubule, also produce certain paracrine regulators, such as growth factors, to influence morphology and functions of Sertoli cells. These cells may also increase the production of transferrin and ABP by the Sertoli cells (8). A potential paracrine agonist produced by the peritubular cells is referred to as PModS (peritubular factor that modulates Sertoli cell function). PModS supposedly mediates the effects of androgens on functions of the Sertoli cells and is even claimed to have a higher impact than that of FSH over Sertoli cells (8,65).

It can be concluded that spermatogenesis greatly relies on testicular cell-cell interactions. LH induces Leydig cell androgen synthesis that promotes a cascade of cellular interactions with testosterone diffusing into Sertoli cells to maintain proper spermatogenesis. Again, FSH acts on the Sertoli cells to trigger cell-cell interactions inducing germinal cell development, differentiation of peritubular myoid and Leydig cell functions. This principal circuit of the interdependent mechanism of action is supported by numerous paracrine regulators defining a complex endocrine and paracrine cross talk in the regulation of spermatogenesis.

5.7 ROLE OF HORMONES IN SPERMIOGENESIS AND SPERMIATION

Spermiogenesis is the most critical postmeiotic spermatid developmental event marking the final step of spermatogenesis. During this phase, the haploid spermatids, through extensive molecular and morphological alterations, produce mature spermatozoa. These spermatozoa then get released from the protective Sertoli cells in the seminiferous epithelium into the tubular lumen by the process of spermiation (27). This phase is characterized by the removal of excess cytoplasm and unnecessary organelles from the maturing spermatozoa. This process requires hydration of the testes and hormonal coordination. LH-induced androgen production by the Leydig cells increases during this phase. This further stimulates the Sertoli cells to aid

the spermiation response. The initiation of spermiation is marked by low sperm count and elevated levels of gonadotropins. Significant sperm production catches up in the next few weeks with gonadotropins level decreasing (1,53).

5.8 CONCLUSION

The intricate hormonal regulation of spermatogenesis is quite complex. There are intertwined actions of hypothalamo-pituitary-testicular hormones and their cross talks with other hormones and factors. Moreover, the testicular cells, such as Leydig, Sertoli and peritubular cells, maintain their local interactions via their own paracrine secretion as well as via the influence of gonadotropins. This chapter has discussed these integrated regulations of spermatogenesis segregating the same in different sections for easy understanding of the mechanism. There are still a lot of unexplored issues in the hormonal control of spermatogenesis which need further research.

REFERENCES

1. O'Shaughnessy PJ. Hormonal control of germ cell development and spermatogenesis. *Semin Cell Dev Biol.* 2014;29:55–65.
2. Holdcraft RW, Braun RE. Hormonal regulation of spermatogenesis. *Int J Androl.* 2004;27(6):335–42.
3. Darbandi M et al. Reactive oxygen species and male reproductive hormones. *Reprod Biol Endocrinol.* 2018;16(1):87.
4. Plant TM, Marshall GR. The functional significance of FSH in spermatogenesis and the control of its secretion in male primates. *Endocrine Rev.* 2001;22(6):764–786.
5. Ramaswamy S, Weinbauer GF. Endocrine control of spermatogenesis: Role of FSH and LH/testosterone. *Spermatogenesis.* 2014;4(2):e996025.
6. Shupe J et al. Regulation of Sertoli-germ cell adhesion and sperm release by FSH and nonclassical testosterone signaling. *Mol Endocrinol.* 2011;25(2):238–252.
7. Simoni M et al. Role of FSH in male gonadal function. *Ann Endocrinol (Paris).* 1999;60(2):102–6.
8. Skinner MK et al. Cell-cell interactions and the regulation of testis function. *Ann NY Acad Sci.* 1991;637(1):354–63.
9. Nistal M et al. Decrease in the number of human Ap and Ad spermatogonia and in the Ap/Ad ratio with advancing age new data on the spermatogonial stem cell. *J Androl.* 1987;8(2):64–8.
10. Schulze C. Morphological characteristics of the spermatogonial stem cells in man. *Cell Tissue Res.* 1979;198(2):191–9.
11. De Rooij D, Van Alphen M, Van de Kant H. Duration of the cycle of the seminiferous epithelium and its stages in the rhesus monkey (*Macaca mulatta*). *Biol Reprod.* 1986;35(3):587–91.
12. Sinha Hikim AP, Swerdloff RS. Hormonal and genetic control of germ cell apoptosis in the testis. *Rev Reprod.* 1999;4(1):38–47.

13. Rodriguez I et al. An early and massive wave of germinal cell apoptosis is required for the development of functional spermatogenesis. *EMBO J.* 1997;16(9):2262–70.

14. Marshall G, Plant T. Puberty occurring either spontaneously or induced precociously in rhesus monkey (*Macaca mulatta*) is associated with a marked proliferation of Sertoli cells. *Biol Reprod.* 1996;54(6):1192–9.

15. Francavilla S et al. Fas expression correlates with human germ cell degeneration in meiotic and postmeiotic arrest of spermatogenesis. *MHR: Basic Sci Reprod Med.* 2002;8(3):213–20.

16. Shaha C, Tripathi R, Mishra DP. Male germ cell apoptosis: Regulation and biology. *Phil Trans R Soc B: Biol Sci.* 2010;365(1546):1501–15.

17. Walczak-Jedrzejowska R et al. During seminiferous tubule maturation testosterone and synergistic action of FSH with estradiol support germ cell survival while estradiol alone has pro-apoptotic effect. *Folia Histochemica et Cytobiologica.* 2007;45(I):59–64.

18. Smith LB, Walker WH. The regulation of spermatogenesis by androgens. *Semin Cell Dev Biol.* 2014;30:2–13

19. Asimakopoulos B. Hypothalamus-pituitary-gonadal axis: It is time for revision. *Hum Genet Embryol.* 2012;2:1000–106.

20. Corradi PF, Corradi RB, Greene LW. Physiology of the hypothalamic pituitary gonadal axis in the male. *Urol Clin.* 2016;43(2):151–62.

21. Dhillo WS et al. Kisspeptin-54 stimulates the hypothalamic-pituitary gonadal axis in human males. *J Clin Endocrinol Metab.* 2005;90(12):6609–15.

22. Simoni M, Gromoll JR, Nieschlag E. The follicle-stimulating hormone receptor: Biochemistry, molecular biology, physiology, and pathophysiology. *Endocr Rev.* 1997;18(6):739–73.

23. Nieschlag E, Behre HM, Nieschlag S. *Testosterone: Action, Deficiency, Substitution.* Cambridge, UK: Cambridge University Press; 2012.

24. Kraemer WJ, Rogol AD. *The Endocrine System in Sports and Exercise.* Vol. 11. New York, NY: John Wiley & Sons; 2008.

25. Ujihara M et al. Subunit-specific sulphation of oligosaccharides relating to charge heterogeneity in porcine lutrophin isoforms. *Glycobiology.* 1992;2(3):225–31.

26. Louvet JP, Harman SM, Ross GT. Effects of human chorionic gonadotropin, human interstitial cell stimulating hormone and human follicle-stimulating hormone on ovarian weights in estrogen-primed hypophysectomized immature female rats. *Endocrinology.* 1975;96(5):1179–86.

27. Rhoades RA, Bell DR. *Medical Physiology: Principles for Clinical Medicine.* Philadelphia, PA: Lippincott Williams & Wilkins; 2012.

28. Channing CP, Tsafriri A. Mechanism of action of luteinizing hormone and follicle-stimulating hormone on the ovary in vitro. *Metabolism.* 1977;26(4):413–68.

29. Strauss JF, Barbieri RL. *Yen & Jaffe's Reproductive Endocrinology E-Book: Physiology, Pathophysiology, and Clinical Management.* New York, NY: Elsevier Health Sciences; 2013.

30. Pitteloud N et al. Inhibition of luteinizing hormone secretion by testosterone in men requires aromatization for its pituitary but not its hypothalamic effects: Evidence from the tandem study of normal and gonadotropin-releasing hormone-deficient men. *J Clin Endocrinol Metab.* 2008;93(3):784–91.

31. Anderson ST, Barclay JL, Fanning KJ, Kusters DH, Waters MJ, Curlewis JD. Mechanisms underlying the diminished sensitivity to prolactin negative feedback during lactation: Reduced STAT5 signaling and up-regulation of cytokine-inducible SH2 domain-containing protein (CIS) expression in tuberoinfundibular dopaminergic neurons. *Endocrinology.* 2006;147(3):1195–1202.

32. Voogt JL et al. Regulation of prolactin secretion during pregnancy and lactation. *Prog Brain Res.* 2001;133:173–85.

33. Purvis K et al. Prolactin and Leydig cell responsiveness to LH/hCG in the rat. *Arch Androl.* 1979;3(3):219–30.

34. Gill-Sharma M. Prolactin and male fertility: The long and short feedback regulation. *Int J Endocrinol.* 2009;2009.

35. Ling N et al. Isolation and partial characterization of a Mr 32,000 protein with inhibin activity from porcine follicular fluid. *Proc Natl Acad Sci.* 1985;82(21):7217–21.

36. Kingsley DM. The TGF-β superfamily: New members, new receptors, and new genetic tests of function in different organisms. *Genes Dev.* 1994;8(2):133–46.

37. De Kretser D, Hedger MP, Loveland KL, Phillips DJ. Inhibins, activins and follistatin in reproduction. *Human Reprod Update.* 2002;8(6):529–41.

38. Tsai M, O'Malley BW. Molecular mechanisms of action of steroid/thyroid receptor superfamily members. *Ann Rev Biochem.* 1994;63(1):451–86.

39. Fix C, Jordan C, Cano P, Walker WH. Testosterone activates mitogen-activated protein kinase and the cAMP response element binding protein transcription factor in Sertoli cells. *Proc Natl Acad Sci.* 2004;101(30):10919–24.

40. O'Donnell L et al. Estrogen and spermatogenesis. *Endocr Rev.* 2001;22(3):289–318.

41. Carreau S. Estrogens and male reproduction. *Folia Histochemica et Cytobiologica.* 2000;38(2):47–52.

42. Steinberger E, Root A, Ficher M, Smith KD. The role of androgens in the initiation of spermatogenesis in man. *J Clin Endocrinol Metab.* 1973;37(5):746–51.

43. Ericsson R, Dutt R. Progesterone and 6α-methyl-17α-hydroxyprogesterone acetate as inhibitors of spermatogenesis and accessory gland function in the ram. *Endocrinology.* 1965;77:203–8.

44. Blache D, Zhang S, Martin G. Fertility in male sheep: Modulators of the acute effects of nutrition on the

reproductive axis of male sheep. *Reprod Suppl.* 2003;61:387–402 .

45. Schneider JE. Energy balance and reproduction. *Physiol Behav.* 2004;81(2):289–317.

46. Mounzih K, Lu R, Chehab FF. Leptin treatment rescues the sterility of genetically obese ob/ob males. *Endocrinology.* 1997;138(3):1190–3.

47. Lampiao F, Agarwal A, du Plessis SS. The role of insulin and leptin in male reproduction. *Arch Med Sci.* 2009;2009(1):54.

48. Bhat GK et al. Influence of a leptin deficiency on testicular morphology, germ cell apoptosis, and expression levels of apoptosis-related genes in the mouse. *J Androl.* 2006;27(2):302–10.

49. Ramos CF, Zamoner A. Thyroid hormone and leptin in the testis. *Front Endocrinol (Lausanne).* 2014;5:198.

50. Li C, Zhou X. Melatonin and male reproduction. *Clin Chim Acta.* 2015;446:175–80.

51. Awad H et al. Melatonin hormone profile in infertile males. *Int J Androl.* 2006;29(3):409–13.

52. La Marca A et al. Anti-Müllerian hormone (AMH) as a predictive marker in assisted reproductive technology (ART). *Hum Reprod Update.* 2010;16(2):113–30.

53. Sofikitis N et al. Hormonal regulation of spermatogenesis and spermiogenesis. *J Steroid Biochem Mol Biol.* 2008;109(3–5):323–30.

54. Trigo RV et al. Altered serum profile of inhibin B, Pro-αC and anti-Müllerian hormone in prepubertal and pubertal boys with varicocele. *Clin Endocrinol (Oxf).* 2004;60(6):758–64.

55. Krajewska-Kulak E, Sengupta P. Thyroid function in male infertility. *Front Endocrinol.* 2013;4:174.

56. Castañeda Cortés DC, Langlois VS, Fernandino JI. Crossover of the hypothalamic pituitary–adrenal/ interrenal–thyroid, and –gonadal axes in testicular development. *Front Endocrinol.* 2014;5:139.

57. Sengupta P, Dutta S. Thyroid disorders and semen quality. *Biomed Pharmacol J.* 2018;11(1):1–10.

58. Aggarwal A, Upadhyay R. *Heat stress and hormones.* In: *Heat Stress and Animal Productivity.* Aggarwal A, Upadhyay R (eds) Springer; 2013, pp. 27–51.67

59. Rhynes W, Ewing L. Testicular endocrine function in Hereford bulls exposed to high ambient temperature 1. *Endocrinology.* 1973;92(2):509–15.

60. Wettemann R, Desjardins C. Testicular function in boars exposed to elevated ambient temperature. *Biol Reprod.* 1979;20(2):235–41.

61. Hansen PJ. Effects of heat stress on mammalian reproduction. *Phil Trans R Soc B: Biol Sci.* 2009;364(1534):3341–50.

62. Megahed G et al. Influence of heat stress on the cortisol and oxidant-antioxidants balance during oestrous phase in buffalo-cows (*Bubalus bubalis*): Thermoprotective role of antioxidant treatment. *Reprod Domest Anim.* 2008;43(6):672–7.

63. Young J, Couzinet B, Chanson P, Brailly S, Loumaye E, Schaison G. Effects of human recombinant luteinizing hormone and follicle-stimulating hormone in patients with acquired hypogonadotropic hypogonadism: Study of Sertoli and Leydig cell secretions and interactions. *J Clin Endocrinol Metab.* 2000;85(9):3239–44.

64. Griswold MD. 50 years of spermatogenesis: Sertoli cells and their interactions with germ cells. *Biol Reprod.* 2018;99(1):87–100.

65. Oliveira PF, Alves MG. Modulation of Sertoli cell metabolism. In: *Sertoli Cell Metabolism and Spermatogenesis.* Oliveira, Pedro F., Alves, Marco G. (eds) New York, NY: Springer; 2015, pp. 57–71.

GH–IGF1 axis in spermatogenesis and male fertility

ANTONIO MANCINI, CARMINE BRUNO, ANDREA PALLADINO, EDOARDO VERGANI, AND ELENA GIACCHI

HIGHLIGHTS

- Growth hormone (GH) has a pivotal role in reproduction, via direct and indirect mechanisms. Many actions are mediated by local production of insulin-like growth factor-1 (IGF-1).
- Different experimental models with manipulation of the GH–IGF-1 axis confirm its role in fertility; similarly, human diseases with growth hormone deficiency (GHD) or GH resistance exhibit lower testicular volume and decreased sperm count, and therefore reduced fertility.
- At present, no clear advantage of GH treatment in idiopathic infertility is reported; however, the diagnosis of acquired adult GHD can be the rationale for the treatment in a specific subset of infertile patients.

6.1 INTRODUCTION

Infertility is defined as the inability of a couple to conceive after a year of unprotected intercourse. Approximately 15% of all couples are recognized as infertile, and the "responsibility" is attributable in half of the cases to the male partner. The latter estimate is growing because some evidence indicates that the quality of human sperm is decaying over the years (1). Among the causes that may be involved in this problem, there are certainly genitourinary infections, environmental exposure to chemical insults that decrease spermatogenesis, anatomical or physiological obstructions, immunological deficiencies, abnormal morphologies and even hormonal disorders. Spermatogenesis is a rather complex cell development process that requires the presence of pituitary gonadotropins and testosterone that indirectly

regulate this mechanism via autocrine, paracrine and juxtacellular pathways. Growth hormone (GH) and its main factor, the insulin-like growth factor-1 (IGF-1), are only two actors in this scenario, but they reach a significant role considering current evidence (2). The GH, mainly represented by the 22 kDa form, is produced by the anterior pituitary gland and regulates, in addition to growth, the formation of secondary sexual tissues as well as the uterus in the woman and the prostate and seminal vesicles in the man.

It is known that the GH–IGF-1 axis is finely regulated by the hypothalamus, with a dual modality: stimulation by GH releasing hormone (GHRH) and inhibition by somatostatin (SS). The modulation of GH is therefore controlled by different stimuli, such as nutritional status, fasting, stressors, sleep and so on, also resulting in a circadian rhythm with the key impact of the metabolic request of the organism (3).

It is not surprising that such pleiotropic activities are strictly related to reproduction. GH circulates in a complex with a GH binding protein (GHBP) and acid-labile subunit; two isoforms of GHBP are present, and the high-affinity form, corresponding to the extracellular domain of GH liver receptor (GHR), is generated by a metalloproteinase (tumor necrosis factor alpha [TNF-α] converting enzyme), which is another fine mechanism of control of GH activity. In the liver, GH stimulates synthesis and secretion of IGF-1; this, in turn, is transported by binding proteins (IGF-BPs). Among these, IGF-BP3 is regulated by GH and represents a mechanism of controlling free IGF-1 to bind to its own receptor.

Interactions with the hypothalamic-pituitary-gonadal axis are exerted at each level; they have been described as stimulatory, permissive or synergistic (4) in both sexes.

6.2 GROWTH HORMONE AND MALE REPRODUCTIVE SYSTEM

By focusing more on the male, the testes themselves are sites of GH production and action. It has been shown that mice without the GH receptor have diminished (but not completely abolished) fertility; from this it has been possible to declare that physiological circulating levels of GH are pro-fertility, although an excess of the latter can promote neoplastic growth, particularly in the prostate (5). The effects of the GH–IGF-1 axis are exerted in three main areas (development, endocrine function and gametogenesis).

6.2.1 Effects on development

At the testicular level, the growth hormone promotes the growth and development of the gonad, in childhood and puberty, and stimulates the gametogenesis and production of steroid hormones, in puberty and adult age. This mechanism is also supported by the IGF-1 produced in response to circulating GH levels. This is confirmed by studies that have shown the decrease in testicular volume in patients with childhood-onset growth hormone deficiency (Co-GHD) and the consequent increase in the same patients treated with replacement doses of GH (6). GH also promotes the development and differentiation of internal testis structures such as seminiferous tubules.

6.2.2 Effects on steroidogenesis

Regarding the hormonal aspect of testicular function, GH is a potent steroidogenic factor, increasing the production of androgens and estradiol by Leydig cells, *in vitro* (7). Other *in vitro* studies have shown that GH is involved at the beginning of the steroidogenesis process; it stimulates the production of "steroidogenic acute regulatory" proteins (StAR), which appear to mediate cholesterol transport across the inner mitochondrial membrane, and enzymes such as the 3-β hydroxysteroid dehydrogenase that converts pregnenolone into progesterone at the testicular level (8).

Another indirect method by which GH would act on fertility and control of circulating androgens could be the action on sex hormone binding globulin (SHBG), since its production diminished as a function of growth hormone. The latter aspect is still somewhat controversial, especially in the age of development, in which there are discordant studies (9,10).

Another factor closely related to GH in the circulation is IGF-1: it is now known that IGF-1 is present and expressed in the testis, but its regulation in this district seems to be more related to the production of gonadotropins instead of strictly endocrine or autocrine/paracrine production of GH. IGF-1 expression in Sertoli cells and Leydig cells is regulated, respectively, by FSH and LH, and, in an autocrine manner, amplifies their actions.

6.2.3 Effects on spermatogenesis

The effects of GH on testicular growth consequently influence the proliferation of germ cells. This point is particularly delicate, as it is a balance whereby a decrease in GH would lead to a decrease in sperm count, a decrease in semen volume and low sperm motility. It has been shown that an excess of GH has the same consequences (11–13), underlining the importance of correct dosage of possible therapies.

Local IGF-1 production can mimic GH effects on germ cells since IGF-1 improves sperm motility and morphology. Receptors for IGF-1 are expressed in the more mature, haploid cells of spermatogenesis (secondary spermatocytes, spermatids and spermatozoa). However, this should not be misleading: IGF-1 is not the only mediator through which GH performs its functions at the testicular level (indeed in some studies it has been shown how these two actors have, in some cases, effects opposite [14], but GH can also act independently of IGF-1 [15]).

The fact that circulating GH is not readily available to testicular cells due to the blood-testicular barrier, as well as to spermatids and spermatozoa, is not to be underestimated. Despite this, GH is present at the testicular level thanks to the expression of genes coding for the growth hormone active in the cells of this district; in some species, the testis is the only recognized site in which mRNA deriving from genes encoding GH is present (16). Potential regulators of GH on-site expression appear to be expressed in the testis, both human and murine. For example, GHRH can also be expressed at this level, with a structure very similar to placental GHRH. GHRH receptors are widely represented in various tissues of the human body such as, in our specific area, Leydig cells, Sertoli cells, germ cells as well as in the prostate. This could indicate that GHRH would have functions other than GH in the testis (17).

6.2.4 Other functions and mechanisms of regulation

The functions of GH in the reproductive sphere, however, do not end up on the testicle, but on accessory sexual organs. This is demonstrated by the presence of GH receptors also in these: for example, GH seems to be the main factor responsible for the transformation of fetal tissues into prostate and seminal vesicles (18). In the prostate, GH stimulates the growth and development of the organ; this is well demonstrated both by the decrease in the volume of the gland in transgenic mice with GH deficiency, and by the frequent presence of prostatic hyperplasia and/or aberrant structures (such as cysts, nodules or calcifications) in acromegalic patients (19,20). Despite this last evidence, there do not appear to be direct or reverse correlations between acromegaly and prostate cancer risk as well as PSA levels. This must, however, be studied and confirmed by further future epidemiological studies.

Both GH and IGF-1 appear to be involved in penile growth and function; the first seems to be more involved in the regulation of erectile function (mainly autocrine/paracrine), while the latter has more action on fibroblasts and cell proliferation (21). The erection underlies a series of modulations on blood flow and on penile smooth muscle: the GH has actions on both these factors—the venous contraction and the relaxation of the musculature. The concentration of intracavernous GH rises during erection and does not occur in patients with erectile dysfunction (22,23). Nevertheless, it should not be forgotten that probably the action of the growth hormone on these tissues can be biphasic, with problems also deriving from overexposure to GH itself (as happens in acromegalics) (24).

In the complex, still incompletely known is the question of direct and indirect effects of GH, in turn related to systemic and local IGF-1 production (25). The same model of classical cascade GH–IGF-1 axis has been questioned in light of the numerous autocrine and paracrine interactions at the testicular level; the discovery of all components of the system, including GHRH, SS, GH, IGF-1, but also other secretagogues (Ghrelin) has allowed the introduction of the term *testicular minihypophysis* (3).

There is no doubt that GH can be considered a "cogonadotropin" (26), as supported by *in vitro* and *in vivo* studies: GH is released together with LH, by peripubertal rat pituitary cells after stimulation by the potent GnRH stimulator kisspeptin (27); both cells types (gonadotropes and somatotropes) can be stimulated by pituitary adenylate cyclase-activating polypeptide (PACAP) (28) or, in a cellular subpopulation, can secrete both hormones (29). Gonadotropes are provided with receptors for GH and GH-binding proteins (26). Finally, the role of GH in the timing of puberty is well known as previously stated.

Recently, other GH regulators like ghrelin and its receptors have also been identified in the testis (ghrelin seems to be able to alter testosterone synthesis and other testicular parameters) (30,31). Ghrelin is a 28-aminoacid peptide, mainly produced in the stomach as proghrelin and furtherly processed by post-translational mechanisms. Two circulating isoforms are described: an acylated form (AG) and a deaceylated form (DAG), which, in different models, can act as synergic or antagonist factors. Ghrelin represent the endogenous ligand of the GH-secretagogue receptor

(GHSR$_{Ia}$). Both ghrelin and GHSR$_{Ia}$ are expressed in the testis in experimental animals (32). Their physiological role is still unknown; this system seems to modulate the sensitivity to FSH in spermatogenic cells. In human testis, on the contrary, ghrelin is expressed especially in Leydig cells and negatively correlates with circulating testosterone levels in normozoospermic individuals (33). Recently, the presence of ghrelin was investigated in testicular tissue of patients who had undergone microscopic testicular sperm extraction (micro-TESE) for idiopathic nonobstructive azoospermia (NOA). Also, in this case, a negative correlation with testosterone was shown, suggesting an important role in spermatogenesis, on one side, but also an endocrine-mediated mechanism of action (34). Finally, ghrelin exerts actions at the hypothalamic-pituitary level, linking GH secretion to stress and nutritional status. While at hypothalamic levels it has been shown to reduce GH pulsatility, also interacting with other modulatory systems like kisspeptin in a negative way on gonadotropin release, at pituitary levels it seems to increase the gonadotropin response to GnRH (32).

Finally, the discovery of Klotho, a protein involved in antiaging effects in mice phenotypes, has thrown light on connections between peripheral organs and pituitary. In humans Klotho is mainly expressed in the kidney but also in the endothelium, where it induces nitric oxide (NO) production. Klotho is a regulator of GH secretion, as shown in both animals and humans, inhibiting negative IGF-1 feedback on GH release; its levels are low in GH-deficient subjects; however, the complex relationships with the GH axis are still to be clarified (35). A schematic representation of the GH–IGF-1 axis is reported in Figure 6.1.

6.3 EFFECTS OF ALTERED GROWTH HORMONE SECRETION ON MALE FERTILITY

Males with GHD exhibit lower testicular volume and decreased sperm count, and therefore reduced fertility (36). Decrease of serum IGF-1 is also associated with lower sperm count, despite the same correlation did not being demonstrated when seminal IGF-1 concentration was considered. However, as previously stated, due to the multiple and reciprocal influences between somatotropic and gonadotropic axes, a number of studies have been performed to define this complex picture. A positive correlation between seminal GH and IGF-1 has been described, but only in patients with asthenozoospermia, accompanied by at least one abnormal semen parameter (37). Seminal IGF-1 has been found to be higher in infertile patients with varicocele than in controls and decreased after varicocelectomy, without any correlation with varicocele grade and sperm quality (22). Therefore, the question remains open. Moreover, IGF-2 has also been claimed to influence spermatogenesis and to be modulated by epigenetic mechanisms (38); however, the regulation of IGF-2 is more complex than that of IGF-1. A review of the IGF

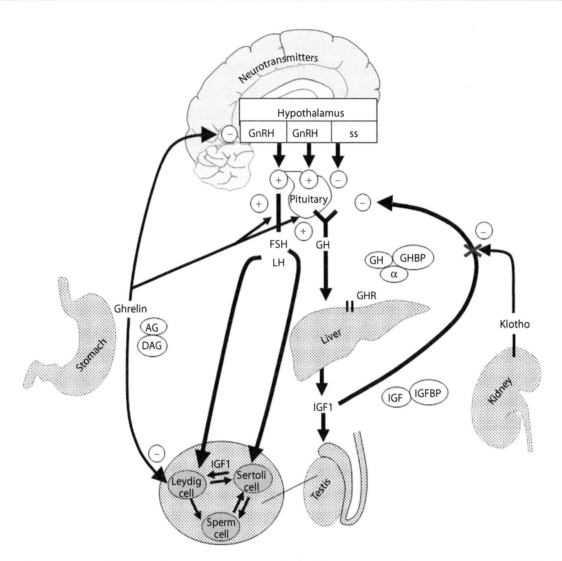

Figure 6.1 The interactions between the GH–IGF-1 axis and gonadotropic-testicular axis. GH is controlled by the hypothalamus via a dual mechanism—stimulation by GH-releasing hormone (GHRH) and inhibition by somatostatin (SS). GH, released by the pituitary gland, circulates in a complex linked to a binding protein (GH-BP), which is a fragment of the GH receptor (GHR), and an acid-labile subunit (α). After binding to GHR in the liver, it stimulates synthesis of the IGF-1 protein, which is the main mediator of GH action at the peripheral organs, including the testis. IGF-1 is bound by IGF-BPs and exerts a negative feedback effect on pituitary GH release. IGF-1 is also produced in the testis, where it exerts paracrine and autocrine actions; testicular IGF-1 is mainly regulated by gonadotropins and augments gonadotropin effects on both Leydig and Sertoli cells. On this principal axis, other recently discovered mechanisms exert a modulation: the protein Klotho, produced in the kidney and involved in antiaging in mice phenotypes, stimulates GH interrupting the IGF-1 negative feedback; the hormone ghrelin, produced by parietal gastric cells (P/D1), directly stimulates GH via specific receptors; subtle actions are exerted on GnRH release (which seems to be blunted) and at pituitary levels (in this case the response of gonadotropes to GnRH is increased); finally it also acts at the testicular level, where it interferes by still unknown mechanisms with testosterone production. The two forms of circulating ghrelin, acetylated (AG) and deacetylated (DAG), are shown, and this post-translational modification of the peptide can modify its influence on the gonadotropin axis.

system on testicular differentiation and function, in different experimental animal species and in human models, is presented in the same paper (38).

To address the question of an altered GH/IGF-1 axis on infertility, two approaches were followed. First, a number of studies have been performed with genetic manipulation of the axis and exploring the effects on fertility. Table 6.1 resumes main studies in rodents, and the comparison with the human model of GH receptor mutations, Laron dwarfing (5,39–70). It is interesting to underline that partial IGF-1 deficiency can be associated with sperm quality alteration. However, polymorphism of the GH receptor gene does not seem to be associated with sperm abnormalities (69).

The second approach was the evaluation of GH dynamics in infertile patients.

Table 6.1 Experimental models of genetic manipulation of somatotropic axis

Model	IGF/hormone status	Testicular/spermatogenic effects	Other effects
GHRH-R deficiency (lit/lit) (39–53)	Decreased IGF-1 and PRL	Normal spermatogenesis and testosterone; hypofertility due to sexual deficiency	Delayed sexual development
GH deficit (dw/dw, rats) (44–46)	Reduced IGF-1, normal LH e FSH	Normal spermatogenesis and androgen levels; subfertility	Increased PRL
GH deficit (rdw/rdw rats) (47–51)	Reduced levels of PRL and thyroid hormones. Normal gonadotropins	Infertility	Infertility
GH deficit (Snell dw/dw, Ames df/df mice) (52–54)	Reduced or undetectable IGF-1, reduced LH and FSH, blunted response to GnRH	Reduction of Leydig cells and testosterone levels; reduced sperm count, infertility	Infertility
IGF-1 null, −/− mutant mice (55)	Reduced IGF-1	Reduced spermatogenesis; decreased number and delayed maturation of Leydig cells; reduced secretion of testosterone; infertility	Uterus hypoplasia, especially in myometrium, failure of gonadotropins to induce ovulation
IGF-1 null mutation (mouse) (56)	Reduced IGF-1 levels	Failure of androgenization, lack of Leydig cell maturation, reduced testosterone due to disproportionate expression of T biosynthetic and metabolizing enzymes	
GHR KO (mice) (5,57–61)	Reduced or absent IGF-1, delayed puberty, blunted response to GnRH, increased PRL	Decreased LH and PRL-R in testis, ↓ testicular volume, ↓ 17BHSD (A=, T↓), reduced fertility	Fertile, but reduced number of preovulatory follicles and corpora lutea
Loss of function allele of collagen receptor gene Ddr2 (mice) (62)	Normal circulating IGF-1, but lower expression of IGF1 mRNA in the liver	Lack of spermatogenesis	Anovulation
Heterozygous IGF (±) (63)	Partial IGF-1 deficiency	Damage of blood-testis barrier, altered testicular structure and testicular function-related gene expression	
IGFBP-1 overexpression (mice) (64,65)	Low free IGF-1	Reduced T secretion; reduced spermatogenesis	Suppressed LH; altered follicular growth
Laron, mutated GHR (66–68)	Absent IGF-1	Delayed puberty	Delayed puberty
Polymorphism GH receptor gene (Exon 3 deletion, GHrd3/d3) (69)	Twofold increase in IGF-1 levels	Trend to larger semen volume, higher inhibin B serum levels	
15q chromosome structural abnormalities (70)	Decreased IGF-1-R gene expression; undetectable IGF-1-R activity	Low testis volume, severe oligoasthenozoospermia, with cryptorchidism and gynecomastia (one patient) and precocious puberty (another patient)	

Source: Adapted from Chandrashekar V et al. *Biol Reprod* [Internet]. 2004 Jul 1 [cited 2018 Oct 31];71(1):17–27. Available from: https://academic.oup.com/biolreprod/article-lookup/doi/10.1095/biolreprod.103.027060.

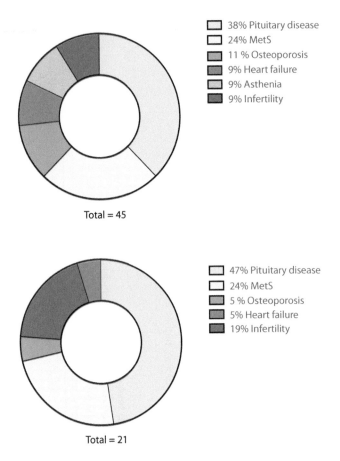

Total = 45

- 38% Pituitary disease
- 24% MetS
- 11 % Osteoporosis
- 9% Heart failure
- 9% Asthenia
- 9% Infertility

Total = 21

- 47% Pituitary disease
- 24% MetS
- 5 % Osteoporosis
- 5% Heart failure
- 19% Infertility

Figure 6.2 Retrospective evaluation for the indication to dynamic GH evaluation in our cohort of 45 males affected by adult-onset GHD and in the subgroup of males aged 20–45 years.

Shimonovitz et al. (72) explored the GH response to clonidine in infertile males. They found a blunted response in 91% of azoospermic men and 18% in oligozoospermic men. However, the groups were small. This blunted response was not confirmed by Carani et al. (73) in hypogonadotropic hypogonadism both before and after replacement therapy. Other authors reported normal GH response to hypoglycemia (74) or lower GH response to arginine (75); also in these cases the number of patients tested was low. Moreover, these GH dynamic tests are not entirely reproducible. Therefore,

a real prevalence of growth hormone deficiency in infertile man has not been clarified.

In our experience, the diagnosis of GHD is underestimated. When evaluating retrospectively a group of 45 male subjects affected by GHD, confirmed by GHRH+arginine test, under treatment with rhGH, we found that infertility, unexplained or unresponsive to gonadotropin, was the main reason to perform the dynamic test in 9% of patients. However, in the subgroup of males aged 20–45 years, this percentage rose to 19% (Figure 6.2). It must be emphasized that the evaluation of IGF-1 levels alone was not predictive of GHD, as explained in Figure 6.3. Only 21% of GHD males exhibited IGF-1 levels under the 2.5 percentile for age (according to our laboratory range provided by LIASON) (Figure 6.3). Therefore, male infertility not clearly attributable to specific causes, especially in case of oligozoospermia or small testes, could be an indication to perform dynamic evaluation of GH (76).

6.4 THERAPEUTIC USE OF GROWTH HORMONE FOR MALE INFERTILITY

The administration of GH has been performed as a possible treatment for infertility, due to the just mentioned capacity to increase seminal volume and sperm motility (77), but the evidence that it can ameliorate sperm quality in patients with astenozoospermia and oligozoospermia is still lacking.

Most studies were performed in the 1990s, as shown in Table 6.2, but they are still inconclusive due to the small number of patients, the heterogeneity of cohorts and the lack of diagnosis of GHD in some studies (74,78–82).

More recently the effects of rhGH administration in GHD patients with childhood-onset (CoGHD) and with delayed puberty have been described, showing a correlation between the age of starting of therapy and puberty onset; moreover, final testicular volume was correlated with the duration of treatment, even if penile size and the testicular volume remained lower than normal range (83). GH has also been administered in a small group of patients with short stature, not related to GHD, and constitutional puberty delay, obtaining normal testicular volume when reaching final puberty and normalization of seminal parameters (in seven out of eight patients) (71).

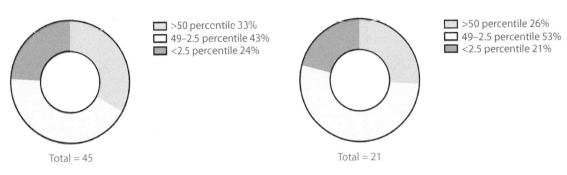

Total = 45

- >50 percentile 33%
- 49–2.5 percentile 43%
- <2.5 percentile 24%

Total = 21

- >50 percentile 26%
- 49–2.5 percentile 53%
- <2.5 percentile 21%

Figure 6.3 Percentage of GHD patients with low IGF-1 (<2.5 percentile), low-normal (under the median for age and sex) and normal IGF-1 levels at the time of diagnosis of GHD.

Table 6.2 Studies on GH administration in infertile patients

Authors	Patients (#)	Seminal picture	Duration	Effects
Radicioni et al. 1994 (78)	10	Severe oligozoospermia	Short-term	5/10 responders
Lee et al. 1995 (74)	12	Oligozoospermia	5 months	No effects
Ovessen et al. 1996 (75)	9	Oligozoospermia Asthenozoospermia	12 weeks	Increased motility Increased motility (3 pregnancies) Increased seminal IGF-1
Giagulli 1999 (80)	4	Azoospermia in HH	6 months	Increased testis volume Persistent azoospermia
Shoham et al. 1992 (81)	7	HH unresponsive to Gn	12 weeks	3/4 augmented T 2/4 augmented sperm count (1 pregnancy)
Zalel et al. 1996(82)	4	OTA patients normoGn	12 weeks	No seminal effects

6.5 CONCLUSIONS

Despite the great number of studies showing the physiological role of the somatotropic axis in male reproduction, the therapeutic implications are still unclear. The GH treatment has been proposed in small groups of infertile males, but no controlled trials exist. However, in our experience, the diagnosis of adult GHD is underestimated; it cannot be based only on the measurement of circulating IGF-1 levels but requires provocative tests. In case of reduced GH secretion, the replacement therapy can be proposed, especially in patients with oligozoospermia and low testicular volume, unresponsive to gonadotropin administration. The role of GH as a modulator of growth, metabolism and protection against oxidative stress are still interesting fields to be explored.

REFERENCES

1. Auger J, Kunstmann JM, Czyglik F, Jouannet P. Decline in semen quality among fertile men in Paris during the past 20 years. N Engl J Med [Internet]. 1995 Feb 2 [cited 2018 Oct 29];332(5):281–5. Available from: http://www.nejm.org/doi/abs/10.1056/NEJM199502023320501
2. Lee HS, Park Y-S, Lee JS, Seo JT. Serum and seminal plasma insulin-like growth factor-1 in male infertility. Clin Exp Reprod Med [Internet]. 2016 Jun [cited 2018 Oct 29];43(2):97–101. Available from: http://synapse.koreamed.org/DOIx.php?id=10.5653/cerm.2016.43.2.97
3. Hull KL, Harvey S. Growth hormone and reproduction: A review of endocrine and autocrine/paracrine interactions. Int J Endocrinol [Internet]. 2014 [cited 2018 Oct 31];2014:1–24. Available from: http://www.hindawi.com/journals/ije/2014/234014/
4. Chandrashekar V, Zaczek D, Bartke A. The consequences of altered somatotropic system on reproduction. Biol Reprod [Internet]. 2004 Jul 1 [cited 2018 Oct 31];71(1):17–27. Available from: https://academic.oup.com/biolreprod/article-lookup/doi/10.1095/biolreprod.103.027060
5. Chandrashekar V, Bartke A, Coschigano KT, Kopchick JJ. Pituitary and testicular function in growth hormone receptor gene knockout mice. Endocrinology. 1999;140(3):1082–8.
6. Albin AK, Ankarberg-Lindgren C, Tuvemo T, Jonsson B, Albertsson-Wikland K, Ritzén EM. Does growth hormone treatment influence pubertal development in short children? Horm Res Paediatr. 2011;76(4):262–72.
7. Sirotkin AV. Control of reproductive processes by growth hormone: Extra- and intracellular mechanisms. Vet J. 2005;170:307–17.
8. Kanzaki M, Morris PL. Growth hormone regulates steroidogenic acute regulatory protein expression and steroidogenesis in Leydig cell progenitors. Endocrinology. 1999;140(4):1681–6.
9. Gafny M, Silbergeld A, Klinger B, Wasserman M, Laron Z. Comparative effects of GH, IGF-I and insulin on serum sex hormone binding globulin. Clin Endocrinol (Oxf). 1994;41(2):169–75.
10. Juul A, Andersson AM, Pedersen SA, Jørgensen JOL, Christiansen JS, Groome NP et al. Effects of growth hormone replacement therapy on IGF-related parameters and on the pituitary-gonadal axis in GH-deficient males. A double-blind, placebo-controlled crossover study. Horm Res. 1998;49(6):269–78.
11. Satoh K, Ohyama K, Nakagomi Y, Ohta M, Shimura Y, Sano T et al. Effects of growth hormone on testicular dysfunction induced by cyclophosphamide (CP) in GH-deficient rats. Endocr J [Internet]. 2002;49(6):611–9. Available from: http://www.ncbi.nlm.nih.gov/pubmed/12625410
12. Nouri HS, Azarmi Y, Movahedin M. Effect of growth hormone on testicular dysfunction induced by methotrexate in rats. Andrologia. 2009;41(2):105–10.
13. Figueiredo MA, Fernandes RV, Studzinski AL, Rosa CE, Corcini CD, Varela Junior AS et al. GH overexpression decreases spermatic parameters and reproductive success in two-years-old transgenic zebrafish males. Anim Reprod Sci. 2013;139(1–4):162–7.
14. Miao ZR, Lin TK, Bongso TA, Zhou X, Cohen P, Lee KO. Effect of insulin-like growth factors (IGFs) and

IGF-binding proteins on in vitro sperm motility. *Clin Endocrinol (Oxf)*. 1998;49(2):235–9.

15. Miura C, Shimizu Y, Uehara M, Ozaki Y, Young G, Miura T. Gh is produced by the testis of Japanese eel and stimulates proliferation of spermatogonia. *Reproduction*. 2011;142(6):869–77.

16. Filby AL, Tyler CR. Cloning and characterization of cDNAs for hormones and/or receptors of growth hormone, insulin-like growth factor-I, thyroid hormone, and corticosteroid and the gender-, tissue-, and developmental-specific expression of their mRNA transcripts in fathead minnow (*Pimephales promelas*). *Gen Comp Endocrinol [Internet]*. 2007 Jan 1 [cited 2018 Oct 31];150(1):151–63. Available from: http://www.ncbi.nlm.nih.gov/pubmed/16970945

17. Gallego Gómez R, Pintos E, García-Caballero T, Raghay K, Boulanger L, Beiras A et al. Cellular distribution of growth hormone-releasing hormone receptor in human reproductive system and breast and prostate cancers. *Histol Histopathol*. 2005;20(3):697–706.

18. Nguyen AP, Chandorkar A, Gupta C. The role of growth hormone in fetal mouse reproductive tract differentiation. *Endocrinology*. 1996;137(9):3659–66.

19. Reiter E, Kecha O, Hennuy B, Lardinois S, Klug M, Bruyninx M et al. Growth hormone directly affects the function of the different lobes of the rat prostate. *Endocrinology*. 1995;136(8):3338–45.

20. Colao A, Marzullo P, Spiezia S, Lombardi G. Acromegaly and prostate cancer. *Growth Horm IGF Res [Internet]*. 2000 Apr [cited 2018 Oct 31];10(Suppl A):S37–8. Available from: http://www.ncbi.nlm.nih.gov/pubmed/10984287

21. Lee SW, Kim SH, Kim JY, Lee Y. The effect of growth hormone on fibroblast proliferation and keratinocyte migration. *J Plast Reconstr Aesthetic Surg*. 2010;63(4).

22. Naderi G, Mohseni Rad H, Tabassomi F, Latif A. Seminal insulin-like growth factor-I may be involved in the pathophysiology of infertility among patients with clinical varicocele. *Hum Fertil (Camb) [Internet]*. 2015 Jun 3 [cited 2018 Oct 31];18(2):92–5. Available from: http://www.tandfonline.com/doi/full/10.3109/14647273.2014.965759

23. Becker AJ, Ückert S, Stief CG, Scheller F, Knapp WH, Hartmann U et al. Cavernous and systemic plasma levels of norepinephrine and epinephrine during different penile conditions in healthy men and patients with erectile dysfunction. *Urology*. 2002;59(2):281–6.

24. Jadresic A, Banks LM, Child DF, Diamant L, Doyle FH, Fraser TR et al. The acromegaly syndrome: Relation between clinical features, growth hormone values and radiological characteristics of the pituitary tumours. *QJM*. 1982;51(2):189–204.

25. Hull KL, Harvey S. Growth hormone: Roles in male reproduction. *Endocrine [Internet]*. 2000 Dec [cited 2018 Oct 31];13(3):243–50. Available from: http://www.ncbi.nlm.nih.gov/pubmed/11216634

26. Hull KL, Harvey S. GH as a co-gonadotropin: The relevance of correlative changes in GH secretion and reproductive state. *J Endocrinol [Internet]*. 2002 Jan [cited 2018 Oct 31];172(1):1–19. Available from: http://www.ncbi.nlm.nih.gov/pubmed/11786370

27. Gutiérrez-Pascual E, Martínez-Fuentes AJ, Pinilla L, Tena-Sempere M, Malagón MM, Castaño JP. Direct pituitary effects of kisspeptin: Activation of gonadotrophs and somatotrophs and stimulation of luteinising hormone and growth hormone secretion. *J Neuroendocrinol [Internet]*. 2007 Jul [cited 2018 Oct 31];19(7):521–30. Available from: http://doi.wiley.com/10.1111/j.1365-2826.2007.01558.x

28. Vaudry D, Gonzalez BJ, Basille M, Yon L, Fournier A, Vaudry H. Pituitary adenylate cyclase-activating polypeptide and its receptors: From structure to functions. *Pharmacol Rev [Internet]*. 2000 Jun [cited 2018 Oct 31];52(2):269–324. Available from: http://www.ncbi.nlm.nih.gov/pubmed/10835102

29. Childs GV. Growth hormone cells as co-gonadotropes: Partners in the regulation of the reproductive system. *Trends Endocrinol Metab [Internet]*. 2000 Jul [cited 2018 Oct 31];11(5):168–75. Available from: http://www.ncbi.nlm.nih.gov/pubmed/10856917

30. Barreiro ML, Tena-Sempere M. Ghrelin and reproduction: A novel signal linking energy status and fertility? Vol. 226, *Mol Cell Endocrinol*. 2004:226:1–9.

31. Tena-Sempere M. Exploring the role of ghrelin as novel regulator of gonadal function. *Growth Horm IGF Res*. 2005;15:83–8.

32. Sominsky L, Hodgson DM, McLaughlin EA, Smith R, Wall HM, Spencer SJ. Linking stress and infertility: A novel role for Ghrelin. *Endocr Rev*. 2017;38:432–67.

33. Ishikawa T, Fujioka H, Ishimura T, Takenaka A, Fujisawa M. Ghrelin expression in human testis and serum testosterone level. *J Androl*. 2007;28:320–4.

34. Ozkanli S, Basar MM, Selimoglu S, Erol B, Ozkanli O, Nurili F et al. The ghrelin and orexin activity in testicular tissues of patients with idiopathic non-obstructive azoospermia. *Kaohsiung J Med Sci*. 2018;34:564–8.

35. Caicedo D, Díaz O, Devesa P, Devesa J. Growth hormone (GH) and cardiovascular system. *Int J Mol Sci*. 2018;19.

36. Magon N, Saxena A, Singh S, Sahay R. Growth hormone in male infertility. *Indian J Endocrinol Metab [Internet]*. 2011 [cited 2018 Oct 29];15(7):248. Available from: http://www.ijem.in/text.asp?2011/15/7/248/84877

37. Simopoulou M, Philippou A, Maziotis E, Sfakianoudis K, Nitsos N, Bakas P et al. Association between male infertility and seminal plasma levels of growth hormone and insulin-like growth factor-1. *Andrologia [Internet]*. 2018 May 28 [cited 2018 Oct 31];50(7):e13048. Available from: http://doi.wiley.com/10.1111/and.13048

38. Cannarella R, Condorelli RA, La Vignera S, Calogero AE. Effects of the insulin-like growth factor system on testicular differentiation and function: A review of

the literature. *Andrology [Internet]*. 2018 Jan [cited 2018 Oct 31];6(1):3–9. Available from: http://doi.wiley.com/10.1111/andr.12444

39. Chubb C, Nolan C. Animal models of male infertility: Mice bearing single-gene mutations that induce infertility. *Endocrinology*. 1985;117(1):338–46.

40. Chubb C. Sexual behavior and fertility of little mice. *Biol Reprod [Internet]*. 1987;37(3):564–9. Available from: http://www.biolreprod.org/content/37/3/564.short

41. Donahue LR, Beamer WG. Growth hormone deficiency in "little" mice results in aberrant body composition, reduced insulin-like growth factor-I and insulin-like growth factor-binding protein-3 (IGFBP-3), but does not affect IGFBP-2, -1 or -4. *J Endocrinol [Internet]*. 1993 Jan [cited 2018 Oct 31];136(1):91–104. Available from: http://www.ncbi.nlm.nih.gov/pubmed/7679139

42. Eicher EM, Beamer WG. Inherited ateliotic dwarfism in mice: Characteristics of the mutation, little, on chromosome 6. *J Hered*. 1976;67(2):87–91.

43. Hammer RE, Palmiter RD, Brinster RL. Partial correction of murine hereditary growth disorder by germ-line incorporation of a new gene. *Nature*. 1984;311(5981):65–7.

44. Bartlett JM, Charlton HM, Robinson IC, Nieschlag E. Pubertal development and testicular function in the male growth hormone-deficient rat. *J Endocrinol [Internet]*. 1990 Aug [cited 2018 Oct 31];126(2):193–201. Available from: http://www.ncbi.nlm.nih.gov/pubmed/2119413

45. Vickers MH, Casey PJ, Champion ZJ, Gravance CG, Breier BH. IGF-I treatment increases motility and improves morphology of immature spermatozoa in the GH-deficient dwarf (dw/dw) rat. *Growth Horm IGF Res [Internet]*. 1999 Aug [cited 2018 Oct 31];9(4):236–40. Available from: http://linkinghub.elsevier.com/retrieve/pii/S1096637499901144

46. Carmignac DF, Bennett PA, Robinson IC. Effects of growth hormone secretagogues on prolactin release in anesthetized dwarf (dw/dw) rats. *Endocrinology [Internet]*. 1998 Aug [cited 2018 Oct 31];139(8):3590–6. Available from: https://academic.oup.com/endo/article-lookup/doi/10.1210/endo.139.8.6148

47. Charlton HM, Clark RG, Robinson IC, Goff AE, Cox BS, Bugnon C et al. Growth hormone-deficient dwarfism in the rat: A new mutation. *J Endocrinol [Internet]*. 1988 Oct [cited 2018 Oct 31];119(1):51–8. Available from: http://www.ncbi.nlm.nih.gov/pubmed/3193048

48. Umezu M, Kawada K, Miwa A, Ishii S, Masaki J. [Pituitary and plasma levels of growth hormone (GH), follicle stimulating hormone (FSH) and luteinizing hormone (LH) in hereditary dwarf rats (rdw/rdw)]. *Jikken Dobutsu [Internet]*. 1991 Oct [cited 2018 Oct 31];40(4):511–5. Available from: http://www.ncbi.nlm.nih.gov/pubmed/1748168

49. Umezu M, Fujimura T, Sugawara S, Kagabu S. Pituitary and serum levels of prolactin (PRL), thyroid stimulating hormone (TSH) and serum thyroxine (T4) in hereditary dwarf rats (rdw/rdw). *Jikken Dobutsu [Internet]*. 1993 Apr [cited 2018 Oct 31];42(2):211–6. Available from: http://www.ncbi.nlm.nih.gov/pubmed/8519297

50. Ono M, Harigai T, Furudate S. Pituitary-specific transcription factor Pit-1 in the rdw rat with growth hormone- and prolactin-deficient dwarfism. *J Endocrinol [Internet]*. 1994 Dec [cited 2018 Oct 31];143(3):479–87. Available from: http://www.ncbi.nlm.nih.gov/pubmed/7836893

51. Jiang JY, Umezu M, Sato E. Improvement of follicular development rather than gonadotrophin secretion by thyroxine treatment in infertile immature hypothyroid rdw rats. *J Reprod Fertil [Internet]*. 2000 Jul [cited 2018 Oct 31];119(2):193–9. Available from: http://www.ncbi.nlm.nih.gov/pubmed/10864830

52. Chatelain PG, Sanchez P, Saez JM. Growth hormone and insulin-like growth factor I treatment increase testicular luteinizing hormone receptors and steroidogenic responsiveness of growth hormone deficient dwarf mice. *Endocrinology [Internet]*. 1991 Apr [cited 2018 Oct 31];128(4):1857–62. Available from: http://www.ncbi.nlm.nih.gov/pubmed/2004605

53. Chandrashekar V, Bartke A. Induction of endogenous insulin-like growth factor-I secretion alters the hypothalamic-pituitary-testicular function in growth hormone-deficient adult dwarf mice. *Biol Reprod [Internet]*. 1993 Mar [cited 2018 Oct 31];48(3):544–51. Available from: http://www.ncbi.nlm.nih.gov/pubmed/8452930

54. Matsushima M, Kuroda K, Shirai M, Ando K, Sugisaki T, Noguchi T. Spermatogenesis in Snell dwarf, little and congenitally hypothyroid mice. *Int J Androl [Internet]*. 1986 Apr [cited 2018 Oct 31];9(2):132–40. Available from: http://www.ncbi.nlm.nih.gov/pubmed/3793256

55. Baker J, Hardy MP, Zhou J, Bondy C, Lupu F, Bellvé AR et al. Effects of an Igf1 gene null mutation on mouse reproduction. *Mol Endocrinol [Internet]*. 1996 Jul [cited 2018 Oct 31];10(7):903–18. Available from: https://academic.oup.com/mend/article-lookup/doi/10.1210/mend.10.7.8813730

56. Wang G-M, O'Shaughnessy PJ, Chubb C, Robaire B, Hardy MP. Effects of insulin-like growth factor I on steroidogenic enzyme expression levels in mouse Leydig cells. *Endocrinology [Internet]*. 2003 Nov [cited 2018 Oct 31];144(11):5058–64. Available from: https://academic.oup.com/endo/article-lookup/doi/10.1210/en.2003-0563

57. Zhou Y, Xu BC, Maheshwari HG, He L, Reed M, Lozykowski M et al. A mammalian model for Laron syndrome produced by targeted disruption of the mouse growth hormone receptor/binding protein gene (the Laron mouse). *Proc Natl Acad Sci USA*. 1997 Nov 25;94(24):13215–20.

58. Keene DE, Suescun MO, Bostwick MG, Chandrashekar V, Bartke A, Kopchick JJ. Puberty is delayed in male growth hormone receptor gene-disrupted mice. *J Androl [Internet]*. [cited 2018 Oct 31];23(5):661–8. Available from: http://www.ncbi.nlm.nih.gov/pubmed/12185100

59. Chandrashekar V, Bartke A, Awoniyi CA, Tsai-Morris CH, Dufau ML, Russell LD et al. Testicular endocrine function in GH receptor gene disrupted mice. *Endocrinology [Internet]*. 2001 Aug [cited 2018 Oct 31];142(8):3443–50. Available from: https://academic.oup.com/endo/article-lookup/doi/10.1210/endo.142.8.8298

60. Bachelot A, Monget P, Imbert-Bolloré P, Coshigano K, Kopchick JJ, Kelly PA et al. Growth hormone is required for ovarian follicular growth. *Endocrinology [Internet]*. 2002 Oct [cited 2018 Nov 1];143(10):4104–12. Available from: http://www.ncbi.nlm.nih.gov/pubmed/12239122

61. Zaczek D, Hammond J, Suen L, Wandji S, Service D, Bartke A et al. Impact of growth hormone resistance on female reproductive function: New insights from growth hormone receptor knockout mice. *Biol Reprod [Internet]*. 2002 Oct [cited 2018 Oct 31];67(4):1115–24. Available from: http://www.ncbi.nlm.nih.gov/pubmed/12297526

62. Kano K, Marín de Evsikova C, Young J, Wnek C, Maddatu TP, Nishina PM et al. A novel Dwarfism with gonadal dysfunction due to loss-of-function allele of the collagen receptor gene, *Ddr2*, in the mouse. *Mol Endocrinol [Internet]*. 2008 Aug [cited 2018 Oct 31];22(8):1866–80. Available from: https://academic.oup.com/mend/article-lookup/doi/10.1210/me.2007-0310

63. Castilla-Cortázar I, Gago A, Muñoz Ú, Ávila-Gallego E, Guerra-Menéndez L, Sádaba MC et al. Mechanisms underlying testicular damage and dysfunction in mice with partial IGF-1 deficiency and the effectiveness of IGF-1 replacement therapy. *Urology [Internet]*. 2015 Dec [cited 2018 Oct 31];86(6):1241.e1–9. Available from: https://linkinghub.elsevier.com/retrieve/pii/S0090429515008912

64. Bienvenu G, Seurin D, Grellier P, Froment P, Baudrimont M, Monget P et al. Insulin-like growth factor binding protein-6 transgenic mice: Postnatal growth, brain development, and reproduction abnormalities. *Endocrinology [Internet]*. 2004 May [cited 2018 Oct 31];145(5):2412–20. Available from: https://academic.oup.com/endo/article-lookup/doi/10.1210/en.2003-1196

65. Froment P, Seurin D, Hembert S, Levine JE, Pisselet C, Monniaux D et al. Reproductive abnormalities in human IGF binding protein-1 transgenic female mice. *Endocrinology [Internet]*. 2002 May [cited 2018 Nov 1];143(5):1801–8. Available from: https://academic.oup.com/endo/article-lookup/doi/10.1210/endo.143.5.8815

66. Laron Z, Sarel R. Penis and testicular size in patients with growth hormone insufficiency. *Acta Endocrinol (Copenh) [Internet]*. 1970 Apr [cited 2018 Nov 1];63(4):625–33. Available from: http://www.ncbi.nlm.nih.gov/pubmed/5468284

67. Laron Z, Sarel R, Pertzelan A. Puberty in Laron type dwarfism. *Eur J Pediatr [Internet]*. 1980 Jun [cited 2018 Nov 1];134(1):79–83. Available from: http://www.ncbi.nlm.nih.gov/pubmed/7408914

68. Laron Z, Klinger B. Effect of insulin-like growth factor-I treatment on serum androgens and testicular and penile size in males with Laron syndrome (primary growth hormone resistance). *Eur J Endocrinol [Internet]*. 1998 Feb [cited 2018 Nov 1];138(2):176–80. Available from: http://www.ncbi.nlm.nih.gov/pubmed/9506862

69. Andreassen M, Jensen RB, Jørgensen N, Juul A. Association between GH receptor polymorphism (exon 3 deletion), serum IGF1, semen quality, and reproductive hormone levels in 838 healthy young men. *Eur J Endocrinol [Internet]*. 2014 Apr [cited 2018 Oct 31];170(4):555–63. Available from: https://eje.bioscientifica.com/view/journals/eje/170/4/555.xml

70. Cannarella R, Mattina T, Condorelli RA, Mongioì LM, Pandini G, La Vignera S et al. Chromosome 15 structural abnormalities: Effect on IGF1R gene expression and function. *Endocr Connect [Internet]*. 2017 Oct [cited 2018 Oct 31];6(7):528–39. Available from: https://ec.bioscientifica.com/view/journals/ec/6/7/EC-17-0158.xml

71. Radicioni AF, Paris E, De Marco E, Anzuini A, Gandini L, Lenzi A. Testicular function in boys previously treated with recombinant-human growth hormone for non-growth hormone-deficient short stature. *J Endocrinol Invest [Internet]*. 2007 Dec 9 [cited 2018 Oct 31];30(11):931–6. Available from: http://www.ncbi.nlm.nih.gov/pubmed/18250614

72. Shimonovitz S, Zacut D, Ben Chetrit A, Ron M. Growth hormone status in patients with maturation arrest of spermatogenesis. *Hum Reprod [Internet]*. 1993 Jun [cited 2018 Oct 31];8(6):919–21. Available from: http://www.ncbi.nlm.nih.gov/pubmed/8345085

73. Carani C, Mantovani R, Procopio M, Del Rio G, Rossetto R, Granata AR. GH/IGF-I axis in azoospermia in primary and secondary hypogonadism: A study before and during replacement therapy. *Int J Androl [Internet]*. 1999 Jun [cited 2018 Oct 31];22(3):184–9. Available from: http://www.ncbi.nlm.nih.gov/pubmed/10367239

74. Lee KO, Ng SC, Lee PS, Bongso AT, Taylor EA, Lin TK et al. Effect of growth hormone therapy in men with severe idiopathic oligozoospermia. *Eur J Endocrinol [Internet]*. 1995 Feb [cited 2018 Oct 31];132(2):159–62. Available from: http://www.ncbi.nlm.nih.gov/pubmed/7858733

75. Ovesen P, Jørgensen JO, Kjaer T, Ho KK, Orskov H, Christiansen JS. Impaired growth hormone secretion and increased growth hormone-binding protein levels in subfertile males. *Fertil Steril [Internet]*. 1996 Jan [cited 2018 Oct 31];65(1):165–9. Available from: http://www.ncbi.nlm.nih.gov/pubmed/8557135

76. Mancini A, Olivieri G, Bruno C, Vergani E, Palladino A, Brunetti A. Infertility as an indication for provocative testing of growth hormone. *World Congr Gynecol Endocrinol.* 6–7.

77. Kalra S, Kalra B, Sharma A. Growth hormone improves semen volume, sperm count and motility in men with idiopathic normogonadotropic infertility. *Endocr Abstr.* 2008;16:P613.

78. Radicioni A, Paris E, Dondero F, Bonifacio V, Isidori A. Recombinant-growth hormone (rec-hGH) therapy in infertile men with idiopathic oligozoospermia. *Acta Eur Fertil [Internet].* [cited 2018 Oct 31];25(5):311–7. Available from: http://www.ncbi.nlm.nih.gov/pubmed/7660721

79. Ovesen P, Jørgensen JO, Ingerslev J, Ho KK, Orskov H, Christiansen JS. Growth hormone treatment of subfertile males. *Fertil Steril [Internet].* 1996 Aug [cited 2018 Oct 31];66(2):292–8. Available from: http://www.ncbi.nlm.nih.gov/pubmed/8690119

80. Giagulli VA. Absence of effect of recombinant growth hormone to classic gonadotropin treatment on spermatogenesis of patients with severe hypogonadotropic hypogonadism. *Arch Androl [Internet].* [cited 2018 Oct 31];43(1):47–53. Available from: http://www.ncbi.nlm.nih.gov/pubmed/10445104

81. Shoham Z, Conway GS, Ostergaard H, Lahlou N, Bouchard P, Jacobs HS. Cotreatment with growth hormone for induction of spermatogenesis in patients with hypogonadotropic hypogonadism. *Fertil Steril [Internet].* 1992 May [cited 2018 Oct 31];57(5):1044–51. Available from: http://www.ncbi.nlm.nih.gov/pubmed/1572472

82. Zalel Y, Manor M, Zadik Z, Shoham Z. Successful induction of spermatogenesis in a patient with hypogonadotropic hypogonadism following co-treatment with growth hormone. *Gynecol Endocrinol [Internet].* 1996 Feb [cited 2018 Oct 31];10(1):29–31. Available from: http://www.ncbi.nlm.nih.gov/pubmed/8737189

83. Smuel K, Kauli R, Lilos P, Laron Z. Growth, development, puberty and adult height before and during treatment in children with congenital isolated growth hormone deficiency. *Growth Horm IGF Res [Internet].* 2015 Aug [cited 2018 Oct 31];25(4):182–8. Available from: https://linkinghub.elsevier.com/retrieve/pii/S1096637415300010

Retinoic acid signaling in spermatogenesis and male (in)fertility

DARIO SANTOS AND RITA PAYAN-CARREIRA

HIGHLIGHTS

- Retinoids and retinoic acid (RA) are essential players in biological signaling pathways.
- RA has a vital role in spermatogenesis and male fertility.
- RA is involved in sperm metabolism and oxidative stress.
- Disturbed RA signaling contributes to human male infertility.

7.1 INTRODUCTION

Spermatogenesis is a complex, highly tuned and orderly process occurring in the seminiferous tubules in male testes. During spermatogenesis, diploid germ cells timely engage in the process of multiplication and differentiation that ends with the release of spermatozoa (a haploid cell) into the lumen of the seminiferous tubules (1). One round of spermatogenesis encompasses three stages: (a) the mitotic proliferation of spermatogonia (SPG), often named as spermatocytogenesis; (b) the reductional meiosis by spermatocytes (SPCs); and (c) the differentiation of spermatids (SPD), an unique maturational process during which an initial round cell transforms into a highly specialized flagellated cell with tightly condensed chromatin and an acrosome—the spermatozoon (2,3). The sequential progress of these three stages is tightly regulated in both time and space, under the orchestrated control of Sertoli cells, Leydig cells and the germ cells themselves (2), fostering a stage-related environment to the developing germ cells.

Postpubertal seminiferous tubules contain numerous generations of germ cells. Spermatogenesis in mammals relies on a pool of undifferentiated spermatogonial stem cells (SSCs) residing in particular locations of the seminiferous tubules named niches that foster cell self-renewal (3). Niches are particular sites within the seminiferous tubules where the contribution from surrounding cells (e.g., Sertoli, myoid and Leydig cells) contributes to the creation of a particular environment that sustains SSC differentiation into a pathway of self-renewal or proliferation (4,5). In niches, SSCs have the unique capability to enroll in two different, exclusive pathways: self-renewal (originating new spermatogonial stem cells) or proliferation into more differentiated progeny (proliferating spermatogonia A).

In the case of self-renewal, complete cytokinesis occurs with the formation of two single cells, while in the proliferative differentiated SPG incomplete cytokinesis results in the formation of two cells connected by cytoplasmatic bridges (6). Novel generations of sperm cells arise from spermatogonia that are stimulated to differentiate into a proliferative profile without waiting for the preceding generations to complete their development and be released into the tubules (1), thereby ensuring that spermatogenesis is maintained throughout the male life span (7). The germ cells originating from an undifferentiated spermatogonium maintain a coordinated rate of differentiation, which is possible due to its syncytial arrangement during spermatogenesis (2).

SSC recruitment into the differentiation pathway and meiosis occur at time intervals, starting asynchronously through the seminiferous tubule (8), at space intervals, contributing to spermatozoal production *in a continuum* (1,3). This particularity underlies the phenomena known as the spermatogenic wave, which has been demonstrated to exist in a large number of mammalian species (1). Recruitment of SSCs into the proliferative pathway supports two distinct events, as from that division, one of the cells returns to a quiescent, nonproliferative stage, allowing for the replenishment of the spermatogonial population, while the other further mitotically divide, committing to meiosis (1,7).

The importance of vitamin A and retinoic acid (RA) as potential regulators of spermatogenesis and sperm maturation through the epididymis has long been recognized (9,10). Insufficient vitamin A intake has been associated with infertility due to loss of most germ cells from the seminiferous tubules. Even though vitamin A or retinoid administration may revert most symptoms of vitamin A deficiency, the dynamics of spermatogenesis may be recovered, albeit in a synchronous pattern that disrupts the typical wave of spermatogenesis (10). Despite treatment unblocking the spermatogonial differentiation and meiosis, it triggers a simultaneous differentiation of undifferentiated spermatogonia and therefore synchronous spermatogenesis (11); it also often increases the number of degenerated cells (12). Solid studies support the evidence that RA affects gene expression in the seminiferous epithelium, in a stage-specific pattern. Any stimuli impairing RA signaling will negatively impact spermatogenesis and may lead to azoospermia (2). It has been shown that the trigger of SSCs into mitosis is rigidly timed and under the control of a peak in RA, whose testicular levels are strictly controlled (2,6). This molecule has also been associated with the initiation of the meiotic process and spermiogenesis (3). Furthermore, RA is crucial for the first cycle of the seminiferous epithelium at puberty.

In this chapter, we review the role played by RA on spermatogenesis and discuss the current understanding of RA signaling pathways in Sertoli cells and germ cells.

7.2 VITAMIN A AND RETINOIDS

Vitamin A is a term usually used as a generic descriptor for all molecules with the biological activity of retinol (ROL) (13). Six isoforms of retinol are reported with biologic activity (14), but the all-*trans*-retinol (generally named retinol, ROL) is the most common and best studied in animal tissues. RA and retinyl esters (REs) are derivatives of ROL and are often collectively referred as vitamin A (15). However, the term *vitamin A* should refer only to all-*trans*-retinol, a compound that, when sufficiently present in the diet, satisfies all the vitamin A requirements for proper development and growth (16). Vitamin A–active compounds presenting the biological activity of ROL, comprise retinoids (ROL, retinaldehyde and RA) and provitamin A (carotenoids). Vitamin A is essential for vision and the immune system as well as indispensable for the formation and maintenance of several animal tissues (17,18). Vitamin A, after conversion to RA, also plays a role in reproduction and embryonic growth and development (19), affecting embryonic development and organogenesis, tissue homeostasis, cell proliferation, differentiation and apoptosis (20,21).

7.2.1 Retinoid metabolism

Most animals cannot synthesize vitamin A. It is an essential micronutrient that must be acquired from the diet either in the form of provitamin A carotenoids, occurring in vegetables and fruits, or as preformed retinoids (REs and ROL the most abundant forms) present in animal source foods (13). Animals cleave absorbed carotenoids to form retinal (21). Alternatively, animals can obtain ROL by eating animal tissues that have already converted carotenoids to retinoids such as ROL and REs (14). Absorbed retinoids are secreted from enterocytes into the lymph either as chylomicrons (containing carotenoids, REs, small amounts of free ROL) or ROL and transported either to target tissues or hepatocytes for storage (15). RE is the primary form stored in the liver of mammals, birds and fish (21).

The REs are hydrolyzed at the hepatocyte cell membrane and free ROL, which is then bound to a ROL binding protein (RBP). RBPs are carrier proteins for ROL that, together with transthyretin, facilitate the transport of fat-soluble ROL in the bloodstream and the interstitial compartment of target tissues (22). In vitamin A–sufficient states, the retinol-RBP (holo-RBP) complex is secreted and associated with transthyretin and transferred from hepatocytes to the stellate cells of the liver. Here it is esterified by LRAT to form mainly retinyl palmitate. The stellate cells contain 90%–95% of hepatic vitamin A as cytoplasmatic lipid droplets (23).

ROL is delivered from the liver to target cells bound to RBP (holo-RBP) and transthyretin (24). Holo-RBP binds to cell surface RBP receptor STRA6 that mediates ROL uptake from holo-RBP into cytoplasmatic CRBPI (25). CRBP is a cellular high-affinity ROL binding protein, which facilitates its transport into the nucleus or its metabolism in different cells (26). ROL is delivered to the intramembrane system (endoplasmatic reticulum) where ROL is esterified by leci- thin ROL acyltransferase (LRAT) to RE or oxidized by alco- hol dehydrogenases (ADHs) to retinal (RAL). Finally, RAL is oxidized to RA by cytoplasmatic retinaldehyde dehydro- genase (RALDH), or they are reduced back to ROL by reti- naldehyde reductases (RalRD) in the internal membranes (27). In addition, RA could derive from β-carotene (CAR) uptaken by the cells, cleaved into two molecules of retinal- dehyde by BCMO-1 (β, β-carotene-15,15′-monooxygenase) and then oxidized into RA (27,28).

In the cell, RA binds to CRABPI or CRABPII and is transferred by holo-CRABPII to the nucleus to activate transcription (autocrine), transported to a nearby target cell (paracrine) or delivered to endoplasmatic CYP enzymes by holo-CRABPI for further degradation (27). Tissue RA con- centrations are regulated both by enzymes that generate RA (ROL and retinal dehydrogenases) and by enzymes that metabolize RA to fewer active metabolites, including cyto- chrome P450 enzymes from the CYP26 family (CYP26A1, CYP26B, CYP26C1) (29,30).

7.2.2 Tissue targeting and retinoic acid signaling

In the classic signaling mechanism (canonical pathway), RA effects are mediated through binding to specific nuclear receptors (retinoid receptors) followed by changes of tran- scription of several genes (31,32). Retinoid receptors can be divided into two subgroups, RA receptors (RARs) and reti- noid X receptors (RXRs) (33). The RAR has three isotypes (RARα, RARβ and RARγ) (34), and each is capable of het- erodimerizing with a retinoid X receptor isotype (RXRα, RXRβ or RXRγ). The RAR–RXR heterodimer binds on the chromosome to sequence stretches called RA-response ele- ments (RAREs) and functions as a transcriptional activator in the presence of its hormonal ligand and as a repressor in the absence of RA (35). Retinoid X receptor (RXR) interacts with RAR, allowing RXR to function as a master controller for signals from various hormonal pathways. In the nucleus, RAR and RXR form heterodimers bound to RAREs and associate with a co-repressor complex.

According to the canonical model of gene regulation by RARs (Figure 7.1), in the absence of RA, the DNA-bound RAR subtype represses target gene expression through the recruit- ment of co-repressors such as nuclear receptor co-repressor (NCoR) or silencing mediator of RA and thyroid hormone receptor (SMRT). Several studies suggested that SMRT would be the RAR-favored co-repressor (36,37), which serves as a molecular adaptor recruiting histone deacetylase (HDAT) (38). The co-repressor complex deacetylates lysine residues in the N-terminal tails of histones and induces chromatin condensation and repressed state over the target promoter (39,40). Binding of RA induces a conformational change of the RAR/RXR heterodimer that results in the release of co-repressors and creates a new interaction surface for co- activators, which include p160 subfamily of steroid receptor coactivators (SRCs), namely, SRC-1, SRC-2 and SRC-3 (29,41).

The p160 coactivators have intrinsic histone acetyltransferase (HAT) activity and acetylate several lysine residues in H3 and H4, initiating gene transcription (42).

Over 500 genes have been put forth as being regulatory targets of RA. In some cases, direct regulation was demon- strated driven by ligand RAR/RXR heterodimers bound to RAREs (43). RA induces the transcription of many genes encoding proteins that are involved in cell differentiation and a variety of biochemical processes (19,44). The first RAR target genes to be discovered were RARβ, laminin B1, CRBP and CRABP (29). Moreover, proteins involved in RA metabolism, such as CYP26, are also directly regulated by RA (43). The Hox gene, one of the most well-known target genes of RARs, is a key regulator of pattern formation in vertebrates during development (45). RARs also regulate factors involved in metabolism (29).

In addition to its canonical effects (gene-mediated), RA has some nongenomic (gene-independent) functions. Noncanonical retinoid signaling is independent of gene tran- scription mediated by RAR/RXR heterodimers (27). Some of these nongenomic effects are the result of RA binding to retinoid receptors but can often occur in the absence of reti- noid receptors. RAR has also been implicated in mediating RA nongenomic actions (46). Evidence indicates that RA also utilizes other nongenomic pathways: phospholipase C-PKC, phosphatidylinositol-3-kinase (PI3 K)-Akt (47), RAF-ERK- MAPK pathway or v-src sarcoma (SRC) tyrosine kinase acti- vation (46,48). PI3 K activates PDK1, which in turn activates Akt. This kinase mediates the mammalian target of rapamy- cin (mTor) activity, a serine/threonine protein kinase. mTor is the catalytic subunit of the mTORC-1 protein complex, inte- grating nutrient signals and mitogen promoting cell survival, growth and proliferation (49). The RA activated-dependent PI3 K/Akt pathway leads to phosphorylation of the tuber- ous sclerosis protein (TSC1), resulting in mTORC-1 activa- tion. The downstream effectors of mTORC-1 are translational modulators within the protein synthesis pathway, ribosomal S6 kinase 1 (S6K1) and initiation factor 4E (eIF4E)-binding protein 1 (4E-BP1), which are stimulated by mTORC1-medi- ated phosphorylation, enhancers of protein synthesis, cell growth and proliferation (49). AKT also contributes to cell cycle progression and inhibition of apoptosis by increasing the expression of cyclins and antiapoptotic Bcl-2 family mem- bers, mediating hyperphosphorylation of proapoptotic BAD, leading to the mitochondrial-dependent apoptosis (intrinsic apoptosis pathway) (50). Additionally, RA activates the ERK- MAPK signaling cascade and regulates mTORC-1 activity: ERK phosphorylates and activates kinase RSK1 that in turn phosphorylates and inhibits TSC1/2, followed by increased activity of mTORC-1 (29,47).

7.3 EFFECTS OF RA ON SPERMATOGENESIS

Several studies revealed that several crucial germ cell differ- entiation steps occur at a particular stage of spermatogen- esis, and all of them are driven by periodic increases in RA

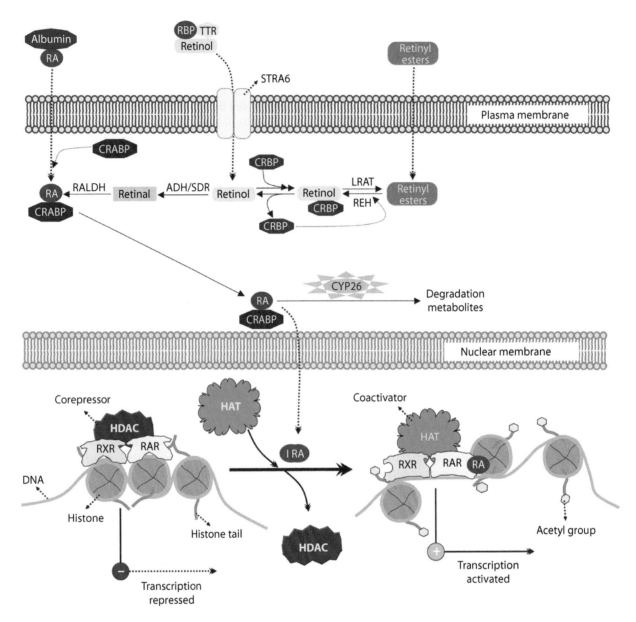

Figure 7.1 Gene regulation by retinoic acid nuclear receptors. The inactive heterodimer RAS-RXR is located in the nucleus and binds DNA. In the absence of retinoic acid, RAR-RXR is complexed with a co-repressor HDAC, which prevents gene transcription. In the presence of retinoic acid, the heterodimer suffers conformational modification, decreasing its affinity for HDAC (that is released) and increasing the affinity for the coactivator HAT, activating the target gene expression. (ADH, alcohol dehydrogenase; CRABP, cellular retinoic acid binding protein; CRBP, cellular retinol binding protein; CYP26, cytochrome P450 family 26; HAT, histone acetyltransferase; HDAC, histone deacetylase; LRAT, lecithin retinol acyltransferase; RA, retinoic acid; RALDH, retinaldehyde dehydrogenase; RAR, retinoic acid receptor; RBP, retinol binding protein; REH, retinyl ester hydrolase; RXR, retinoid X receptor; STRA6, stimulated by retinoic acid gene 6; TTR, transthyretin.)

levels (e.g., stages VII–XII in the mouse model) (51). It has been shown that the occurrence of all those steps is concentrated in the same spermatogenic steps, such as the differentiation of spermatogonia, meiotic initiation, acquisition of SPD polarity and spermiation (51–53). From this point on, this review concentrates on the effects of RA in those particular events of spermatogenesis. Most of the available information on the RA effects on spermatogenesis was gathered from rodent species. There is still a lot to explore about RA signaling pathways in other species.

7.3.1 Evidence of retinoid acid effects in spermatogenesis

The first study supporting vitamin A requirements for normal spermatogenesis was published in 1925. This study showed that vitamin A deficiency induces an early arrest of spermatogenesis, which was later associated with degeneration of germ cells and defective testosterone secretion. These changes could be reversed by either vitamin A or RA administration (22). Using transgenic animals, several experiments described the disruption of spermatogonial differentiation and further downstream effects of RA. Along with excess and depleted RA models, those studies allowed for clarification of some RA signaling pathways and RA effects on spermatogenesis (11,22).

In vitamin A–deficient (VAD) animals, the complete arrest of undifferentiated spermatogonia that failed to enter the proliferative pathway that starts spermatogenesis were described. This arrest could be reversed by administration of ROL, but its administration only allowed for synchronization of spermatogenesis and the loss of the wave dynamics typical of the spermatogenic process (54).

Studies in postnatal knockout mice showed that dietary depletion of vitamin A originates meiotic arrest due to the loss of the gene *Stra8* expression (55), which is indispensable to switch from mitosis to meiosis (30). The accumulation of undifferentiated spermatogonia also found in those animals (8) further aggravates the effects of the meiotic arrest on the loss of spermatogenesis.

Models using both genetic and metabolic impairment of RA signaling, particularly those resulting in changes (inhibition or stimulation) of RA receptors, suggested that there are different pathways involved in retinoids signaling in spermatogenesis, which differ between testicular somatic cells and germ cells, and even between different populations of germ cells (10). In normal tissue, these diverse pathways and players contribute to the finely tuned spermatogenic process, but when the mainstream RA signaling is disrupted, the negative effects on sperm production and male fertility are also potentialized.

7.3.2 Expression of retinoids and retinoid receptors in the mammalian testis

In the testis, all the main cellular types (peritubular myoid cells, Sertoli cells, germ cells and Leydig cells) respond to retinoids (22). Peritubular cells capture ROL, coupling it with cellular retinol binding protein (CRBP) and secrete it bound to a new RBP toward the Sertoli cells. Sertoli cells are able to take up and store ROL, either from the blood circulation or the peritubular cells, and convert it into RA. RA production and storage within Sertoli cells vary with the stage of the seminiferous epithelium, associated with changes in FSH secretion (11). Inside Sertoli cells, RA is made available to germ cells and Sertoli cell functions, while the RBP-bound ROL can also be used by spermatocytes to synthesize RA (Figure 7.2). Besides the Sertoli cells, SPDs and testicular and epididimal spermatozoa can store retinoids (11). In the interstitium, Leydig cells can capture RBP-bound ROL secreted by the peritubular cells (22).

Cell compartmentalization of enzymes and proteins involved in RA synthesis, degradation and storage, kept testicular RA levels tightly regulated—both temporally and spatially. In the seminiferous tubules, pulses or RA are produced in a stage-dependent manner, allowing for the adaptation of RA levels to particular stages of sperm cell development. The peritubular myoid cell layer acts as a catabolic barrier, preventing RA from entering the seminiferous tubules. Also, late pachytene and diplotene SPCs can synthesize RA, providing the germ cells developing in the adluminal compartment with a complementary RA

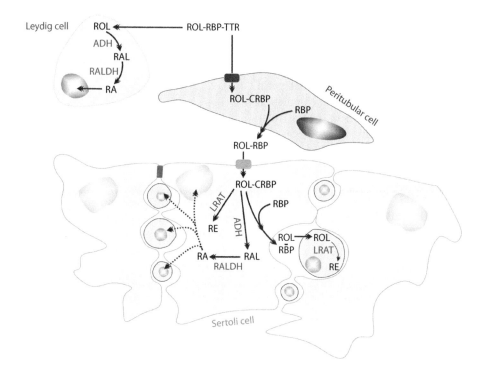

Figure 7.2 Regulation of testicular functions by retinoids. (ADH, alcohol dehydrogenase; CRBP, cellular retinol binding protein; LRAT, lecithin retinol acyltransferase; RA, retinoic acid; RALDH, retinaldehyde dehydrogenase; RAR, retinoic acid receptor; RBP, retinol binding protein; RE, retinyl ester; ROL, retinol; TTR, transthyretin.)

Table 7.1 Location of retinoid receptors and proteins in the testicular tissue

Testicular cells		Molecule
Sertoli cells		CRBP-I
		CRABP-II [Foetal and early postnatal]
		RAR-α1, RAR-α2
		RAR-β
		RXR-β
Peritubular myoid cells		CRBP-I
		RAR-α
Germ cells	Gonocytes	CRABP-I
	SPG	CRBP-I
		CRABP-I
		RAR-α
		RAR-γ
	SPC-I	CRBP-I
		RAR-α1 [SPC-pach]
		RAR-γ [SPC-pach]
	SPD-r	RAR-α1
		RXR-α
		RXR-γ
Leydig cells		CRBP-I
		CRABP-I
		CRABP-II [Foetal and early postnatal]
		RAR-α
		RAR-γ
		RXR-β
		RXR-γ

Abbreviations: CRABP, cellular retinoic acid binding protein; CRBP, cellular retinol binding protein; RAR, retinoic acid receptor; RXR, retinoid X receptor; SPC-pach, pachytene spermatocytes; SPD-r, round spermatids; SPG, spermatogonia.

source (52,56). It has also been demonstrated that germ cells express RA receptors according to their developmental stage (56). A summary of the RA receptors in the testicular cells of mammals are listed in Table 7.1.

7.3.3 RA signaling pathways in male germ cells and spermatogenesis

7.3.3.1 RA IN FETAL AND PREPUBERTAL SUSPENSION OF SPERMATOGENESIS

Albeit spermatogenesis often refers to the process of spermatozoa production that starts at puberty in the male, one could consider that it should also respect the embryonic period, when primordial germ cells (PGCs) migrate into the differentiating genital ridge (Figure 7.3). PGCs actively proliferate until they associate with somatic cells. Soon after the somatic sex differentiation in the gonad, the proliferating primordial germ cells gradually lose their mitotic ability and enter a quiescent phase that is maintained until puberty (5,57). The arrest of the proliferative ability and the inhibition to enter meiosis contrast with that observed in the

female gonad (58) and has been related to inhibition of the RA signaling cascades (59).

Evidence showed that in male gonads, after the indifferent gonad acquires a male-like morphological pattern under the influence of SRY, the RA of mesonephric origin is sequestrated (metabolized) mainly by Sertoli cells. Consequently, the levels of RA are too low to trigger the production of STA8, which do not permit germ cells to initiate meiosis (59,60). Several studies demonstrated that, in Sertoli cells, CYP26B1 degrades all-*trans*-RA into inactive metabolites, thereby locally regulating the RA levels (cf. [59]). Similarly, in cultures of male fetal mouse gonads treated with CYP26B1 inhibitors, primordial germ cells enter meiosis, like it occurs in the female gonad (61).

Gonocytes are the sole source of the functional SSCs pool in the postnatal testis (60). While maintenance of the SSC begins shortly after birth and continues through the extent of adulthood, as a result of the self-renewal ability demonstrated by SSCs, spermatogonial differentiation from those undifferentiated cells starts at the onset of puberty (Figure 7.3) (57).

7.3.3.2 RA AND THE ASYNCHRONOUS SPERMATOGONIA RECRUITMENT

Spermatogonial differentiation (or its exit from the stem cell pool) is one of the pivotal transitions in spermatogenesis (51). Once the pool of SSCs is established, in adult testes, differentiation of those cells can involve two types of processes, as already said: the self-renewal pathway that produces progenitor cells, or the one originating differentiating spermatogonia (62,63). The second type of differentiation process depends on RA signaling, which results in the expression of c-Kit, in the differentiated SPG (57,62). When this type of differentiation occurs, the differentiated SPG leaves the niche and commits to spermatogenesis (57). The proliferation of differentiated spermatogonia is originated by binding of the stem cell factor (SCF), produced by Sertoli cells, to the SPG existing c-Kit, and allowing for the amplification of the number of cells acquiring the competency to enter meiosis (63). In mice, WNT-family polypeptides accelerate SSC proliferation (64).

Proliferation and differentiation of SSCs are regulated by intrinsic factors (the stem cell itself) and extrinsic factors (the niche environment). The intrinsic regulation of the SSC fate remains poorly understood (63), but it may be possible that it would command the ability of SSCs to respond to environmental cues to differentiation. Regarding the extrinsic factors, it is now accepted that within the niche, endogenous, locally controlled RA gradients or pulses trigger the periodic differentiation of male germ cells (8,53,63), according to an asynchronous pattern of SSC differentiation that fosters a continuum of spermatozoa production through the male adult life.

The RA pulses result from its storage after synthesis from ROL by RDH or DHRS enzymes (53) in Sertoli and peritubular myoid cells. Activation of RDH or DHRS enzymes occurs in a stage-specific manner (Figure 7.4), contributing

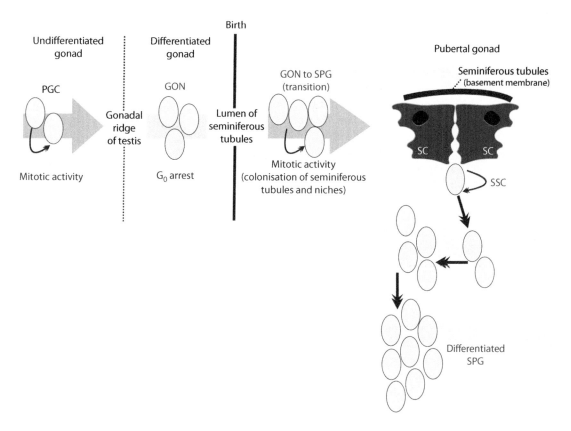

Figure 7.3 Overview of mitotic germ cell development in mammals. (GON, gonocytes; PGC, primordial germ cells; SE, Sertoli cell; SPG, spermatogonia; SSC, spermatogonial stem cells.)

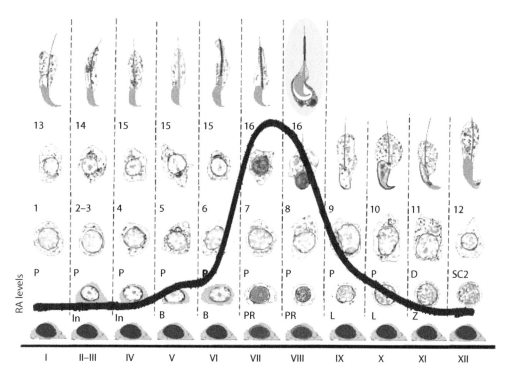

Figure 7.4 The proposed RA relative levels (in blue) through the cycle of the seminiferous epithelium in mice, as per the pulse theory. Red color signals the critical RA-dependent transitions reported in germ cells (spermatogonial differentiation from SSCs, meiotic competency and acquisition of polarity in spermatids), which culminate in spermiation when mature elongated spermatids are freed to the lumen of the seminiferous tubules as single cells.

to the spatiotemporal control of RA biosynthesis. RA chaperoned by CRABP binds to its receptors. According to Mecklenburg and Hermann (63), it is not clear whether RARs or RXRs are the retinoid receptors involved in the cellular changes induced by RA in progenitor spermatogonia. In consequence, the nuclear response includes the translation of mRNAs encoding the KIT tyrosine kinase and STRA8, through a mechanism involving P13 K/AKT/mTOR (65) and ERK signaling pathways (62).

While in the niche, SSCs are exposed to changes in the gradients of growth factors and cytokines, among other molecules, promoting the maintenance of the actual and potential germline stem cells in their undifferentiated state (57,63). By leaving the niche, the differentiated SPG eludes their influences and engages in proliferation.

7.3.3.3 RA IN THE INITIATION OF MEIOSIS

During spermatogenesis, the switch from mitosis to meiosis is dependent on the activation of the *Stra8* gene (8,61,66), an early RA responsive gene. STRA8 protein has been evidenced in preleptotene SPCs and is being considered crucial to the transition from type B spermatogonia/preleptotene to leptotene SPCs, and support progression of later stages of the meiotic prophase (67). Despite its dependence on RA, it seems that the *Stra8* gene may also be under an epigenetic control that would contribute to its responsivity to RA stimulation (66). *Stra8* has been shown to be depressed by bHLH transcription factors, such as SOHLHs, *Nanos* (66) and DMRTs (68,69), which are obtained by limiting all RA-induced transcription in general. However, Toyoda and collaborators (70) demonstrated that *Sohlh2* would interact with *Sohlh1* to control *Kit* synthesis (a marker of spermatogonia differentiation into preleptotene SPCs) through the transcriptional regulation of E-box, but they did not find marked changes in *Stra8* transcription.

Stra8 is crucial to the SPC transition to the zygotene/pachytene stages. According to Ma et al. (66), *Stra8* regulates, directly or indirectly, the transcription of multiple genes, which relate to premeiotic DNA replication, double-strand break formation, chromosomal rearrangements and pairing, chromosomal synapsis, meiotic recombination processes and telomers binding.

Albeit the most accepted theory considers that *Stra8* is necessary and sufficient for initiation of meiosis in male germ cells, it has been recently suggested that other RA-induced players may be involved in the process (59). Kouhova and colleagues (71) demonstrated that RA-dependent meiotic initiation uses both the *Stra8* and the *Rec8* independent pathways, both of them requiring the germ cells to express *Dazl*. *Rec8* is incorporated in the cohesin meiotic complex, essential during chromosome segregation and chiasmata formation.

Increased *Stra8* gene expression has been hypothesized to be triggered, in the germ cells, by the canonic signaling pathway of RAR/RXR-RA and RARE (71). However, the RA-induced mechanisms of *Rec8* expression remained elusive.

7.3.3.4 RA IN SPERMATID DEVELOPMENT

RA signaling through RARα is essential for SPD polarization and orientation within the tubules. Failure in this pathway leads to a temporary arrest on SPD development (72) and an increase in apoptosis of elongating SPD (73).

It has been demonstrated that the actin filament bundles maintain SPD polarity at the Sertoli cell–elongating/elongated SPD interface at the apical ectoplasmic specializations (74), which first appears when SPD starts polarization and elongation.

Rai14 is a RA-induced protein and an actin-binding protein that participates in the organization of actin cytoskeleton filaments in the seminiferous epithelium. This protein has been implicated in the integrity of actin-based tight junctional complexes, in the basal ectoplasmic specializations, that participate in the blood-testis barrier (75).

Disruption of Rai14 expression led to defects in the SPD polarity, SPD elongation and spermiation. Moreover, elongating and elongated SPD are also often found entrapped deeper in the seminiferous epithelium, at an inappropriate location for spermiation. It has been shown that disturbance of Rai14 would compromise the proper F-actin organization, mediated by the binding to paladin, and consequently would impair the proper transport of SPD across the spermatogenic epithelium (76). Such defects in F-actin organization were described either at the Sertoli-spermatid interface or at the blood-testis barrier. Furthermore, RARα signaling participates in the control of cell adhesion. Hasegawa and Saga (77), in mice, demonstrated that RAR-mediated RA signaling is associated with a stage-dependent organization of the blood-testis barrier.

It has been shown that spermiation depends on RA signaling via the RARα/RXRβ heterodimer expressed in Sertoli cells (78). In consequence, it occurs after the reorganization of the actin filaments into highly branched networks forming the tubulobulbar complexes, transient endocytic structures through which the excess of SPD cytoplasm is removed, contributing to the final disengagement of SPDs from Sertoli cells (79).

7.3.3.5 RA AND THE BLOOD-TESTIS BARRIER

The spatial arrangement of the germ cells within the tubules is crucial to spermatogenesis. This arrangement results in the particular junctional system created by both inter-Sertoli cell interactions and germ–Sertoli cell interactions. These different junctions create different functional compartments within the seminiferous tubules that serve the need for particular environmental conditions throughout germ cell development while also creating an immune privileged site for the development of haploid germ cells. Peer et al. (3) found RA signaling through RARα cross talk with Sertoli cells controlled the junctional processes that ensure the migration of germ cells from one compartment to another (52). This transmigration is accomplished by breaking the inter-Sertolian tight junctions ahead of them and reforming the junctions behind, creating a transient compartment (80). Like in spermiation, an involvement of Rai14 has been proposed.

7.3.4 Influence of RA on sperm metabolism and oxidative stress

Free radicals and other reactive oxygen species (ROS) are continuously generated as by-products of normal cellular metabolism. Cells accommodate ROS using scavenger molecules, including vitamin A. Retinoids are potent scavengers of ROS (81), playing a crucial function in the cellular redox balance in different tissues and situations.

Research on biological systems has shown that ROS are far more than the unavoidable by-products of oxygen metabolism and that they play essential roles, when in low, controlled levels, as signaling molecules regulating biological processes (82).

Normal physiologic levels of ROS are essential for fertilization, through their involvement in processes such as capacitation, acrosome reaction, gamete chemotaxis, binding to the zona pellucida and sperm-oocyte fusion (83–85). Increasing levels of P-Tyr proteins characterize sperm capacitation. Protein phosphorylation results from an increased activity of protein kinase A (PKA), activated by cAMP, which is driven by stimulation of adenylate cyclase (AC) in the presence of physiological ROS levels, specifically superoxide radicals. High levels of P-Tyr proteins may also result from an inhibitory effect of ROS over the phosphotyrosine phosphatase (PTPase) (83,86).

In spermatozoa, the normal ROS values are controlled by the cellular antioxidant system that consists of catalase (CAT), superoxide dismutase (SOD), glutathione peroxidase and vitamin E (87,88). SOD has been detected in the sperm of several species, including humans, rabbits and mice (89,90). Sustained SOD activity triggers increased levels of H_2O_2, which in turn has been implicated in ROS signaling, namely, in the activity of protein phosphatases (PTPs), non-receptor protein tyrosine kinases (PTKs), protein kinase C (PKC), mitogen-activated protein kinases (MAPKs) and transcriptional factors (TFs)—all of them critical intracellular pathways of normal spermatozoa function (85,91,92).

Excessive production of ROS has been associated with sperm dysfunction (81,85,93). Lipid and protein peroxidation of sperm membranes, DNA damage and cell death (apoptosis) follow the increase in ROS concentrations, consequently affecting sperm concentration, motility and morphology (94–99). In brief, they compromise male fertility, which agrees with the finding that superoxide dismutase activity is lower in the seminal plasma of infertile patients (100).

RA has been shown to mitigate tissue susceptibility to oxidative stress by acting on some oxidative stress enzymes, such as SOD, CAT and glutathione reductase (101,102). RA impacts oxidative stress–mediated apoptosis in several tissues (103–105) and embryo differentiation (106). Redox-mediated apoptosis could be reverted in those tissues by the administration of all-*trans*-retinoic acid (ATRA). RA modulates antioxidant mechanisms also in spermatozoa (107). The action of RA in cell physiology is mediated by nuclear RA receptors and retinoid X receptors. Additionally, it has been described as a cytoplasmatic localization of receptors in bull and dog sperm, probably playing an active role in the cross talk with other signal transduction pathways (108).

Evidence showed that a broad spectrum of RA physiological effects might result from both a receptor- and a non-receptor-dependent mechanism (109). RA at physiological concentrations inhibits the decrease in SOD activity and significantly reduces hyperglycemia-induced oxidative stress, protects neurons from oxidative stress and prevents a reduction in SOD levels in rats after heart overload with pressure (110,111). Besides, RA mitigated changes in SOD protein levels decreasing the rate of SOD protein degradation in staurosporine-induced oxidative stress in neonatal rat hippocampus cells (102).

7.4 ABNORMAL RA SIGNALING AND HUMAN MALE INFERTILITY

Supported by the crucial role of RA in spermatogenesis, it has been hypothesized that infertile men have insufficient RA levels to sustain spermatogenesis due to impaired biosynthesis of RA (112). Reduced aldehyde dehydrogenase enzymes were found in testicular samples of men with idiopathic infertility associated with oligospermia or azoospermia (113). The decrease in ALDH was accompanied by a reduction of germ cells in the testicular tissue, particularly of the cells in postmeiotic stages of development (113). Later, it was shown that the intratesticular levels of 13-*cis*-retinoic acid were lower in men with oligoasthenozoospermia compared to healthy subjects, albeit the intratesticular ATRA levels remained at similar levels (112). The administration of 13-*cis*-retinoic acid (20 mg/day twice a day for 20 weeks) improved the total sperm counts and the sperm morphology, while the motile sperm count per ejaculate was only slightly improved (114).

Besides, RAR or RXR loss of function in Sertoli cells has been related to spermiation failure and desquamation of immature germ cells, as well as with increased germ cell apoptosis, while the Sertoli cells lose their stage-dependent gene expression (115).

Although there are studies supporting the assumption that certain types of infertility seem to correlate with lower concentrations of intratesticular RA (112,114), a clear association between RA intratesticular levels and sperm impaired motility are yet to be established. It is, however, possible that such effects may be related to an alternative pathway, linking RA signaling to oxidative stress, as previously mentioned. In recent years, it has been shown that ATRA administration ameliorates oxidative stress and apoptosis in diverse conditions mediated by toxicity or inflammation (116,117), including in men varicocele-related infertility (118). Besides the already mentioned interplay with oxidative stress enzymes and oxidative-induced apoptosis, it has been shown that RA affects cell membrane integrity and mitochondrial function (119), as well as DNA integrity (117). Dysregulation of RA signaling could, therefore, help to explain sperm impaired motility defects or excessive DNA damage, often associated with oxidative stress imbalance. This particular topic, however, has not yet been addressed when studying RA effects on sperm.

7.5 CONCLUDING REMARKS

Spermatogenesis is a highly complicated cellular differentiation process and a crucial determinant of male fertility. Spermatogenesis is regulated through a complex, multilevel process, whereby diverse molecules play a critical role and engage in cross talk designed to ensure the continual production of spermatozoa. RA is one of those molecules, and its importance has been highlighted in the last decades. Available information on RA signaling pathways is derived mostly from studies developed in rodent species. Despite that, there is still much to learn; the progress made so far challenges researchers to find and develop a method that can support *in vitro* spermatogenesis. In particular, the culture of SSCs to be used for colonization of seminiferous tubules would support the development of new techniques in the assisted reproduction area, mainly directed to restore fertility in young males submitted to chemotherapy. In addition, it would enhance knowledge of the mechanisms controlling spermatogenesis.

The relationship between RA imbalance and fertility remains elusive, but it may be related to the disruption of the oxidative stress balance, particularly in post-testicular or ejaculated spermatozoa. Further research on this topic is necessary. Due to the particularities of the spermatozoon chromatin, it is possible that the molecular pathways involved in RA signaling are different from those reported to act in other cells.

We hope with this chapter to provide the reader with a concise reference on the RA signaling pathways in spermatogenesis and male (in)fertility.

REFERENCES

1. Staub C, Johnson L. Review: Spermatogenesis in the bull. *Animal.* 2018;12(s1):s27–35.
2. Mäkelä J-A, Toppari J. Seminiferous cycle. In: Skinner MK (Ed.), *Encyclopedia of Reproduction* (2nd ed.). Oxford, UK: Academic Press; 2018, pp. 134–44.
3. Peer NR, Law SM, Murdoch B, Goulding EH, Eddy EM, Kim K. Germ cell-specific retinoic acid receptor α functions in germ cell organization, meiotic integrity, and spermatogonia. *Endocrinology.* 2018;159(9):3403–20.
4. Hermo L, Pelletier RM, Cyr DG, Smith CE. Surfing the wave, cycle, life history, and genes/proteins expressed by testicular germ cells. Part 1: Background to spermatogenesis, spermatogonia, and spermatocytes. *Microsc Res Tech.* 2010;73(4):241–78.
5. Law NC, Oatley JM. Spermatogonial stem cell and niche. In: Skinner MK (Ed.), *Encyclopedia of Reproduction* (2nd ed.). Oxford, UK: Academic Press; 2018, pp. 117–23.
6. Potter SJ, DeFalco T. Role of the testis interstitial compartment in spermatogonial stem cell function. *Reproduction.* 2017;153(4):R151–62.
7. de Rooij DG. Organization of the seminiferous epithelium and the cycle, and morphometric description of spermatogonial subtypes (rodents and primates). In: Oatley JM, Griswold MD (Eds.), *The Biology of Mammalian Spermatogonia.* New York, NY: Springer; 2017, pp. 3–20.
8. Snyder EM, Small C, Griswold MD. Retinoic acid availability drives the asynchronous initiation of spermatogonial differentiation in the mouse. *Biol Reprod.* 2010;83(5):783–90.
9. Packer AI, Wolgemuth DJ. Genetic and molecular approaches to understanding the role of retinoids in mammalian spermatogenesis. In: Nau H, Blaner WS (Eds.), *Retinoids: The Biochemical and Molecular Basis of Vitamin A and Retinoid Action.* Berlin, Heidelberg: Springer; 1999. pp. 347–68.
10. Wolgemuth DJ, Chung SS. Retinoid signaling during spermatogenesis as revealed by genetic and metabolic manipulations of retinoic acid receptor alpha. *Soc Reprod Fertil Suppl.* 2007;63:11–23.
11. Beedle M-T, Hogarth CA, Griswold MD. Role of retinoic acid signaling in the differentiation of spermatogonia. In: Oatley JM, Griswold MD (Eds.), *The Biology of Mammalian Spermatogonia.* New York, NY: Springer; 2017, pp. 133–46.
12. van Beek ME, Meistrich ML. Spermatogenesis in retinol-deficient rats maintained on retinoic acid. *J Reprod Fertil.* 1992;94(2):327–36.
13. Combs GF Jr. *The Vitamins—Fundamental Aspects in Nutrition and Health.* 3rd. ed. New York, NY: Academic Press; 2007.
14. Napoli JL. Biochemical pathways of retinoid transport, metabolism, and signal transduction. *Clin Immunol Immunopathol.* 1996;80(3 Pt 2):S52–62.
15. Blaner WS, Li Y. Vitamin A metabolism, storage and tissue delivery mechanisms. In: Dollé P, Neiderreither K (Eds.), *The Retinoids: Biology, Biochemistry, and Disease.* New York, NY: Wiley; 2015, pp. 1–34.
16. Chytil F. Retinoic acid: Biochemistry and metabolism. *J Am Acad Dermatol.* 1986;15(4 Pt 2):741–7.
17. Ball GFM. *Vitamins: Their Role in the Human Body.* Oxford, UK: Blackwell; 2004.
18. Parker RO, Crouch RK. Retinol dehydrogenases (RDHs) in the visual cycle. *Exp Eye Res.* 2010;91(6):788–92.
19. Clagett-Dame M, Knutson D. Vitamin A in reproduction and development. *Nutrients.* 2011;3(4):385–428.
20. Morriss-Kay GM, Ward SJ. Retinoids and mammalian development. *Int Rev Cytol.* 1999;188:73–131.
21. Blomhoff R, Blomhoff HK. Overview of retinoid metabolism and function. *J Neurobiol.* 2006;66(7):606–30.
22. Livera G, Rouiller-Fabre V, Pairault C, Levacher C, Habert R. Regulation and perturbation of testicular functions by vitamin A. *Reproduction.* 2002;124(2):173–80.

23. Vogel S, Gamble MV, Blaner WS. Biosynthesis, absorption, metabolism and transport of retinoids. In: Nau H, Blaner WS (Eds.), *Retinoids: The Biochemical and Molecular Basis of Vitamin A and Retinoid Action.* Berlin, Heidelberg: Springer; 1999, pp. 31–95.

24. Li Y, Wongsiriroj N, Blaner WS. The multifaceted nature of retinoid transport and metabolism. *Hepatobiliary Surg Nutr.* 2014;3(3):126–39.

25. Kawaguchi R, Yu J, Honda J, Hu J, Whitelegge J, Ping P et al. A membrane receptor for retinol binding protein mediates cellular uptake of vitamin A. *Science.* 2007;315(5813):820–5.

26. Napoli JL. Functions of intracellular retinoid binding-proteins. *Subcell Biochem.* 2016;81:21–76.

27. Theodosiou M, Laudet V, Schubert M. From carrot to clinic: An overview of the retinoic acid signaling pathway. *Cell Mol Life Sci.* 2010;67(9):1423–45.

28. Goodman DS. Overview of current knowledge of metabolism of vitamin A and carotenoids. *J Natl Cancer Inst.* 1984;73(6):1375–9.

29. Niederreither K, Dollé P. Retinoic acid in development: Towards an integrated view. *Nat Rev Genet.* 2008;9(7):541–53.

30. Griswold MD, Hogarth CA, Bowles J, Koopman P. Initiating meiosis: The case for retinoic acid. *Biol Reprod.* 2012;86(2):35.

31. Giguere V, Ong ES, Segui P, Evans RM. Identification of a receptor for the morphogen retinoic acid. *Nature.* 1987;330(6149):624–9.

32. Petkovich M, Brand NJ, Krust A, Chambon P. A human retinoic acid receptor which belongs to the family of nuclear receptors. *Nature.* 1987;330(6147):444–50.

33. Chambon P. A decade of molecular biology of retinoic acid receptors. *FASEB J.* 1996;10(9):940–54.

34. Kastner P, Chambon P, Leid M. Role of nuclear retinoic acid receptors in the regulation of gene expression. In: Blomhoff R (Eds.), *Vitamin A in Health and Disease.* Boca Raton: CRC Press; 1994,pp.189–238.

35. Zechel C, Shen XQ, Chambon P, Gronemeyer H. Dimerization interfaces formed between the DNA binding domains determine the cooperative binding of RXR/RAR and RXR/TR heterodimers to DR5 and DR4 elements. *EMBO J.* 1994;13(6):1414–24.

36. Cohen RN, Brzostek S, Kim B, Chorev M, Wondisford FE, Hollenberg AN. The specificity of interactions between nuclear hormone receptors and corepressors is mediated by distinct amino acid sequences within the interacting domains. *Mol Endocrinol.* 2001;15(7):1049–61.

37. Dilworth FJ, Chambon P. Nuclear receptors coordinate the activities of chromatin remodeling complexes and coactivators to facilitate initiation of transcription. *Oncogene.* 2001;20:3047.

38. Perissi V, Jepsen K, Glass CK, Rosenfeld MG. Deconstructing repression: Evolving models of co-repressor action. *Nat Rev Genet.* 2010;11(2):109–23.

39. Rosenfeld MG, Lunyak VV, Glass CK. Sensors and signals: A coactivator/corepressor/epigenetic code for integrating signal-dependent programs of transcriptional response. *Genes Dev.* 2006;20(11):1405–28.

40. Kouzarides T. Chromatin modifications and their function. *Cell.* 2007;128(4):693–705.

41. Lefebvre P, Martin PJ, Flajollet S, Dedieu S, Billaut X, Lefebvre B. Transcriptional activities of retinoic acid receptors. *Vitam Horm.* 2005;70:199–264.

42. Allis CD, Berger SL, Cote J, Dent S, Jenuwien T, Kouzarides T et al. New nomenclature for chromatin-modifying enzymes. *Cell.* 2007;131(4):633–6.

43. Balmer JE, Blomhoff R. Gene expression regulation by retinoic acid. *J Lipid Res.* 2002;43(11):1773–808.

44. Mark M, Ghyselinck NB, Chambon P. Function of retinoic acid receptors during embryonic development. *Nucl Recept Signal.* 2009;7:e002.

45. Langston AW, Gudas LJ. Retinoic acid and homeobox gene regulation. *Curr Opin Genet Dev.* 1994;4(4):550–5.

46. Liao YP, Ho SY, Liou JC. Non-genomic regulation of transmitter release by retinoic acid at developing motoneurons in Xenopus cell culture. *J Cell Sci.* 2004;117(Pt 14):2917–24.

47. Masiá S, Alvarez S, de Lera AR, Barettino D. Rapid, nongenomic actions of retinoic acid on phosphatidylinositol-3-kinase signaling pathway mediated by the retinoic acid receptor. *Mol Endocrinol.* 2007;21(10):2391–402.

48. Liou JC, Ho SY, Shen MR, Liao YP, Chiu WT, Kang KH. A rapid, nongenomic pathway facilitates the synaptic transmission induced by retinoic acid at the developing synapse. *J Cell Sci.* 2005;118(Pt 20):4721–30.

49. Hemmings BA, Restuccia DF. PI3K-PKB/Akt pathway. *Cold Spring Harb Perspect Biol.* 2012;4(9):a011189.

50. Noy N. Between death and survival: Retinoic acid in regulation of apoptosis. *Annu Rev Nutr.* 2010;30:201–17.

51. Endo T, Romer KA, Anderson EL, Baltus AE, de Rooij DG, Page DC. Periodic retinoic acid-STRA8 signaling intersects with periodic germ-cell competencies to regulate spermatogenesis. *Proc Natl Acad Sci USA.* 2015;112(18):E2347–56.

52. Hogarth C. Retinoic acid metabolism, signaling, and function in the adult testis. In: Griswold MD (Ed.), *Sertoli Cell Biology* (2nd ed.). Oxford, UK: Academic Press; 2015, pp. 247–72.

53. Hogarth CA, Arnold S, Kent T, Mitchell D, Isoherranen N, Griswold MD. Processive pulses of retinoic acid propel asynchronous and continuous murine sperm production. *Biol Reprod.* 2015;92(2):37.

54. van Pelt AM, de Rooij DG. Retinoic acid is able to reinitiate spermatogenesis in vitamin A-deficient rats and high replicate doses support the full development of spermatogenic cells. *Endocrinology.* 1991;128(2):697–704.

55. Li H, Palczewski K, Baehr W, Clagett-Dame M. Vitamin A deficiency results in meiotic failure and accumulation of undifferentiated spermatogonia in prepubertal mouse testis. *Biol Reprod.* 2011;84(2):336–41.

56. Vernet N, Dennefeld C, Rochette-Egly C, Oulad-Abdelghani M, Chambon P, Ghyselinck NB et al. Retinoic acid metabolism and signaling pathways in the adult and developing mouse testis. *Endocrinology.* 2006;147(1):96–110.

57. Payne CJ. Cycling to and from a stem cell niche: The temporal and spatial odyssey of mitotic male germ cells. *Int J Dev Biol.* 2013;57(2–4):169–77.

58. Frydman N, Poulain M, Arkoun B, Duquenne C, Tourpin S, Messiaen S et al. Human foetal ovary shares meiotic preventing factors with the developing testis. *Hum Reprod.* 2017;32(3):631–42.

59. Bowles J, Koopman P. Retinoic acid, meiosis and germ cell fate in mammals. *Development.* 2007;134(19):3401–11.

60. Wu J, Ding X, Wang J. Stem cells in mammalian gonads. *Results Probl Cell Differ.* 2016;58:289–307.

61. Koubova J, Menke DB, Zhou Q, Capel B, Griswold MD, Page DC. Retinoic acid regulates sex-specific timing of meiotic initiation in mice. *Proc Natl Acad Sci USA.* 2006;103(8):2474–9.

62. Mei XX, Wang J, Wu J. Extrinsic and intrinsic factors controlling spermatogonial stem cell self-renewal and differentiation. *Asian J Androl.* 2015;17(3):347–54.

63. Mecklenburg JM, Hermann BP. Mechanisms regulating spermatogonial differentiation. *Results Probl Cell Differ.* 2016;58:253–87.

64. Chapman KM, Medrano GA, Chaudhary J, Hamra FK. NRG1 and KITL signal downstream of retinoic acid in the germline to support soma-free syncytial growth of differentiating spermatogonia. *Cell Death Discov.* 2015;1.

65. Busada JT, Chappell VA, Niedenberger BA, Kaye EP, Keiper BD, Hogarth CA et al. Retinoic acid regulates Kit translation during spermatogonial differentiation in the mouse. *Dev Biol.* 2015;397(1):140–9.

66. Ma HT, Niu CM, Xia J, Shen XY, Xia MM, Hu YQ et al. Stimulated by retinoic acid gene 8 (Stra8) plays important roles in many stages of spermatogenesis. *Asian J Androl.* 2018;20(5):479–87.

67. Rossi P, Dolci S. Paracrine mechanisms involved in the control of early stages of mammalian spermatogenesis. *Front Endocrinol (Lausanne).* 2013;4:181.

68. Matson CK, Murphy MW, Griswold MD, Yoshida S, Bardwell VJ, Zarkower D. The mammalian doublesex homolog DMRT1 is a transcriptional gatekeeper that controls the mitosis versus meiosis decision in male germ cells. *Dev Cell.* 2010;19(4):612–24.

69. Zhang T, Murphy MW, Gearhart MD, Bardwell VJ, Zarkower D. The mammalian doublesex homolog DMRT6 coordinates the transition between mitotic and meiotic developmental programs during spermatogenesis. *Development.* 2014;141(19):3662–71.

70. Toyoda S, Miyazaki T, Miyazaki S, Yoshimura T, Yamamoto M, Tashiro F et al. Sohlh2 affects differentiation of KIT positive oocytes and spermatogonia. *Dev Biol.* 2009;325(1):238–48.

71. Koubova J, Hu YC, Bhattacharyya T, Soh YQ, Gill ME, Goodheart ML et al. Retinoic acid activates two pathways required for meiosis in mice. *PLOS Genet.* 2014;10(8):e1004541.

72. Chung SS, Wolgemuth DJ. Role of retinoid signaling in the regulation of spermatogenesis. *Cytogenet Genome Res.* 2004;105(2–4):189–202.

73. Hogarth CA, Griswold MD. Driving asynchronous spermatogenesis: Is retinoic acid the answer. *Anim Reprod.* 2012;9(4):742–50.

74. Su W, Mruk DD, Cheng CY. Regulation of actin dynamics and protein trafficking during spermatogenesis-insights into a complex process. *Crit Rev Biochem Mol Biol.* 2013;48(2):153–72.

75. Qian X, Mruk DD, Cheng CY. Rai14 (retinoic acid induced protein 14) is involved in regulating f-actin dynamics at the ectoplasmic specialization in the rat testis. *PLOS ONE.* 2013;8(4):e60656.

76. Qian X, Mruk DD, Cheng Y-H, Cheng CY. RAI14 (retinoic acid induced protein 14) is an F-actin regulator: Lesson from the testis. *Spermatogenesis.* 2013;3(2):e24824.

77. Hasegawa K, Saga Y. Retinoic acid signaling in Sertoli cells regulates organization of the blood-testis barrier through cyclical changes in gene expression. *Development.* 2012;139(23):4347–55.

78. O'Donnell L, Nicholls PK, O'Bryan MK, McLachlan RI, Stanton PG. Spermiation: The process of sperm release. *Spermatogenesis.* 2011;1(1):14–35.

79. Kumar A, Raut S, Balasinor NH. Endocrine regulation of sperm release. *Reprod Fertil Dev.* 2018;30.

80. Su W, Mruk DD, Cheng CY. Regulation of actin dynamics and protein trafficking during spermatogenesis—Insights into a complex process. *Crit Rev Biochem Mol Biol.* 2013;48(2):153–72.

81. Ko E, Sabanegh E, Agarwal A. Male infertility testing: Reactive oxygen species and antioxidant capacity. *Fertil Steril.* 2014;102(6):1518–27.

82. Bartosz G. Reactive oxygen species: Destroyers or messengers? *Biochem Pharmacol.* 2009;77(8):1303–15.

83. de Lamirande E, Jiang H, Zini A, Kodama H, Gagnon C. Reactive oxygen species and sperm physiology. *Rev Reprod.* 1997;2(1):48–54.

84. Guthrie HD, Welch GR. Effects of reactive oxygen species on sperm function. *Theriogenology.* 2012;78(8):1700–8.

85. Du Plessis SS, Agarwal A, Halabi J, Tvrda E. Contemporary evidence on the physiological role of reactive oxygen species in human sperm function. *J Assist Reprod Genet.* 2015;32(4):509–20.

86. Donà G, Fiore C, Tibaldi E, Frezzato F, Andrisani A, Ambrosini G et al. Endogenous reactive oxygen species content and modulation of tyrosine phosphorylation during sperm capacitation. *Int J Androl.* 2011;34(5 Pt 1):411–9.

87. Zini A, de Lamirande E, Gagnon C. Reactive oxygen species in semen of infertile patients: Levels of superoxide dismutase- and catalase-like activities in seminal plasma and spermatozoa. *Int J Androl.* 1993;16(3):183–8.

88. Smith R, Vantman D, Ponce J, Escobar J, Lissi E. Total antioxidant capacity of human seminal plasma. *Hum Reprod.* 1996;11(8):1655–60.

89. Mennella MR, Jones R. Properties of spermatozoal superoxide dismutase and lack of involvement of superoxides in metal-ion-catalysed lipid-peroxidation and reactions in semen. *Biochem J.* 1980;191(2):289–97.

90. Nissen HP, Kreysel HW. Superoxide dismutase in human semen. *Klin Wochenschr.* 1983;61(1):63–5.

91. Wang Y, Branicky R, Noë A, Hekimi S. Superoxide dismutases: Dual roles in controlling ROS damage and regulating ROS signaling. *J Cell Biol.* 2018;217(6):1915–28.

92. Alvarez JG, Storey BT. Lipid peroxidation and the reactions of superoxide and hydrogen peroxide in mouse spermatozoa. *Biol Reprod.* 1984;30(4):833–41.

93. Aitken RJ, Gibb Z, Baker MA, Drevet J, Gharagozloo P. Causes and consequences of oxidative stress in spermatozoa. *Reprod Fertil Dev.* 2016;28(1-2):1–10.

94. Agarwal A, Mulgund A, Sharma R, Sabanegh E. Mechanisms of oligozoospermia: An oxidative stress perspective. *Syst Biol Reprod Med.* 2014;60(4):206–16.

95. Kuroda S, Yumura Y, Mori K, Yasuda K, Takeshima T, Kawahara T et al. Negative correlation between presence of reactive oxygen species and Sperm Motility Index in whole semen samples of infertile males. *Revista Internacional de Andrología.* 2017;15(3):84–9.

96. Agarwal A, Tvrda E, Sharma R. Relationship amongst teratozoospermia, seminal oxidative stress and male infertility. *Reprod Biol Endocrinol.* 2014;12:45.

97. Yumura Y, Iwasaki A, Saito K, Ogawa T, Hirokawa M. Effect of reactive oxygen species in semen on the pregnancy of infertile couples. *Int J Urol.* 2009;16(2):202–7.

98. Sharma RK, Agarwal A. Role of reactive oxygen species in male infertility. *Urology.* 1996;48(6):835–50.

99. Kemal Duru N, Morshedi M, Oehninger S. Effects of hydrogen peroxide on DNA and plasma membrane integrity of human spermatozoa. *Fertil Steril.* 2000;74(6):1200–7.

100. Murawski M, Saczko J, Marcinkowska A, Chwiłkowska A, Gryboś M, Banaś T. Evaluation of superoxide dismutase activity and its impact on semen quality parameters of infertile men. *Folia Histochem Cytobiol.* 2007;45 Suppl 1:S123–6.

101. Chiu H, Fischman D, Hammerling U. Vitamin A depletion causes oxidative stress, mitochondrial dysfunction, and PARP-1-dependent energy deprivation. *FASEB J.* 2008;22(11):3878–87.

102. Ahlemeyer B, Bauerbach E, Plath M, Steuber M, Heers C, Tegtmeier F et al. Retinoic acid reduces apoptosis and oxidative stress by preservation of SOD protein level. *Free Radic Biol Med.* 2001;30(10):1067–77.

103. Kitamura M, Ishikawa Y, Moreno-Manzano V, Xu Q, Konta T, Lucio-Cazana J et al. Intervention by retinoic acid in oxidative stress-induced apoptosis. *Nephrol Dial Transplant.* 2002;17 Suppl 9:84–7.

104. Molina-Jijón E, Rodríguez-Muñoz R, Namorado MeC, Bautista-García P, Medina-Campos ON, Pedraza-Chaverri J et al. All-trans retinoic acid prevents oxidative stress-induced loss of renal tight junction proteins in type-1 diabetic model. *J Nutr Biochem.* 2015;26(5):441–54.

105. Jiang H, Dan Z, Wang H, Lin J. Effect of ATRA on contents of liver retinoids, oxidative stress and hepatic injury in rat model of extrahepatic cholestasis. *J Huazhong Univ Sci Technolog Med Sci.* 2007;27(5):491–4.

106. Castro-Obregón S, Covarrubias L. Role of retinoic acid and oxidative stress in embryonic stem cell death and neuronal differentiation. *FEBS Lett.* 1996;381(1–2):93–7.

107. Griveau JF, Dumont E, Renard P, Callegari JP, Le Lannou D. Reactive oxygen species, lipid peroxidation and enzymatic defence systems in human spermatozoa. *J Reprod Fertil.* 1995;103(1):17–26.

108. Kasimanickam VR, Kasimanickam RK, Rogers HA. Immunolocalization of retinoic acid receptor-α, -β, and -γ, in bovine and canine sperm. *Theriogenology.* 2013;79(6):1010–8.

109. Radominska-Pandya A, Chen G, Czernik PJ, Little JM, Samokyszyn VM, Carter CA et al. Direct interaction of all-trans-retinoic acid with protein kinase C (PKC). Implications for PKC signaling and cancer therapy. *J Biol Chem.* 2000;275(29):22324–30.

110. Guleria RS, Pan J, Dipette D, Singh US. Hyperglycemia inhibits retinoic acid-induced activation of Rac1, prevents differentiation of cortical neurons, and causes oxidative stress in a rat model of diabetic pregnancy. *Diabetes.* 2006;55(12):3326–34.

111. Choudhary R, Palm-Leis A, Scott RC, Guleria RS, Rachut E, Baker KM et al. All-trans retinoic acid prevents development of cardiac remodeling in aortic banded rats by inhibiting the renin-angiotensin system. *Am J Physiol Heart Circ Physiol.* 2008;294(2):H633–44.

112. Nya-Ngatchou JJ, Arnold SL, Walsh TJ, Muller CH, Page ST, Isoherranen N et al. Intratesticular 13-cis retinoic acid is lower in men with abnormal semen analyses: A pilot study. *Andrology.* 2013;1(2):325–31.

113. Amory JK, Arnold S, Lardone MC, Piottante A, Ebensperger M, Isoherranen N et al. Levels of the retinoic acid synthesizing enzyme aldehyde dehydrogenase-1A2 are lower in testicular tissue from men with infertility. *Fertil Steril.* 2014;101(4):960–6.

114. Amory JK. *Isotretinoin Administration Improves Sperm Production in Men with Infertility.* Seattle, WA: University of Washington; 2017. https://digital.lib.washington.edu/researchworks/handle/1773/40669?show=full

115. Mark M, Ghyselinck NB. Retinoic acid receptor signaling in post-natal male germ cell differentiation. In: Dollé P, Neiderreither K (Eds.), *The Retinoids*. Hoboken, New Jersey: John Wiley & Sons, Inc.; 2015,pp.485–504.

116. Bilodeau JF, Chatterjee S, Sirard MA, Gagnon C. Levels of antioxidant defenses are decreased in bovine spermatozoa after a cycle of freezing and thawing. *Mol Reprod Dev*. 2000;55(3):282–8.

117. Tokarz P, Piastowska-Ciesielska AW, Kaarniranta K, Blasiak J. All-trans retinoic acid modulates DNA damage response and the expression of the VEGF-A and MKI67 genes in ARPE-19 cells subjected to oxidative stress. *Int J Mol Sci*. 2016;17(6).

118. Malivindi R, Rago V, De Rose D, Gervasi MC, Cione E, Russo G et al. Influence of all-trans retinoic acid on sperm metabolism and oxidative stress: Its involvement in the physiopathology of varicocele-associated male infertility. *J Cell Physiol*. 2018;233(12):9526–37.

119. de Oliveira MR. Vitamin A and retinoids as mitochondrial toxicants. *Oxid Med Cell Longev*. 2015; 2015:140267.

Testosterone signaling in spermatogenesis, male fertility and infertility

ARIJIT CHAKRABORTY, VERTIKA SINGH, KIRAN SINGH, AND RAJENDER SINGH

HIGHLIGHTS

- Testosterone is critical for spermatogenesis and male fertility.
- The androgen receptor (AR) is located on the Sertoli cells but not on germ cells.
- Estrogen signaling through their receptors ER1 and ER2 in the Sertoli cells acts on the germ cells to complete the signaling initiated by the androgens.
- Classical testosterone signaling involves AR-mediated effects while nonclassical mechanism relies mainly on the triggering of ZIP9 cellular cascade in the Sertoli cells.
- An optimum level of testosterone (>70 nM) is essential to maintain spermatogenesis in rodents.
- Testosterone binding to the AR and subsequent regulation of gene expression response have been shown to saturate at concentrations of 1 nM only.

8.1 INTRODUCTION

Classical androgens such as testosterone and male steroid hormones are prerequisites for the initiation and maintenance of spermatogenesis and overall functioning of the male reproductive system. These hormones exert their functions through the androgen receptors (ARs), and their signaling in the testis is essential for spermatogenesis. Developing germ cell lineages do not express ARs; therefore, testosterone exerts its functions through testicular Sertoli cells via the regulation of an associated transcription factor assembly. Studies on different animal models have shown that intricate mechanistic fine-tuning of spermatogenesis involves a complex interplay of factors, including AR signaling. Successful completion of meiosis, precise maintenance of spermatogonial numbers along with adhesion of spermatids and spermiation are under testosterone supremo, failing which infertility is inevitable. The present chapter aims at providing an up-to-date review of our understanding of the role of testosterone signaling in spermatogenesis.

The androgen receptor (AR) is principally localized on the Leydig, peritubular and Sertoli cells of the testis. Several studies have suggested the absence of the AR in germ cells (1,2). Experimental evidence has identified that even if germ cells express the AR, it is not required for reproductive function. Normal spermatozoa derived from androgen-resistant chimeric male mice are also capable of producing healthy pups (3). Further, AR-deficient germ cells transplanted to azoospermia male mice are also capable of initiating normal spermatogenesis (1). Sertoli cells are known to be the chief targets of testosterone signaling, which is essential for regulating germ cell proliferation, development, and survival. During rat spermatogenesis, the expression of AR protein is predominant during stages VI–VIII, when the level of AR rises dramatically. Similarly, in men, the expression of AR is primarily required during stages VI–IX of spermatogenesis.

8.2 TESTOSTERONE PRODUCTION AND REGULATION OF THE STEROIDOGENIC PATHWAY

Testicular Leydig cells synthesize the male sex steroid hormones, which are low molecular weight compounds derived from cholesterol, under the regulation of LH. While Leydig cells are capable of *de novo* synthesis of cholesterol from acetyl coenzyme A, the main source of cholesterol comes from lipoprotein particles transported through the blood into the Leydig cells. Steroid synthesis commences with the transportation of cytosolic cholesterol from the outer membrane to the inner membrane of the mitochondria, which also serves as the rate-limiting step in the process of steroidogenesis. A number of proteins assist in the transportation of the hydrophobic cholesterol, which is unable to simply diffuse through the membrane on its own. The most important of these proteins is the steroidogenic acute regulatory protein StAR (4), consisting of a family of 37 kDa (precursor) and 30 kDa (mature) mitochondrial proteins (5). It mainly detects the response of Leydig cells against tropic hormones and other external stimuli and helps in transporting free cholesterol inside mitochondria of the Leydig cells, stimulating steroidogenesis.

Steroidogenic enzymes responsible for the biosynthesis of various steroid hormones, including progestins, androgens, and estrogens from cholesterol, are several specific cytochrome P450 enzymes (CYPs), hydroxysteroid dehydrogenases (HSDs) and steroid reductases (6). The steroid hormones of the reproductive system are produced primarily in the gonads, although some steroidogenic chemical reactions are also found at peripheral tissue sites. For the male, the steroidogenic pathway is found in the testes and to some extent, in the adrenal glands. Within the testis, steroidogenesis occurs in the Leydig cell. The Leydig cells are interstitial cells that are interspersed between the seminiferous tubules. Inside the Leydig cells, the steroidogenic pathway begins in the cytoplasm and includes chemical reactions that occur in the mitochondria and smooth endoplasmic reticulum, where the final end-product, i.e., testosterone, is produced (7). Other active androgenic hormones are produced in the testis as well as at the peripheral tissue sites. In the pathway of steroid hormone biosynthesis, there are two major types of enzymes involved, cytochromes P450 and other steroid oxidoreductases.

The steroidogenic enzyme P450scc cleaves the side chain of cholesterol (C27-sterol), resulting in the formation of C21 steroid pregnenolone followed by StAR-mediated transportation to the inner membrane of the mitochondria (8). The knockout of StAR gene has proved to be embryonically lethal, reflecting its essential function beyond steroidogenesis, such as an integral component in apoptosis, which also affects steroid hormone production (9). It has been found that the steroidogenic factor 1 (SF-1/NR5A1) and DAX-1 are critical in StAR gene regulation, especially in the endocrine tissues like the testis and the ovary (5). Subsequently, pregnenolone is released from the mitochondria into the smooth endoplasmic reticulum (SER), other enzymatic reactions take place in the SER (8). Pregnenolone is converted into the precursor of testosterone, androstenedione, by two major pathways, viz. the Δ^5 or Δ^4 steroid pathway through Δ^5 3β-hydroxysteroid and Δ^4 3-ketosteroid intermediates, respectively. The Δ^5 pathway involves the production of 17α -hydroxypregnenolone and di-hydroepiandrosterone (DHEA), while the Δ^4 steroid pathway involves the production of 17α-hydroxyprogesterone, from progesterone and its intermediate (10). The two pathways are also interconnected since the intermediates of Δ^5 simultaneously pass through the Δ^4 pathway. The 3β-hydroxysteroid dehydrogenase (3β-HSD) enzyme acts on three Δ^5 intermediates—pregnenolone, 17α-hydroxypregnenolone and DHEA—and converts 3β-hydroxysteroids to 3-ketosteroids by catalysis of a 3β-hydrogenation and isomerization (11).

Conversion of C21 to C19 involves 17α-hydroxylation and cleavage of the C17–20 bond leading to 17α-hydroxypregnenolone or 17α-hydroxyprogesterone as transient intermediates, which rapidly get converted to DHEA or androstenedione. These conversions are sequentially catalyzed by a microsomal protein located in the endoplasmic reticulum and are, hence, regarded as the qualitative regulator of steroidogenesis (12). The synthesis of testosterone is terminated by the reduction of androstenediol or androstenedione and DHEA to testosterone, which is catalyzed by 17β-HSD. Testosterone then gets converted by the isoenzymes 5α-reductase into dihydrotestosterone (DHT), which is a more potent and active androgen in the target tissues.

8.3 CLASSICAL AND NONCLASSICAL TESTOSTERONE SIGNALING

8.3.1 Classical testosterone signaling

Testosterone has been shown to act primarily through two pathways: the classical and the nonclassical (13). In the classical pathway, testosterone diffuses through the plasma membrane and binds AR that is sequestered by heat shock proteins in the cytoplasm. A conformational change in the AR releases the receptor from the heat shock proteins. AR then translocates to the nucleus where it binds to androgen response elements (AREs) in gene promoter regions, recruits coregulator proteins and regulates gene transcription. Activation of the classical pathway requires at least 30–45 minutes to initiate changes in gene expression (13).

Several microarray studies using various models have been performed to survey testicular gene expression in the presence and absence of testosterone signaling (14). A broad spectrum of genes in the testis was regulated by testosterone, but the number of Sertoli cell–specific genes that are regulated by testosterone make up a small subset only. Furthermore, the genes identified in the microarray studies show relatively little overlap, and the number of genes displaying a twofold or greater change in expression are limited (15). Interestingly, a relatively high percentage of the regulated genes are inhibited by testosterone itself. Although one study determined that 65% of AR-regulated genes were associated with a conserved ARE region within 6 kb of their transcription start sites, only the *Rhox5* (Pem) homeobox transcription factor encoding gene has been shown to be induced in Sertoli cells by androgens through AR binding to the ARE promoter elements (16). Presently, there is no evidence that an explicit AR-regulated gene is critical for the completion of spermatogenesis; however, it is likely that spermatogenesis would be disrupted as a result of the mutation or elimination of multiple AR-regulated genes (17). Further work is required to characterize the AR-regulated genes controlled by testosterone via the classical pathway as being essential or nonessential for spermatogenesis.

Because testosterone and AR are essential for spermatogenesis and male fertility, it is surprising that the gene survey studies have not identified more testosterone-regulated genes expressed in Sertoli cells that are required for spermatogenesis. One explanation for the lack of identified genes responsible for spermatogenesis may lie in the animal models used to obtain the microarray data. To date, gene expression data have been obtained from either prepubertal rats or mice or from AR knockout mice in which AR expression is eliminated before birth. In both models, the testes lack full complements of germ cells, which decreases the complexity of the signals received by Sertoli cells (18). One solution to the problem may be to selectively knockout AR in Sertoli cells in adult mice and obtain gene expression profiles prior to the loss of germ cells. Extensive studies have developed an adult mouse model in which the AR gene can be inducibly extinguished (19). Further confirmation of the importance of AR-regulated genes for maintaining fertility in mice may be obtained in the future through the comparisons of mutated genes found in infertile men.

8.3.2 Nonclassical testosterone signaling

There are possibly two types of pathways through which testosterone signaling can take place within the somatic testicular cells. The most well-studied and widely established pathway that takes hours to take place is called the classical type of testosterone signaling. However, one that is dependent on the calcium efflux and influx is faster and is called nonclassical testosterone signaling. Not much has been studied about the nonclassical type of testosterone signaling, and there have been very few reports so far. However, there is some evidence that the membrane and cytosolic AR are identical, while others propose that the AR on the membrane is a G-protein-coupled receptor (GPCR). Recent investigations by Shihan et al. (20) showed that silencing AR

expression through siRNA did not influence testosterone-induced activation of Erk1/2, CREB or ATF-1, indicating that this pathway is not activated by the classical cytosolic/nuclear AR. However, it was found that consequent suppression of G-protein, leads to the inhibition of Gnα11 along with subsequent inhibition in the activity of those signaling molecules, suggesting that these responses are elicited through a membrane-bound GPCR. Further studies on Sertoli cell lines c93RS2, which lack classical AR, the signaling cascade characterized by the phosphorylation of Erk1/2 and transcription factors CREB and ATF-1, also depicted an activation G-protein-induced signaling cascade under testosterone (21). This study also demonstrated that in Sertoli cells, testosterone acts through the receptor ZIP9 to trigger the nonclassical signaling cascade, resulting in increased claudin expression and tight junction (TJ) formation. Since TJ formation is a prerequisite for the maintenance of the blood-testis barrier, the testosterone/ZIP9 effects might be significant for male physiology and may be considered as a nonclassical mechanism for the testosterone signaling pathway.

8.4 ESTROGEN SIGNALING AND TESTOSTERONE

There are three main endogenous estrogens—17β-estradiol (E2), estrone (E1) and estriol (E3), of which E2 is predominant and most active. E2 is produced from testosterone by aromatase enzyme cytochrome P45019 A1, encoded by the *CYP19* gene (22). Cellular signaling of estrogens is mediated primarily through two estrogen receptors, ESR1 and ESR2 (also known as ERα and ERβ, respectively), both belonging to the nuclear receptor family of transcription factors. Recent studies have shown that in the microenvironment of the seminiferous epithelium, wherein Sertoli cells support germ cells at different stages of development, spermatogenesis involves locally produced autocrine and paracrine factors (23). Sertoli cells are the major source of estrogens in immature rats, although Leydig and germ cells synthesize these hormones in adult animals (24). Follicle-stimulating hormone (FSH) has been shown to increase the rate of proliferation of Sertoli cells, and thyroid hormones alter the period in which proliferation can occur by regulating the maturation of Sertoli cells (25).

E2 at physiological concentration activates translocation of ESRs to the plasma membrane mediated by the SRC family of tyrosine kinases, which results in the phosphorylation of epidermal growth factor receptor (EGFR) and mitogen-activated protein kinase 3/1 (MAPK3/1, also known as ERK1/2). E2-ESRs also induce PI3K-AKT activation (26). E2-ESRs can also induce PI3K-AKT activation to bring about its effects. A study using estrogen nonresponsive ESR1 knock-in (ENERKI) mice, which have a point mutation in the ligand-binding domain of ESR1 that significantly reduces interaction with endogenous estrogens, without affecting ligand-independent ESR1 pathways mediated by growth factors, confirmed that estrogen-dependent

ESR1 signaling is required for germ cell viability, most likely through the support of Sertoli cell function (27). Further studies elucidating the biological role of the membrane-initiated estrogen receptor signaling, either alone or in conjunction with ESR nuclear transcriptional function, are necessary for our inclusive understanding of estrogen receptor biological function in the Sertoli cells. Thus, better knowledge of the role of 17β-estradiol and its receptors in the regulation of the homeostasis and functions of the Sertoli cell will be important for understanding spermatogenesis and male infertility.

8.5 REGULATION OF TESTOSTERONE SIGNALING BY MELATONIN

Melatonin is an indoleamine, which is a major secretory product of the pineal gland. It regulates the circadian cycle and acts as a cytokine, neuromodulator and biological response modifier. This hormone functions as a regulator of the reproductive physiology in response to environmental light in seasonally dependent mammals. It displays both hydrophilic and lipophilic properties and can enter testicular cells by crossing the blood-testis barrier. Multiple studies have demonstrated the localization of melatonin receptors on the reproductive system with primary target sites on the testis, epididymis, vas deferens, prostate and ovary. Melatonin is also suggested to regulate the timing for the release of hormones in the female reproductive system. It can act through several receptors such as melatonin receptor 1 (MT1), melatonin receptor 2 (MT2) and retinoid acid receptor–related orphan receptor A (RORα) (28). MT1 and MT2 interact with G-protein to regulate testosterone synthesis by modulating cAMP signal transduction (29). Research suggests that RORα directly activates the aromatase to accelerate the conversion of androgens into estrogens (30).

Numerous studies have highlighted an antigonadotrophic function of melatonin on the mammalian reproductive system via the neuroendocrine-reproductive axis. However, the effect of melatonin on reproductive hormones is variable, depending on the physiological condition of the species (31). In seasonal breeders, such as rodents, during the long day period, melatonin decreases the expression of the androgen receptor and androgen binding protein (32). In Syrian hamsters, injection of melatonin into the testis during the breeding period significantly reduces the testosterone level, testicular volume and androgen synthesis (33). Nevertheless, a persistent supplementation of melatonin to the short-day breeding animals stimulates the gonadal functions (34). In Sika deer, long-term treatment with melatonin stimulates early testicular development (35). Also, in goats, subcutaneous injections of melatonin ameliorate testosterone levels (36). Furthermore, melatonin levels are positively correlated with androgen concentration in short-day period of the seasonal breeding animals. A study recently reported that melatonin treatment in sheep results in a two-fold higher concentration of testosterone in the somatic cells

of the testes (37). Studies on animal models and cultured cells have highlighted that the inhibitory effect of melatonin on testosterone production occurs primarily through the inhibition of various proteins and enzymes, such as StAR, P450SCC and 3β-HSD, which are involved in testosterone synthesis (38,39).

8.6 MELATONIN AND HUMAN FERTILITY

Melatonin receptors have been found on human spermatozoa and seminal plasma suggesting their involvement in modulating sperm activity (40,41); however, no association with sperm motility was observed (42). A study reported that long-term administration of melatonin in healthy men resulted in a decline in semen quality (43). However, it is interesting to note that melatonin acts as an effective antioxidant and is a potent physiological scavenger of hydroxyl radicals (44). Recent studies have highlighted that melatonin could protect sperm from DNA damage and apoptosis induced by ROS (41,45,46). Additionally, melatonin levels have been shown to improve the number of motile spermatozoa in human semen (47). However, despite this evidence, the association between melatonin and male infertility is still controversial and ambiguous.

8.7 ABERRANT TESTOSTERONE SIGNALING AND MALE INFERTILITY

It is well known that androgens and the androgen receptor (AR) play important roles in male fertility, although the detailed mechanisms, particularly how androgen/AR influences spermatogenesis in particular cell types and the molecular entities involved, remain unclear. Literary reports have documented that exposure to testosterone elicits upregulation of numerous genes and proteins directly (48), whereas few genes are also induced by AR binding to the promoter elements in Sertoli cell types (49). There are some observations that conclude that alternative mechanisms of testosterone activity exist to counteract classical AR actions on Sertoli cell types. One of these is that optimum levels of testosterone are required by the Sertoli cells for the maintenance of spermatogenesis (>70 nM); however, testosterone binding to the AR and subsequent gene expression response have been shown to be saturated at concentrations of 1 nM only (50). Another point may be that the levels of intracellular calcium are very high in primary Sertoli cells shortly after androgen stimulation, negating the AR-DNA interactions and initiation of gene expression (49). Taken together, these results suggest that testosterone may act in the Sertoli cells through both alternative pathways as well as classical mechanisms to regulate spermatogenesis.

Androgen insensitivity syndrome (AIS) is a disorder in which there is alteration in the androgen function due to a nonfunctional androgen receptor (AR). This is an X-linked recessive disorder with a 46,XY karyotype. We previously reported a number of mutations in the AR gene that cause AIS (51). Hundreds of such mutations have been tabulated in the Androgen Receptor Gene Mutations Database (52). There are mechanistic studies demonstrating that S-AR$^{-/y}$ mice have defects in the expression of anti-Müllerian hormone, androgen-binding protein, cyclin A1 and sperm-1, which play important roles in the control of spermatogenesis and/or steroidogenesis. Hence, it was shown that Sertoli cell–specific AR knockout mice provide *in vivo* evidence of the need for functional AR in the Sertoli cells to maintain normal spermatogenesis and testosterone production and to ensure normal male fertility (53). In certain diseases like AIS, spinal bulbar muscular atrophy (SBMA), benign prostatic hyperplasia (BPH) and prostate cancer, abnormalities in the function of androgen receptor have been identified. Recently, novel therapeutic interventions using miRNAs in prostate cancer have been proposed that specifically target the transactivation function of the AR at post-transcriptional stages (54).

8.8 TESTOSTERONE THERAPY FOR AZOOSPERMIC MEN

Oligoasthenoteratozoospermia (OAT) and nonobstructive azoospermia (NOA) are correlated with male infertility. Based on the approximate 40%–60% sperm retrieval rate from NOA, half of NOA patients have some quantitative disorder; however, the majority of NOA pathophysiology involves qualitative damage at different spermatogenic steps ranging from the Sertoli cell to the late maturation arrest. To date, the ability of hormonal therapy to increase sperm production in men with NOA has never been demonstrated in a randomized controlled trial. However, the information obtained from gonadotropin therapy for OAT would at least in part apply to the NOA cases.

NOA represents a failure of spermatogenesis within the testis and, from a controlling perspective, is due to either a lack of appropriate stimulation by gonadotropins or an intrinsic testicular impairment. These groups of patients have been diagnosed with hypogonadotropic-hypogonadism, and they benefit from specific hormonal therapy showing a remarkable recovery of spermatogenic function with exogenously administered gonadotropins or gonadotropin-releasing hormone. In the other, larger category of NOA, gonadotropin levels are very high; hence, most of the medical therapies including hormonal supplements have been found to be ineffective for substantial improvement of spermatogenesis as the receptors concerned for gonadotropins are generally downregulated (55). Shiraishi (56) found a mechanism for hormonal treatment of NOA men by optimizing intratesticular testosterone levels, as these patients have low testosterone levels and improper testosterone-to-estradiol ratios. In a case report by Zhao et al. (57), letrozole, an aromatase inhibitor, was used for the duration of 3 months for activation of spermatogenesis in NOA men with elevated FSH level, resulting in normal spermatogenesis.

In conditions of low testosterone levels such as in Klinefelter syndrome, patients receiving medical therapy

to enhance testosterone production had a better chance of sperm retrieval (58). Buchter et al. (59) suggested GnRH as an effective therapy in achieving spermatogenesis and pregnancy in patients with hypothalamic disorders having an intact pituitary function. It was found that pulsatile administration of 5–20 mg gonadotropin at intervals of 2 hours via an infusion pump was preferred over intravenous or invasive supplement of GnRH for convenience with improved compliance. Prolonged use of this procedure in azoospermic men for over 12–24 months resulted in a significant increase in the presence of spermatozoa (60). In another study, it was found that coexposure of gonadotropin and hCG, with or without FSH, also lead to sperm production within 3–6 months (61). Studies with human chorionic gonadotropin with testosterone supplementation at a dose 1,000–3,000 IU three times weekly were found to achieve a near eugonadal state, though highly purified FSH was required in conjugation in some cases. The dose duration was extended up to several months, if necessary, to achieve adequate spermatogenesis or to return sperm to the ejaculate (62). Administration of FSH is required to complete spermatogenesis in certain men with acquired or congenital hypogonadism where there is impairment of the normal pituitary feedback loop mechanism.

8.9 CONCLUSION AND FUTURE DIRECTIONS

Adequate testosterone has been shown to qualitatively initiate, maintain and reinitiate spermatogenesis to sustain fertility status. The classical testosterone signaling involves AR-mediated effects, while the nonclassical mechanism relies mainly on the triggering of the ZIP9 cellular cascade in the Sertoli cells. Melatonin hormone has also been found to be a critical regulator of testosterone signaling acting via its receptors widely present in the testis. Extensive studies on testosterone and its association with male fertility have unveiled the molecular mechanisms by which testosterone supports spermatogenesis. The identification of testosterone-regulated genes in the Sertoli cells has led to the discovery of precise targets at testosterone-specific sites of action and allowed a better understanding of its role in the regulation of the complex process of spermatogenesis. However, as the molecular mechanisms of testosterone signaling continue to be revealed, it could help in the development of therapies intended for the treatment of specific male infertility conditions or provide new targets for hormone-independent, reversible male contraception.

REFERENCES

1. Chang C, Lee SO, Wang RS, Yeh S, Chang TM. Androgen receptor (AR) physiological roles in male and female reproductive systems: Lessons learned from AR-knockout mice lacking AR in selective cells. *Biol Reprod.* 2013 Jul 1;89(1):21.

2. Singh R, Singh L, Thangaraj K. Phenotypic heterogeneity of mutations in androgen receptor gene. *Asian J Androl*. 2007 Mar;9(2):147–79.

3. Wang RS, Yeh S, Tzeng CR, Chang C. Androgen receptor roles in spermatogenesis and fertility: Lessons from testicular cell-specific androgen receptor knockout mice. *Endocr Rev*. 2009 Apr 1;30(2):119–32.

4. Stocco DM. Steroidogenic acute regulatory (StAR) protein: What's new? *BioEssays*. 1999;21(9):768–75.

5. King SR, Stocco DM. Steroidogenic acute regulatory protein expression in the central nervous system. *Front Endocrinol*. 2011 Nov 10;2:72.

6. Miller WL. Early steps in androgen biosynthesis: From cholesterol to DHEA, *Baillieres Clin Endocrinol Metab*. 1999;12:67–81.

7. Stocco DM. StAR protein and the regulation of steroid hormone biosynthesis. *Annu Rev Physiol*. 2001;63:193–213.

8. Zirkin BR, Chen H. Regulation of Leydig cell steroidogenic function during aging. *Biol Reprod*. 2000;63:977–81.

9. Papadopoulos V, Amri H, Boujrad N et al. Peripheral benzodiazepine receptor in cholesterol transport and steroidogenesis. *Steroids*. 1997;62:21–28.

10. Sherbet DP, Tiosano D, Kwist KM, Hochberg Z, Auchus RJ. CYP17 mutation E305G causes isolated 17, 20-lyase deficiency by selectively altering substrate binding. *J Biol Chem*. 2003;278 (49):48563–9.

11. de Launoit Y, Simard J, Durocher F, Labrie F. Androgenic 17 β-hydroxy steroid dehydrogenase activity of expressed rat type I 3β-hydroxysteroid dehydrogenase/Δ5-Δ4 isomerase. *Endocrinology*. 1992;130:553–5.

12. Hughes IA. Minireview: Sex differentiation. *Endocrinology*. 2001;142(8)3281–7.

13. Walker WH. Testosterone signaling and the regulation of spermatogenesis. *Spermatogenesis*. 2011 Apr 1;1(2):116–20.

14. Verhoeven G, Willems A, Denolet E, Swinnen JV, De Gendt K. Androgens and spermatogenesis: Lessons from transgenic mouse models. *Philos Trans R Soc Lond B Biol Sci*. 2010;365:1537–56.

15. Petrusz P, Jeyaraj DA, Grossman G. Microarray analysis of androgen-regulated gene expression in testis: The use of the androgen-binding protein (ABP)-transgenic mouse as a model. *Reprod Biol Endocrinol*. 2005 Dec;3(1):70.

16. Hazra R, Corcoran L, Robson M, McTavish KJ, Upton D, Handelsman DJ, Allan CM. Temporal role of Sertoli cell androgen receptor expression in spermatogenic development. *Mol Endocrinol*. 2013 Jan 1;27(1):12–24.

17. Liu S, Kumari S, Hu Q et al. A comprehensive analysis of coregulator recruitment, androgen receptor function and gene expression in prostate cancer. *Elife*. 2017 Aug 18;6:e28482.

18. Zhou W, Wang G, Small CL, Liu Z, Weng CC, Yang L, Griswold MD, Meistrich ML. Gene expression alterations by conditional knockout of androgen receptor in adult Sertoli cells of Utp14b jsd/jsd (jsd) mice. *Biol Reprod*. 2011 Feb;84(2):400–8.

19. McJunkin K, Mazurek A, Premsrirut PK, Zuber J, Dow LE, Simon J, Stillman B, Lowe SW. Reversible suppression of an essential gene in adult mice using transgenic RNA interference. *Proc Natl Acad Sci USA*. 2011 Apr 26;108(17):7113–8.

20. Shihan M, Bulldan A, Scheiner-Bobis G. Non-classical testosterone signaling is mediated by a G-protein-coupled receptor interacting with Gnα11. *Biochim Biophys Acta*. 2014 Jun 1;1843(6):1172–81.

21. Bulldan A, Dietze R, Shihan M, Scheiner-Bobis G. Non-classical testosterone signaling mediated through ZIP9 stimulates claudin expression and tight junction formation in Sertoli cells. *Cell Signal*. 2016 Aug 1;28(8):1075–85.

22. Boon WC, Chow JD, Simpson ER. The multiple roles of estrogens and the enzyme aromatase. In: L. Martini (Ed.). *Progress in Brain Research* (Vol. 181). New York, NY: Elsevier, 2010 Jan 1, pp. 209–232.

23. Sharpe RM, McKinnell C, Kivlin C, Fisher JS. Proliferation and functional maturation of Sertoli cells, and their relevance to disorders of testis function in adulthood. *Reproduction*. 2003 Jun 1;125(6):769–84.

24. Serge C, Hess RA. Oestrogens and spermatogenesis. *Phil Trans R Soc*. 2010;365(1546):1517–35.

25. Carreau S, De Vienne C, Galeraud-Denis I. Aromatase and estrogens in man reproduction: A review and latest advances. *Adv Med Sci*. 2008 Dec 1;53(2).

26. Lucas TF, Pimenta MT, Pisolato R, Lazari MF, Porto CS. 17β-estradiol signaling and regulation of Sertoli cell function. *Spermatogenesis*. 2011 Oct 1;1(4):318–24.

27. Munro S, Lewin S, Swart T, Volmink J. A review of health behaviour theories: How useful are these for developing interventions to promote long-term medication adherence for TB and HIV/AIDS? *BMC Public Health*. 2007 Dec;7(1):104.

28. Sanchez-Barcelo EJ, Mediavilla MD, Vriend J, Reiter RJ. Constitutive photomorphogenesis protein 1 (COP 1) and COP 9 signalosome, evolutionarily conserved photomorphogenic proteins as possible targets of melatonin. *J Pineal Res*. 2016;61:41–51.

29. Cipolla-Neto J, Amaral FG, Afeche SC, Tan DX, Reiter RJ. Melatonin, energy metabolism, and obesity: A review. *J Pineal Res*. 2014;56:371–381.

30. Odawara H, Iwasaki T, Horiguchi J et al. Activation of aromatase expression by retinoic acid receptor-related orphan receptor (ROR) α in breast cancer cells: Identification of a novel ROR response element. *J Biol Chem*. 2009;284:17711–9.

31. Reiter RJ, Tan D-X, Rosales-Corral S, Manchester LC. The universal nature, unequal distribution and antioxidant functions of melatonin and its derivatives. *Mini Rev Med Chem*. 2013;13:373–84.

32. Ahmad R, Haldar C. Effect of intra-testicular melatonin injection on testicular functions, local and general immunity of a tropical rodent *Funambulus pennanti*. *Endocrine*. 2010;37:479–88.

33. Qin F, Zhang J, Zan L, Guo W, Wang J, Chen L, Cao Y, Shen O, Tong J. Inhibitory effect of melatonin on testosterone synthesis is mediated via GATA-4/SF-1 transcription factors. *Reprod Biomed Online*. 2015;31:638–46.

34. Mura MC, Luridiana S, Bodano S, Daga C, Cosso G, Diaz ML, Bini PP, Carcangiu V. Influence of melatonin receptor 1A gene polymorphisms on seasonal reproduction in Sarda ewes with different body condition scores and ages. *Anim Reprod Sci*. 2014;149:173–7.

35. Wang L, Zhuo Z-Y, Shi W-Q, Tan DX, Gao C, Tian XZ et al. Melatonin promotes superovulation in sika deer (*Cervus nippon*). *Int J Mol Sci*. 2014;15:12107–18.

36. Rekik M, Taboubi R, Ben Salem I, Fehri Y, Sakly C, Lassoued N et al. Melatonin administration enhances the reproductive capacity of young rams under a southern Mediterranean environment. *Anim Sci J*. 2015;86:666–72.

37. Deng SL, Chen SR, Wang ZP, Zhang Y, Tang JX, Li J, Wang XX. Melatonin promotes development of haploid germ cells from early developing spermatogenic cells of Suffolk sheep under in vitro condition. *J Pineal Res*. 2016;60:435–47.

38. Frungieri MB, Mayerhofer A, Zitta K, Pignataro OP, Calandra RS, Gonzalez-Calvar SI. Direct effect of melatonin on Syrian hamster testes: Melatonin subtype 1a receptors, inhibition of androgen production, and interaction with the local corticotropin-releasing hormone system. *Endocrinology*. 2005;146:1541–52.

39. Mukherjee A, Haldar C. Photoperiodic regulation of melatonin membrane receptor (MT1R) expression and steroidogenesis in testis of adult golden hamster, *Mesocricetus auratus*. *J Photochem Photobiol B Biol*. 2014;140:374–80.

40. Bornman MS, Oosthuizen JMC, Barnard HC, Schulenburg GW, Boomker D, Reif S. Melatonin and sperm motility/melatonin und spermatozoenmotilität. *Andrologia*. 1989;21:483–485.

41. Sharbatoghli M, Valojerdi MR, Bahadori MH, Salman Yazdi R, Ghaleno LR. The relationship between seminal melatonin with sperm parameters, DNA fragmentation and nuclear maturity in intra-cytoplasmic sperm injection candidates. *Cell J*. 2015;17:547.

42. van Vuuren RJJ, Pitout MJ, van Aswegen CH, Theron JJ. Putative melatonin receptor in human spermatozoa. *Clin Biochem*. 1992;25:125–7.

43. Luboshitzky R, Shen-Orr Z, Nave R, Lavi S, Lavie P. Melatonin administration alters semen quality in healthy men. *J Androl*. 2002;23:572–8.

44. Hardeland R, Reiter RJ, Poeggeler B, Tan D-X. The significance of the metabolism of the neurohormone melatonin: Antioxidative protection and formation of bioactive substances. *Neurosci Biobehav Rev*. 1993;17:347–57.

45. Espino J, Bejarano I, Ortiz Á, Lozano GM, García JF, Pariente JA, Rodríguez AB. Melatonin as a potential tool against oxidative damage and apoptosis in ejaculated human spermatozoa. *Fertil Steril*. 2010;94:1915–7.

46. Espino J, Ortiz Á, Bejarano I, Lozano GM, Monllor F, García JF, Rodríguez AB, Pariente JA. Melatonin protects human spermatozoa from apoptosis via melatonin receptor– and extracellular signal–regulated kinase-mediated pathways. *Fertil Steril*. 2011;95:2290–6.

47. Ortiz A, Espino J, Bejarano I, Lozano GM, Monllor F, García JF, Pariente JA, Rodríguez AB. High endogenous melatonin concentrations enhance sperm quality and short-term in vitro exposure to melatonin improves aspects of sperm motility. *J Pineal Res*. 2011;50:132–9.

48. Kokontis JM, Liao S. Molecular action of androgen in the normal and neoplastic prostate. In: *Vitamins and Hormones* (Vol. 55). New York, NY: Academic Press: 1998 Jan 1, pp. 219–307.

49. Fix C, Jordan C, Cano P, Walker WH. Testosterone activates mitogen-activated protein kinase and the cAMP response element binding protein transcription factor in Sertoli cells. *Proc Natl Acad Sci USA*. 2004 Jul 27;101(30):10919–24.

50. Sharpe RM. Regulation of spermatogenesis. *Physiol Reprod*. 1994;1:1363–434.

51. Singh R, Shastry PK, Rasalkar AA, Singh L, Thangaraj K. A novel androgen receptor mutation resulting in complete androgen insensitivity syndrome and bilateral Leydig cell hyperplasia. *J Androl*. 2006 Jul 8;27(4):510–6.

52. Gottlieb B, Beitel LK, Nadarajah A, Paliouras M, Trifiro M. The Androgen Receptor Gene Mutations Database: 2012 update. *Hum Mutat*. 2012 May;33(5):887–94.

53. Chang C, Chen YT, Yeh SD, Xu Q, Wang RS, Guillou F, Lardy H, Yeh S. Infertility with defective spermatogenesis and hypotestosteronemia in male mice lacking the androgen receptor in Sertoli cells. *Proc Natl Acad Sci USA*. 2004 May 4;101(18):6876–81.

54. Shukla GC, Plaga AR, Shankar E, Gupta S. Androgen receptor-related diseases: What do we know? *Andrology*. 2016 May;4(3):366–81.

55. Kumar R. Medical management of non-obstructive azoospermia. *Clinics*. 2013;68:75–9.

56. Shiraishi K. Hormonal therapy for non-obstructive azoospermia: Basic and clinical perspectives. *Reprod Med Biol*. 2015 Apr 1;14(2):65–72.

57. Zhao D, Pan L, Zhang F, Pan F, Ma J, Zhang X, Liu Y. Successful use of aromatase inhibitor letrozole in NOA with an elevated FSH level: A case report. *Andrologia*. 2014 May;46(4):456–7.

58. Ramasamy R, Ricci JA, Palermo GD, Gosden LV, Rosenwaks Z, Schlegel PN. Successful fertility treatment for Klinefelter's syndrome. *J Urol*. 2009 Sep;182(3):1108–13.

59. Buchter D, Behre HM, Kliesch S, Nieschlag E. Pulsatile GnRH or human chorionic gonadotropin/human menopausal gonadotropin as effective treatment for men with hypogonadotropic hypogonadism: A review of 42 cases. *Eur J Endocrinol.* 1998;139:298–303.

60. Pitteloud N, Hayes FJ, Dwyer A, Boepple PA, Lee H, Crowley WF Jr. Predictors of outcome of long-term GnRH therapy in men with idiopathic hypogonadotropic hypogonadism. *J Clin Endocrinol Metab.* 2002;87: 4128–36.

61. Burgues S, Calderon MD. Subcutaneous self-administration of highly purified follicle stimulating hormone and human chorionic gonadotrophin for the treatment of male hypogonadotrophic hypogonadism. Spanish Collaborative Group on Male Hypogonadotropic Hypogonadism. *Hum Reprod.* 1997;12:980–6.

62. Bhasin S. Approach to the infertile man. *J Clin Endocrinol Metab.* 2007;92: 1995–2004.

Wnt signaling in spermatogenesis and male infertility

VERTIKA SINGH, MEGHALI JOSHI, KIRAN SINGH, AND RAJENDER SINGH

HIGHLIGHTS

- Regulated Wnt signaling is required at multiple stages of spermatogenesis and testicular development.
- Nineteen Wnt proteins have been identified in the developing or adult testes of male rodents or humans.
- Wnt antagonists such as Dkk1 and Sfrp1 promote spermatogenesis and testis formation.
- Wnt signaling plays an important part in epididymal sperm maturation.
- Altered Wnt signaling is associated with human male infertility.

9.1 INTRODUCTION

The Wnt signaling pathway is a highly conserved cell-to-cell communication mechanism during development (1). It has essential functions in tissue homeostasis, and dysregulation of Wnt signaling could lead to several pathological states (2). It is categorized into canonical (Wnt/β-catenin) and noncanonical branches. In this chapter, we mainly focus on the canonical pathway, which is commonly known as the Wnt/β-catenin signaling pathway (3). Wnt proteins (ligands), which are secreted cysteine-rich proteins, initiate the Wnt signaling (4). The process of spermatogenesis is regulated by various factors including the extrinsic and intrinsic regulators. Hormones and paracrine factors are extrinsic regulators, whereas intrinsic regulators are the genetic factors. Among the paracrine regulators, Wnt signaling plays a key role in germ cell development (4). There are 19 Wnt proteins

secreted in vertebrates, out of which Wnt1 (5), Wnt3 (6), Wnt3a (7), Wnt4 (8), Wnt5a (9), Wnt7a (10), Wnt10b (11) and Wnt11 (12) have been identified in the developing or adult testes of male rodents or humans.

The Wnt ligands bind to the seven-pass transmembrane receptor FZD, which leads to the phosphorylation of disheveled proteins (DVL) and inhibition of the activity of GSK3 and CK1 to phosphorylate their substrates (13). In the absence of Wnt proteins, β-catenin is phosphorylated by GSK3 and CK1 and is degraded through the ubiquitin pathway by β-TrCP, the E3 ubiquitin ligase (13,14). In the active state, DVL, Axin and GSK3 form a complex with the LRP receptor, thus releasing the unphosphorylated β-catenin from the Axin complex, which on accumulation in the cytoplasm enters the nucleus. In the nucleus, β-catenin interacts with the transcription factor TCF/LEF and in turn activates the target genes (14).

Recently, many studies have unveiled the role of the Wnt signaling pathway in testicular development. In the seminiferous tubule, undifferentiated spermatogonia proliferate to maintain their number, some of which differentiate to produce spermatocytes. It is important to have a fine balance between the two populations (dividing and differentiating) in order to ensure continuous sperm production (15). A number of evolutionarily conserved pathways are reported to be crucial in the maintenance and differentiation of stem cells; for instance, fibroblast growth factor, notch, the transforming growth factor superfamily, Hedgehog and Wnt signaling (16). Among all, Wnt signaling plays the most important role in self-renewal and differentiation of adult stem cells (17,18). The development of primordial germ cells involves the activation of Wnt signaling (19). Wnt signaling was reported to stimulate self-renewal of the SCCs and proliferation of the progenitor cell population (7,9). However, there are limited number of studies showing the involvement of Wnt signaling in germ cell development and differentiation in adult testis.

9.2 CANONICAL WNT SIGNALING PATHWAY

Canonical Wnt signaling involves the accumulation of β-catenin in the cytoplasm and its subsequent translocation into the nucleus (Figure 9.1). When there is no ligand, a destruction complex is formed, which consists of a group of proteins, mainly Axin, adenomatous polyposis coli (APC), casein kinase 1α (CK1α) and glycogen synthase kinase 3 (GSK-3). β-Vatenin is phosphorylated by casein kinase 1α (CK1α) at Ser[45], followed by phosphorylation by GSK-3 at Thr[41], Ser[37] and Ser[33]. Phosphorylated β-catenin becomes ubiquitylated and is targeted for proteasomal degradation (20). On binding of Wnt to a receptor complex, which is composed of members of the Frizzled (Fz) family of seven-transmembrane, low-density lipoprotein receptor-related protein (LRP), serpentine receptors, the Axin-APC-CK1α-GSK-3 complex is inhibited. This inhibition stops phosphorylation of β-catenin by CK1α and GSK-3, further inhibiting its proteasomal degradation. This unphosphorylated β-catenin accumulates in the cytoplasm and is translocated into the nucleus where it interacts with the T-cell-specific transcription factor/lymphoid enhancer-binding factor 1 (TCF/LEF) family of transcription factors and regulates the expression of the target genes (21).

9.2.1 Wnt/Receptor interactions

Frizzled receptors like GPCRs are seven-transmembrane proteins acting as the primary receptors for Wnt signaling. The Fz receptor consists of an extracellular cysteine-rich domain (CRD), which is the site of interaction with Wnt proteins (22). There are 10 FZD genes present in humans, numbered from FZD1 to FZD10. FZD proteins are divided into five subgroups: FZD1/2/7, FZD3/6, FZD5/8, FZD9/10

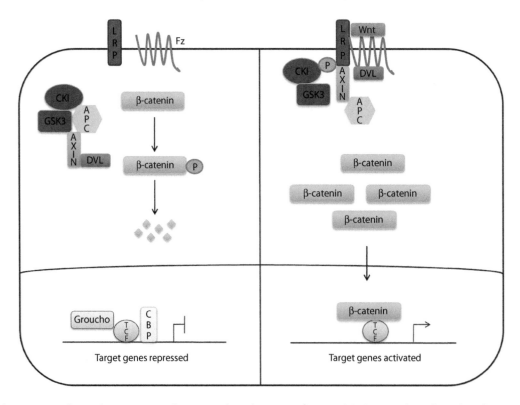

Figure 9.1 The canonical Wnt/β-catenin pathway. In the absence of Wnt, GSK3 complex phosphorylates β-catenin and induces its proteasomal degradation, resulting in the inhibition of target gene transcription. The binding of Wnt to the receptors Frizzled (Fz) and LRP6 leads to the inhibition of β-catenin degradation. β-Catenin, in turn, interacts with members of the TCF/Lef-1 family of transcription factors to coactivate target gene transcription.

and FZD4 (23). Another family of receptors is called low-density lipoprotein-related receptors (LRPs), which are single-pass transmembrane proteins and are over 1,600 amino acids in size (24,25). LRP5 and LRP6 are the homologs of *Drosophila* Arrow protein (26). They are also important for signal transduction along with FZD receptors. This raised the possibility that FZD and LRP function as coreceptors for Wnt proteins. An interaction between Wnt and LRP has been seen, and a ternary complex is formed between Wnt and extracellular domains of FZD and LRP in mouse (25). It has been reported that the overexpression of the intracellular domain of LRP6 can activate the Wnt signaling constitutively, suggesting that the extracellular domain plays a regulatory role in controlling signal transduction. There are multiple phosphorylation sites present on the intracellular domain of LRP5/6. The phosphorylation of these sites is important for the initiation of the signal transduction through Wnt/β-catenin signaling. LRP6 is phosphorylated by many kinases either in a Wnt-dependent (G protein receptor kinase 5/6) or Wnt-independent (protein kinase A, PFTAIRE protein kinase 1) manner (27).

9.2.2 Signal relay in the cytoplasm

There is an event taking place in the cytoplasm, which bridges the activation of FZD/LRP receptors and the inhibition of β-catenin destruction complex. A key protein involved in this process is Dishevelled (DVL1–3 in human, Dsh in *Drosophila*), which is a cytosolic phosphoprotein working upstream of Axin-APC-CSK1α-GSK-3 inhibition in both fly and mammalian cells (23). It is 700 amino acids in size and consists of three main domains, each composed of about 80–90 amino acids: DIX (Dishevelled, Axin), PDZ (Postsynaptic density 95, disc large, zona occudens-1) and DEP (Dishevelled, Egl-10, Pleckstrin) (28). The PDZ domain is the key domain for signal transduction as it interacts directly with the intracellular domain of Frizzled (20). After the successful binding of Wnt to FZD, the first intracellular step is the activation of DVL proteins, which phosphorylate the intracellular domain of LRP5/6. While the requirement of Dishevelled in Wnt signaling has long been known, the molecular events involved in the activation of Dsh by Frizzled and the manner in which it transduces the Wnt signal to the inhibitory complex need to be explored. There are several reports on the physical association between FZD and Dsh and the Wnt-dependent phosphorylation of Dsh (29). Another protein that plays a key role in linking receptor activation to inhibition of the β-catenin destruction complex is Axin, which is a member of the destruction complex itself. It was shown that Axin binds directly to the intracellular domain of LRP in response to Wnt reception (30). The phosphorylation of LRP on key residues by the kinases CK1 and GSK-3 leads to the recruitment of Axin to LRP (31). Overexpression of the membrane-bound form of the LRP intracellular domain can lead to β-catenin accumulation, even in the absence of FZD and DVL, indicating that the recruitment of Axin to the intracellular domain of LRP is sufficient to activate Wnt signaling (32).

9.2.3 Nuclear activity of β-catenin

In the nucleus, β-catenin activates the transcription of target genes through interaction with the members of the TCF/LEF family of transcription factors (33,34). In the absence of nuclear β-catenin, TCF interacts with the repressor protein Groucho and histone deacetylases and forms a repressive complex, thereby blocking the transcription of Wnt target genes (35,36). Upon the activation of Wnt signaling, β-catenin gets accumulated in the cytoplasm. The accumulated β-catenin gets into the nucleus, where it interacts with the TCF transcription factor, replacing Groucho and converting the complex to a transcriptional activator, activating the transcription of Wnt target genes (37).

9.3 WNT SIGNALING IN TESTIS DETERMINATION AND DEVELOPMENT

In the early embryo, mammalian gonads are indifferent. The development of Müllerian or Wolffian ducts results in the female or male reproductive system, respectively. Sry (sex determining gene Y) regulates the production of the anti-Müllerian hormone (AMH) or the Müllerian inhibiting substance (MIS) by aggregated pre–Sertoli cells, which results in the regression of the Müllerian duct and the development of the Wolffian duct. Once the sexual duct is determined and formed, the germ cells differentiate into the corresponding gametes (sperm or ova) depending on the molecular milieu. This bidirectional differentiation is finely tuned by an interplay of various signaling pathways.

The Wnt/β-catenin pathway is particularly known to promote ovarian development, whereas the activation of the Sry/Sox9/FGF9 pathway is involved in testis determination. Sry activates Sox9 by binding to testis-specific enhancer (TES) on Sox9 promoter with SF1 to enhance SOX9 expression in undifferentiated gonads of XY embryos in humans and mice (38). Sox9 is considered as the master regulator of testis determination and is capable of self-activation by binding to its enhancer (39). Testicular Sox9 regulation is considered indispensable for the reproductive capacity of the species (40). Deletions (41) and complete loss of function mutations (42) in Sox9 result in male-to-female sex reversal (XY female), and the duplication (43) of Sox9 or its ectopic expression results in female-to-male sex reversal (XX male).

Sox9 can trigger the expression of its downstream targets, FGF9 and PGDS (prostaglandin D synthase) (40). Both FGF9 and PGDS promote the proliferation and differentiation of the Sertoli cells, thus promoting the masculinization of the testis (40). A shift of balance from Sox9/FGF9 to Wnt/β-catenin signaling can result in a transition from male to female in various species (44,45). In-frame missense and splicing mutations in the MAP kinase pathway gene MAP3K1 tilt the balance from the male to the female sex-determining pathway, resulting in the 46,XY disorder of sex development. These MAP3K1 mutations arbitrate this balance by enhancing the β-catenin activity and WNT/β-catenin/FOXL2 expression and by reducing the expression of SOX9/FGF9/FGFR2/SRY (46). In summary, Wnt signaling plays a major inhibitory role in testis determination.

As Wnt signaling plays an inhibitory role in testis formation, their antagonists have been discovered to promote testis formation (47). Dickkopf-related protein 1 (Dkk1) is an antagonist of the canonical Wnt signaling pathway that belongs to the Dickkopf family of proteins and plays crucial roles in multiple developmental systems by modulating Wnt activity. A study investigated the role of Dkk1 in mouse sex-determination and early gonadal development. They found that Dkk1 mRNA expression was enhanced sex-specifically during testis differentiation, implying that Dkk1 could inhibit Wnt signaling in the developing testis (47). Dkk1 inhibits Wnt/β-catenin by binding to low-density lipoprotein receptor related protein 5/low-density lipoprotein receptor-related protein 6 (LRP5/LRP6) receptors, disrupting the formation of Fzd–LRP5/6 complex (48). Dkk1 expression is elevated at 12.0 dpc (days postcoitus) in mice testis, suggesting its crucial role in testis determination.

Secreted Frizzled-related proteins (Sfrps) are secreted glycoproteins that are well-known antagonists of the canonical and noncanonical Wnt signaling pathways (29). Regulated expression of secreted Frizzled-related protein 1 (sFRP1) is required for spermatid adhesion and sperm release at spermiation (Figure 9.2). sFRP1 is known to regulate spermatid adhesion in testis by dephosphorylation of focal adhesion kinase and the nectin-3 adhesion protein complex (29). Interestingly, Sfrp1 and Sfrp2 null mouse embryos exhibit defects in reproductive tract maturation, gonadal positioning, morphology and external genitalia development (49). Doublesex and mab-3-related transcription factor 1, Dmrt1, is another factor that plays a crucial role in testis determination and differentiation. Dmrt1 has been shown to repress Wnt4 expression in chickens (50). Its high expression in testicular cells of fishes (44) and pigs (51) suggests that it determines the formation of the testis by inhibiting Wnt4. Recently, to investigate the role of dmrt1 in sex determination and gonad development, mutations disrupting this gene were studied in Zebrafish (52). They found that most of the dmrt1 mutant fishes developed as fertile females, suggesting a complete male-to-female sex reversal in mutant animals

that would have otherwise developed as males. Few of the mutant animals developed as sterile males and displayed testicular dysgenesis, suggesting a crucial role of dmrt1 in male sex determination and testis development. Mutant dmrt1 males displayed aberrant gonadal development at the onset of gonad sex differentiation and reduced oocyte apoptosis followed by the development of intersex gonads and failed testis morphogenesis and spermatogenesis. By contrast, female ovaries developed normally (52). In addition, some positive effects of Wnt signaling on testis determination are also known. Wnt4 null gonads show a significant reduction in Sertoli cell numbers (53). Moreover, Wnt4 and Rspo1 null embryos display reduced Sertoli cell numbers, hypoplastic testis and few seminiferous tubules (53), suggesting a significant role of Wnt signaling in testicular development.

Wnt4 is one of the most important ligands that triggers the canonical Wnt signaling pathway for sex determination in mouse and human. The duplication of WNT4 and RSPO1 genes in humans is associated with several gonadal abnormalities including male-to-female sex reversal in XY patients and cryptorchidism (54). In mice, the loss of Wnt4 gene (Wnt4$^{-/-}$) results in the absence of Müllerian duct formation (55). Respondin1 (Rspo1) is another ligand of the canonical Wnt signaling cascade that interacts with Wnt4 to inhibit the development of testis while activating ovarian development (54). β-Catenin is also shown to be involved in sex determination. The stabilization of β-catenin in normal XY mice disrupts the male program, resulting in male-to-female sex reversal. Both the human SRY and mouse sry can repress the Rspo1/Wnt/β-catenin signaling by binding to β-catenin, which results in switching the ovarian development to testis development.

9.4 WNT SIGNALING IN MALE GERM CELL PROLIFERATION AND MATURATION

Spermatogenesis involves the generation of spermatogonial stem cells (SSCs), which are present at the basement of the seminiferous tubules and undergo mitosis and meiosis to finally differentiate into mature spermatozoa that are released into the lumen of the seminiferous tubule (56). In Wnt4 mutant testis, Sertoli cell differentiation was compromised, and this defect occurs downstream of Sry but upstream of Sox9 and desert hedgehog (8). Similarly, the deletion of Wnt7a inhibits the regression of the Müllerian duct. This causes female reproductive tract retention in adult males, which can block sperm passage at ejaculation (57). Constitutive activation of β-catenin in the Müllerian duct mesenchyme also causes the retention of the Müllerian duct in male mice (17). All of these studies highlight the importance of a balanced signaling pathway during fetal life for normal fertility.

Wnt signaling is important for the maintenance of SSCs. Different Wnt ligands and their receptors are seen to take part in SSC maintenance. A study conducted using SSC culture showed that Wnt5a inhibits SSCs apoptosis via

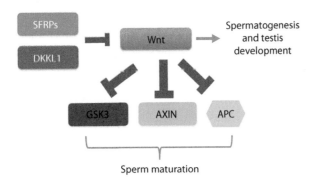

Figure 9.2 Wnt signaling plays an inhibitory role in spermatogenesis. Wnt antagonists such as Dkk1 and Sfrp1 promote spermatogenesis and testis formation.

β-catenin-independent JNK signaling and hence promotes SSC maintenance (9). In another study, it was found that both Wnt3a and Wnt10b promoted the proliferation of the C18–4 cell line through the β-catenin pathway (11). Although Yeh et al. found that Wnt3a leads to an increased SSC number and induced β-catenin dependent signaling in a large subset of germ cells, further investigation revealed that cell populations with increased β-catenin signaling activity contained fewer SSCs. In addition, an increased number of SSCs by Wnt3a was associated with cell aggregations and cell-cell adhesion. Thus, Wnt/β-catenin signaling might be involved in SSCs maintenance indirectly by enhancing the progenitor cells' association (58). It was reported that Wnt4 induces SSC apoptosis *in vivo* through the noncanonical Wnt signaling. However, Wnt4 activates β-catenin in Sertoli cells through the canonical Wnt signaling pathway. Further, it was found that β-catenin promotes Wnt4 expression to cause SSC loss, thus forming a regulatory loop (58). An inactivating mutation in the Wnt pathway inhibitor, naked cuticle homolog 1 (NKD1), leads to increased nuclear β-catenin in elongated spermatids, which caused defective spermatogenesis in the adult mouse (59). Recently, a group of investigators developed a mouse model having germ cell–specific constitutive activation of β-catenin (60). Similar to the controls, the young mutants showed normal germ cell development. However, interestingly, with age, the mutant testis displayed defective spermatogenesis, progressive germ cell loss and abnormal meiotic entry of the spermatogonial cells (60). Using a thymidine analogs-based DNA double labeling technique, they further established a decline in germ cell proliferation and differentiation in the mutant group. Furthermore, the RNA sequencing analysis of testes highlighted significant alterations in the noncoding regions of the mutant mouse genome (60).

9.5 ROLE OF WNT SIGNALING IN DEVELOPMENT AND MAINTENANCE OF SERTOLI CELLS

Sertoli cells are the somatic cells of the testis, located at the periphery of the seminiferous tubules. Besides providing physical support to the developing germ cells, they play a crucial role in the development of testis (61). The Wnt/β-catenin pathway is specifically involved in the proliferation and maturation of Sertoli cells. The β-catenin expression is predominantly observed in the seminiferous cords of the embryonic gonads of male mice, principally in the Sertoli cells. This implied that the Wnt/β-catenin pathway might play a significant role in Sertoli cell proliferation (62).

Results from several studies have provided contradictory evidence regarding the effect of Wnt/β signaling on the Sertoli cells. The deletion of β-catenin did not show any observable effects on Sertoli cells; however, the stabilization of β-catenin is associated with immature, incompletely differentiated Sertoli cells. Its stabilization also results in reduced proliferation and increased apoptosis of germ

cells (4). APC knockout mice with truncated APC protein show impairment of Sertoli and germ cell conjunction via the activation of the Wnt/β-catenin pathway. This highlights the effect of Wnt/β-catenin inhibition on the maturation and proliferation of Sertoli cells. Similarly, Dkk3 (63) mutants also show Sertoli cell defects via Wnt/β-catenin pathway inhibition. Apart from the canonical Wnt signaling molecules, Wnt signaling ligands such as Wnt4 and Wnt11 also regulate Sertoli cell polarity via a noncanonical planar cell polarity (PCP) pathway.

9.6 DEREGULATED WNT SIGNALING AND TESTICULAR TUMOR

The testicular tumor is the most common form of cancer observed in males aged 22–39 years (64). As Wnt signaling is one of the important pathways of development, it has been widely investigated to understand the mechanism of testicular tumor development. Testicular tumors are generally classified into germ cell tumors (GCTs) and Sertoli cell tumors (SCTs). GCTs are further classified into gonadal and extragonadal tumors. Gonadal tumors include seminomas and nonseminomas. While the gonadal tumors generally occur in adolescents and adults, the extragonadal tumors mostly express in infancy and childhood.

Altered expressions of Wnt signaling pathway genes have been found in testicular germ cell tumors (TGCTs) (65). Furthermore, genome-wide expression studies have shown that the Wnt signaling cascade is disrupted in carcinoma in situ (CIS) stage, a common precursor of TGCTs (66). This highlights the involvement of the Wnt signaling pathway in the development of GCTs. The expression of β-catenin has been shown in patients with gonadoblastoma (67). A study indicated that nuclear accumulation of β-catenin parallels with oct3/4 expression in the proliferation of immature germ cells in gonadoblastoma (68). Altered expression of genes such as Wnt5A and Fzd7 and some Wnt target genes such as JUN, FGF4, versican and connexion have been identified in patients with embryonic carcinoma. However, in seminomas, CDX1 and NRCAM show high expression (69). These studies highlight the significance of the Wnt signaling pathway in the transformation of the embryonic carcinomas into differentiated nonseminomas (70).

Besides these, SCTs, another kind of testicular tumor, are sporadic and unifocal. The expression of β-catenin is intense in the nuclei of testicular cells from patients with SCTs (71). Furthermore, deregulated Wnt/β-catenin signaling is associated with the development of postnatal testicular stromal tumors (72). Male mice that express a constitutively active form of β-catenin specifically in the Sertoli cells develop tumors at 1 year of age (73). These studies show a causal link between overactive Wnt/β-catenin signaling and testicular/Sertoli cell tumor development. Further studies are required to confirm these observations and provide a clear insight into the significance of the Wnt/β-catenin pathway in testicular tumor development.

9.7 WNT SIGNALING IN MALE FERTILITY

Wnt signaling is seen to play a role during both early and late spermatogenesis. It was shown by the expression profiling studies that Wnt signaling is active in early spermatogenesis in mice and rainbow trout (74). Conditional knockout mice for APC and β-catenin showed a significant loss of postmitotic germ cells, which included spermatocytes and spermatids, especially the elongated spermatids. Additionally, it was observed that Wnt signaling is active in multiple steps in the mouse, as in the VI pachytene spermatocytes, a nuclear envelope signal for β-catenin was detected. This gradually increased to a more intense nuclear signal in stage IX–XII spermatocytes, and the most intense signal was observed in I–VIII stage of round spermatids (1). There is evidence showing the importance of Wnt/β-catenin signaling in the process of spermiogenesis. The deletion of β-catenin in round spermatids led to germ cell apoptosis, abnormal acrosome formation, defects in chromatin compaction and sperm motility defects (75). An antagonist of the Wnt signaling pathway, DKKL1, was shown to express in spermatocytes and round spermatids (76). It has been observed that DKKL1 interacts with SLY1 (Sycp3-like Y-linked 1), which is an important candidate for spermiogenesis on the Y-chromosome long arm (77), and SLX1 (Sycp3-like X-linked 1), a homolog with SLY and a spermatid cytoplasmic protein (78) in acrosome. All these studies suggest that DKKL1 has an important role in acrosome formation during spermiogenesis. In another study, the expression of Dvl1 mRNA was detected in the pachytene spermatocytes, which further increases in the round and elongated spermatids, and then declines in the mature sperm, suggesting its possible role in spermiogenesis (79,80). Wnt signaling is required not only for germ cell development but also for sperm maturation in the epididymis. Wnt ligands are produced from the epithelial cells in the epididymis and released into the lumen by exosomes. In the epididymis, LRP6 is activated by the Wnt ligands. The activated Wnt signaling inhibits GSK3 to promote sperm maturation in the epididymis through three distinct mechanisms: (a) stabilizing the protein by inhibiting polyubiquitination (Wnt/Stop signaling); (b) promoting Septin 4 polymerization, which is required for the formation of a membrane diffusion barrier at the annulus in sperm head; and (c) inhibiting PP1 (protein phosphatase 1) to activate motility as immature spermatozoa pass through the epididymis (81).

In 2015, a study analyzed and compared the expression of β-catenin in the testicular tissues of obstructive and nonobstructive azoospermic infertile men (82). Interestingly, the study found that the β-catenin was abnormally aggregated in the Leydig cells of nonobstructive azoospermic men; however, the expression of β-catenin did not show any significant difference between the two groups. This study highlighted that the accumulation of β-catenin in the cytoplasm of the Leydig cells can impair spermatogenesis and cause infertility in men (82).

9.8 CONCLUSION AND FUTURE DIRECTIONS

Beginning with gonadal development, Wnt signaling favors the default gonadal development toward ovaries. The testicular master regulators suppress Wnt signaling to deviate the development to testis formation. A compromise in Sertoli cell differentiation in Wnt4 mutant mouse suggested its role in Sertoli cell development. Further studies have suggested the role of Wnt5a in inhibiting and Wnt4 in promoting the apoptosis of SSCs. Thus, Wnt signaling may help in regulating the development and the number of SSCs. The expression of β-catenin in embryonic gonads of male mice suggests the role of Wnt signaling in Sertoli cell proliferation, which determines the testicular size. Nevertheless, the deletion of β-catenin did not show an observable effect on Sertoli cells; however, its stabilization resulted in incompletely differentiated Sertoli cells, suggesting its effect on Sertoli cell maturation and proliferation. It appears that Wnt signaling shows alterations during the seminiferous epithelial cycle of sperm production. Wnt may also play a significant role in the process of spermiogenesis, i.e., sperm differentiation. Wnt ligands are produced and secreted by the epithelial cells of the epididymis, highlighting its importance in sperm maturation during their transit through the epididymis. From this, it appears that Wnt in the infantile gonad is anti-testis but may have important functions in the development and regulation of Sertoli cell and germ cell development in the later stages of testicular development, particularly in the spermatogenically active testes.

Based on the present studies, it is clear that Wnt signaling plays a crucial role in almost every aspect of gonadal development and in making spermatogenesis possible. Furthermore, the evidence has confirmed that Wnt signaling plays its role mostly through the canonical pathway mediated by Wnt4. Presently, several Wnt inhibitors have been discovered to regulate normal testis development, such as Dkk1, Dmrt1 and Sfrp1. Contrarily, a few studies have mentioned that Wnt may also play a positive role in testis determination and development. Hence, it is now essential to analyze the strength of such positive effects, as well as the mechanisms and processes that are involved in mediating such functions. With reference to germ cell development, relatively fewer studies have taken an in-depth analysis of the Wnt signaling functions. Based on the recent evidence, multiple Wnt ligands and various types of Wnt signalings have been discovered to partake PGC specification, proliferation and migration, SSC maintenance and spermatogenesis. However, given the complexity of the role of Wnt signaling in early gonadal/testicular development, SSC proliferation and spermatid differentiation, further studies are required to link Wnt dynamics with particular and specific aspects of spermatogenesis and male fertility.

REFERENCES

1. Kerr GE, Young JC, Horvay K, Abud HE, Loveland KL. Regulated Wnt/β-catenin signaling sustains adult spermatogenesis in mice. *Biol Reprod.* 2014;90:1–3.

2. Cadigan KM, Liu YI. Wnt signaling: Complexity at the surface. *J Cell Sci.* 2006;119:395–402.

3. Logan CY, Nusse R. The Wnt signaling pathway in development and disease. *Annu Rev Cell Dev Biol.* 2004;20:781–810.

4. Lombardi APG, Royer C, Pisolato R, Cavalcanti FN, Lucas TFG, Lazari MFM, Porto CS. Physiopathological aspects of the Wnt/β-catenin signaling pathway in the male reproductive system. *Spermatogenesis.* 2013;3:e23181.

5. Erickson RP, Lai L, Grimes J. Creating a conditional mutation of Wnt-1 by antisense transgenesis provides evidence that Wnt-1 is not essential for spermatogenesis. *Dev Genet.* 1993;14:274–281.

6. Katoh M. Molecular cloning and characterization of human WNT3. *Int J Oncol.* 2001;19:977–982.

7. Yeh JR, Zhang X, Nagano MC. Indirect effects of Wnt3a/β-catenin signalling support mouse spermatogonial stem cells *in vitro. PLOS ONE.* 2012;7:e40002.

8. Jeays-Ward K, Dandonneau M, Swain A. Wnt4 is required for proper male as well as female sexual development. *Dev Biol.* 2004;276:431–40.

9. Yeh JR, Zhang X, Nagano MC. Wnt5a is a cell-extrinsic factor that supports self-renewal of mouse spermatogonial stem cells. *J Cell Sci.* 2011;124:2357–2366.

10. Ikegawa S, Kumano Y, Okui K, Fujiwara T, Takahashi E, Nakamura Y. Isolation, characterization and chromosomal assignment of the human WNT7A gene. *Cytogenet Genome Res.* 1996;74:149–52.

11. Golestaneh N, Beauchamp E, Fallen S, Kokkinaki M, Uren A, Dym M. Wnt signaling promotes proliferation and stemness regulation of spermatogonial stem/progenitor cells. *Reproduction.* 2009;138:151.

12. Wang XN, Li ZS, Ren Y, Jiang T, Wang YQ, Chen M, Zhang J, Hao JX, Wang YB, Sha RN. The Wilms tumor gene, Wt1, is critical for mouse spermatogenesis via regulation of Sertoli cell polarity and is associated with non-obstructive azoospermia in humans. *PLOS Genet.* 2013;9:e1003645.

13. Polakis P. Wnt signaling and cancer. *Genes Dev.* 2000;14:1837–51.

14. Nusse R. Wnt signaling. *Cold Spring Harb Perspect Biol.* 2012;4:a011163.

15. Singh SR, Burnicka-Turek O, Chauhan C, Hou SX. Spermatogonial stem cells, infertility and testicular cancer. *J Cell Mol Med.* 2011;15:468–83.

16. Blank U, Karlsson G, Karlsson S. Signaling pathways governing stem-cell fate. *Blood.* 2008;111:492–503.

17. Tanwar PS, Zhang L, Tanaka Y, Taketo MM, Donahoe PK, Teixeira JM. Focal Müllerian duct retention in male mice with constitutively activated β-catenin expression in the Müllerian duct mesenchyme. *Proc Natl Acad Sci.* 2010;107:16142–7.

18. Reya T, Clevers H. Wnt signalling in stem cells and cancer. *Nature.* 2005;434:843.

19. Ohinata Y, Ohta H, Shigeta M, Yamanaka K, Wakayama T, Saitou M. A signaling principle for the specification of the germ cell lineage in mice. *Cell.* 2009;137:571–84.

20. Foulquier S, Daskalopoulos EP, Lluri G, Hermans KCM, Deb A, Blankesteijn WM. WNT signaling in cardiac and vascular disease. *Pharmacol Rev.* 2018;70:68–141.

21. Molenaar M, van de Wetering M, Oosterwegel M, Peterson-Maduro J, Godsave S, Korinek V, Roose J, Destrée O, Clevers H. XTcf-3 transcription factor mediates β-catenin-induced axis formation in Xenopus embryos. *Cell.* 1996;86:391–9.

22. Janda CY, Waghray D, Levin AM, Thomas C, Garcia KC. Structural basis of Wnt recognition by Frizzled. *Science.* 2012;337:59–64.

23. MacDonald BT, He X. Frizzled and LRP5/6 receptors for Wnt/β-catenin signaling. *Cold Spring Harb Perspect Biol.* 2012;4:a007880.

24. Pinson KI, Brennan J, Monkley S, Avery BJ, Skarnes WC. An LDL-receptor-related protein mediates Wnt signalling in mice. *Nature.* 2000;407:535.

25. Tamai K, Semenov M, Kato Y, Spokony R, Liu C, Katsuyama Y, Hess F, Saint-Jeannet J-P, He X. LDL-receptor-related proteins in Wnt signal transduction. *Nature.* 2000;407:530.

26. Wehrli M, Dougan ST, Caldwell K, O'keefe L, Schwartz S, Vaizel-Ohayon D, Schejter E, Tomlinson A, DiNardo S. Arrow encodes an LDL-receptor-related protein essential for Wingless signalling. *Nature.* 2000;407:527.

27. Niehrs C, Shen J. Regulation of Lrp6 phosphorylation. *Cell Mol Life Sci.* 2010;67:2551–62.

28. Pan WJ, Pang SZ, Huang T, Guo HY, Dianqing WU, Lin LI. Characterization of function of three domains in dishevelled-1: DEP domain is responsible for membrane translocation of dishevelled-1. *Cell Res.* 2004;14:324.

29. Wong EWP, Lee WM, Cheng CY. Secreted Frizzled-related protein 1 (sFRP1) regulates spermatid adhesion in the testis via dephosphorylation of focal adhesion kinase and the nectin-3 adhesion protein complex. *FASEB J.* 2013;27:464–77.

30. Mao J, Wang J, Liu B, Pan W, Farr GH, III, Flynn C, Yuan H, Takada S, Kimelman D, Li L. Low-density lipoprotein receptor-related protein-5 binds to Axin and regulates the canonical Wnt signaling pathway. *Mol Cell.* 2001;7:801–9.

31. Wolf J, Palmby TR, Gavard J, Williams BO, Gutkind JS. Multiple PPPS/TP motifs act in a combinatorial fashion to transduce Wnt signaling through LRP6. *FEBS Lett.* 2008;582:255–61.

32. Brennan K, Gonzalez-Sancho JM, Castelo-Soccio LA, Howe LR, Brown AMC. Truncated mutants of the putative Wnt receptor LRP6/Arrow can stabilize β-catenin independently of Frizzled proteins. *Oncogene.* 2004;23:4873.

33. Brunner E, Peter O, Schweizer L, Basler K. *pangolin* encodes a Lef-1 homologue that acts downstream of Armadillo to transduce the Wingless signal in *Drosophila. Nature.* 1997;385:829.

34. Van Wetering de M, Cavallo R, Dooijes D, van Beest M, van Es J, Loureiro J, Ypma A, Hursh D, Jones T, Bejsovec A. Armadillo coactivates transcription driven by the product of the *Drosophila* segment polarity gene dTCF. *Cell.* 1997;88:789–99.

35. Chen G, Fernandez J, Mische S, Courey AJ. A functional interaction between the histone deacetylase Rpd3 and the corepressor Groucho in *Drosophila* development. *Genes Dev.* 1999;13:2218–30.

36. Cavallo RA, Cox RT, Moline MM, Roose J, Polevoy GA, Clevers H, Peifer M, Bejsovec A. *Drosophila* Tcf and Groucho interact to repress Wingless signalling activity. *Nature.* 1998;395:604.

37. Daniels DL, Weis WI. β-Catenin directly displaces Groucho/TLE repressors from Tcf/Lef in Wnt-mediated transcription activation. *Nat Struct Mol Biol.* 2005;12:364.

38. Kimura R, Murata C, Kuroki Y, Kuroiwa A. Mutations in the testis-specific enhancer of SOX9 in the SRY independent sex-determining mechanism in the genus *Tokudaia. PLOS ONE.* 2014;9:e108779.

39. Li Y, Zheng M, Lau Y-FC. The sex-determining factors SRY and SOX9 regulate similar target genes and promote testis cord formation during testicular differentiation. *Cell Rep.* 2014;8:723–33.

40. Moniot B, Declosmenil F, Barrionuevo F, Scherer G, Aritake K, Malki S, Marzi L, Cohen-Solal A, Georg I, Klattig J. The PGD2 pathway, independently of FGF9, amplifies SOX9 activity in Sertoli cells during male sexual differentiation. *Development.* 2009;136:1813–21.

41. Barrionuevo F, Bagheri-Fam S, Klattig J, Kist R, Taketo MM, Englert C, Scherer G. Homozygous inactivation of Sox9 causes complete XY sex reversal in mice. *Biol Reprod.* 2006;74:195–201.

42. Wagner T, Wirth J, Meyer J, Zabel B, Held M, Zimmer J, Pasantes J, Bricarelli FD, Keutel J, Hustert E. Autosomal sex reversal and campomelic dysplasia are caused by mutations in and around the SRY-related gene SOX9. *Cell.* 1994;79:1111–20.

43. Huang B, Wang S, Ning Y, Lamb AN, Bartley J. Autosomal XX sex reversal caused by duplication of SOX9. *Am J Med Genet.* 1999;87:349–53.

44. Sreenivasan R, Jiang J, Wang X, Bártfai R, Kwan HY, Christoffels A, Orbán L. Gonad differentiation in zebrafish is regulated by the canonical Wnt signaling pathway. *Biol Reprod.* 2014;90:41–5.

45. Nicol B, Yao HH-C. Gonadal identity in the absence of pro-testis factor SOX9 and pro-ovary factor β-catenin in mice. *Biol Reprod.* 2015;93:35.

46. Loke J, Pearlman A, Radi O, Zuffardi O, Giussani U, Pallotta R, Camerino G, Ostrer H. Mutations in MAP3K1 tilt the balance from SOX9/FGF9 to WNT/β-catenin signaling. *Hum Mol Genet.* 2013;23:1073–83.

47. Combes AN, Bowles J, Feng C-W, Chiu HS, Khoo P-L, Jackson A, Little MH, Tam PPL, Koopman P. Expression and functional analysis of Dkk1 during early gonadal development. *Sex Dev.* 2011;5:124–30.

48. Zaytouni T, Efimenko EE, Tevosian SG. GATA transcription factors in the developing reproductive system. *Adv Genet.* 2011;76:93–134.

49. Warr N, Siggers P, Bogani D, Brixey R, Pastorelli L, Yates L, Dean CH, Wells S, Satoh W, Shimono A. Sfrp1 and Sfrp2 are required for normal male sexual development in mice. *Dev Biol.* 2009;326:273–84.

50. Lambeth LS, Raymond CS, Roeszler KN, Kuroiwa A, Nakata T, Zarkower D, Smith CA. Over-expression of DMRT1 induces the male pathway in embryonic chicken gonads. *Dev Biol.* 2014;389:160–72.

51. Bratuś A, Słota E. Comparative cytogenetic and molecular studies of DM domain genes in pig and cattle. *Cytogenet Genome Res.* 2009;126:180–5.

52. Webster KA, Schach U, Ordaz A, Steinfeld JS, Draper BW, Siegfried KR. Dmrt1 is necessary for male sexual development in zebrafish. *Dev Biol.* 2017;422:33–46.

53. Chassot A-A, Bradford ST, Auguste A, Gregoire EP, Pailhoux E, De Rooij DG, Schedl A, Chaboissier M-C. WNT4 and RSPO1 together are required for cell proliferation in the early mouse gonad. *Development.* 2012;139:4461–72.

54. Eggers S, Sinclair A. Mammalian sex determination—Insights from humans and mice. *Chromosom Res.* 2012;20:215–38.

55. Prunskaite-Hyyryläinen R, Skovorodkin I, Xu Q, Miinalainen I, Shan J, Vainio SJ. Wnt4 coordinates directional cell migration and extension of the Müllerian duct essential for ontogenesis of the female reproductive tract. *Hum Mol Genet.* 2015;25:1059–73.

56. Ahmed EA, de Rooij DG. Staging of mouse seminiferous tubule cross-sections. In: Keeney S. (Ed.). *Meiosis: Methods in Molecular Biology.* Springer; 2009, vol. 1, (pp. 263–277), Totowa, NJ: Humana Press.

57. Parr BA, McMahon AP. Sexually dimorphic development of the mammalian reproductive tract requires Wnt-7a. *Nature.* 1998;395:707.

58. Boyer A, Yeh JR, Zhang X, Paquet M, Gaudin A, Nagano MC, Boerboom D. CTNNB1 signaling in Sertoli cells downregulates spermatogonial stem cell activity via WNT4. *PLOS ONE.* 2012;7:e29764.

59. Li Q, Ishikawa T, Miyoshi H, Oshima M, Taketo MM. A targeted mutation of Nkd1 impairs mouse spermatogenesis. *J Biol Chem.* 2005;280:2831–9.

60. Kumar M, Atkins J, Cairns M, Ali A, Tanwar PS. Germ cell-specific sustained activation of Wnt signalling perturbs spermatogenesis in aged mice, possibly through non-coding RNAs. *Oncotarget.* 2016;7:85709.

61. Kaur G, Thompson LA, Dufour JM. Sertoli cells—Immunological sentinels of spermatogenesis. *Semin Cell Dev Biol.* 2014;30:36–44.

62. Takase HM, Nusse R. Paracrine Wnt/β-catenin signaling mediates proliferation of undifferentiated spermatogonia in the adult mouse testis. *Proc Natl Acad Sci.* 2016;201601461.

63. Das DS, Wadhwa N, Kunj N, Sarda K, Pradhan BS, Majumdar SS. Dickkopf homolog 3 (DKK3) plays a crucial role upstream of WNT/β-CATENIN signaling for Sertoli cell mediated regulation of spermatogenesis. *PLOS ONE.* 2013;8:e63603.

64. Richardson LC, Neri AJ, Tai E, Glenn JD. Testicular cancer: A narrative review of the role of socioeconomic position from risk to survivorship. *Urol Oncol.* 2012;30:95–101.

65. Skotheim RI, Monni O, Mousses S, Fosså SD, Kallioniemi O-P, Lothe RA, Kallioniemi A. New insights into testicular germ cell tumorigenesis from gene expression profiling. *Cancer Res.* 2002;62:2359–64.

66. Almstrup K, Leffers H, Lothe RA, Skakkebæk NE, Sonne SB, Nielsen JE, Meyts ER, Skotheim RI. Improved gene expression signature of testicular carcinoma in situ. *Int J Androl.* 2007;30:292–303.

67. Honecker F, Oosterhuis JW, Mayer F, Hartmann JT, Bokemeyer C, Looijenga LHJ. New insights into the pathology and molecular biology of human germ cell tumors. *World J Urol.* 2004;22:15–24.

68. Abeyawardene SA, Plant TM. Reconciliation of the paradox that testosterone replacement prevents the postcastration hypersecretion of follicle-stimulating hormone in male rhesus monkeys (*Macaca mulatta*) with an intact central nervous system but not in hypothalamic-lesioned, gonadotropin-releasing hormone-replaced animals. *Biol Reprod.* 1989;40:578–84.

69. Korkola JE, Houldsworth J, Chadalavada RSV, Olshen AB, Dobrzynski D, Reuter VE, Bosl GJ, Chaganti RSK. Down-regulation of stem cell genes, including those in a 200-kb gene cluster at 12p13. 31, is associated with *in vivo* differentiation of human male germ cell tumors. *Cancer Res.* 2006;66:820–7.

70. Skotheim RI, Lind GE, Monni O, Nesland JM, Abeler VM, Fosså SD, Duale N, Brunborg G, Kallioniemi O, Andrews PW. Differentiation of human embryonal carcinomas *in vitro* and *in vivo* reveals expression profiles relevant to normal development. *Cancer Res.* 2005;65:5588–98.

71. Perrone F, Bertolotti A, Montemurro G, Paolini B, Pierotti MA, Colecchia M. Frequent mutation and nuclear localization of β-catenin in Sertoli cell tumors of the testis. *Am J Surg Pathol.* 2014;38:66–71.

72. Tanwar PS, Commandeur AE, Zhang L, Taketo MM, Teixeira MM. The Müllerian inhibiting substance type 2 receptor suppresses tumorigenesis in testes with sustained β-catenin signaling. *Carcinogenesis.* 2012;33:2351–61.

73. Chang H, Guillou F, Taketo MM, Behringer RR. Overactive β-catenin signaling causes testicular Sertoli cell tumor development in the mouse. *Biol Reprod.* 2009;81:842–9.

74. Nicol B, Guiguen Y. Expression profiling of Wnt signaling genes during gonadal differentiation and gametogenesis in rainbow trout. *Sex Dev.* 2011;5: 318–29.

75. Chang Y-F, Lee-Chang JS, Harris KY, Sinha-Hikim AP, Rao MK. Role of β-catenin in post-meiotic male germ cell differentiation. *PLOS ONE.* 2011;6:e28039.

76. Yan Q, Wu X, Chen C, Diao R, Lai Y, Huang J, Chen J, Yu Z, Gui Y, Tang A. Developmental expression and function of DKKL1/Dkkl1 in humans and mice. *Reprod Biol Endocrinol.* 2012;10:51.

77. Reynard LN, Cocquet J, Burgoyne PS. The multicopy mouse gene Sycp3-like Y-linked (Sly) encodes an abundant spermatid protein that interacts with a histone acetyltransferase and an acrosomal protein. *Biol Reprod.* 2009;81:250–7.

78. Zhuang X, Hou X, Liao S-Y, Wang X-X, Cooke HJ, Zhang M, Han C. SLXL1, a novel acrosomal protein, interacts with DKKL1 and is involved in fertilization in mice. *PLOS ONE.* 2011;6:e20866.

79. Gong W, Pan L, Lin Q, Zhou Y, Xin Y, Yu X, Cui P, Hu S, Yu J. Transcriptome profiling of the developing postnatal mouse testis using next-generation sequencing. *Sci China Life Sci.* 2013;56:1–12.

80. Ma P, Wang H, Guo R, Ma Q, Yu Z, Jiang Y, Ge Y, Ma J, Xue S, Han D. Stage-dependent Dishevelled-1 expression during mouse spermatogenesis suggests a role in regulating spermatid morphological changes. *Mol Reprod Dev Inc Gamete Res.* 2006;73:774–83.

81. Koch S, Acebron SP, Herbst J, Hatiboglu G, Niehrs C. Post-transcriptional Wnt signaling governs epididymal sperm maturation. *Cell.* 2015;163:1225–36.

82. Novin MG, Mirfakhraie R, Nazarian H. Aberrant Wnt/β-catenin signaling pathway in testis of azoospermic men. *Adv Pharm Bull.* 2015;5:373.

MAPK signaling in spermatogenesis and male infertility

ARCHANA DEVI, BHAVANA KUSHWAHA, AND GOPAL GUPTA

HIGHLIGHTS

- The mitogen-activated protein kinase (MAPK) cascade plays a pivotal role in regulating spermatogenesis and spermatozoal functions.
- MAPKs are involved in the junction restructuring of testicular seminiferous epithelium, especially testis-specific adherens junction (AJ) and ectoplasmic specialization (ES).
- MAPKs are key players for triggering apoptosis in germ cells with potential as targets for the development of male contraceptives.

10.1 INTRODUCTION

Spermatogenesis is an orderly series of highly synchronized events, which give rise to the life progenitor, i.e., the sperm. This complex cellular, molecular and biochemical process involves spermatogonial stem cells located at the basal membrane of the seminiferous tubules, which undergo repeated mitotic divisions, and finally, a meiotic division culminating in the production of haploid cells that differentiate into mature spermatozoa (1). Its hormonal regulation involves the gonadotropin-releasing hormone (GnRH) that controls the release of peptide hormones, follicle-stimulating hormone (FSH) and luteinizing hormone (LH), which in turn govern the process of spermatogenesis. The process is further driven by the steroid hormone testosterone produced by the Leydig cells under the influence of LH (2,3). The Sertoli cells are somatic testicular cells that provide a nurturing environment for the developing germ cells and support their growth, division, migration and release into the lumen of seminiferous tubules. They

also form an immunological barrier for protection of the germ cells, which remain associated with them throughout spermatogenesis (4,5). For this, the Sertoli cells form several junctions, such as tight junctions, adherens junctions, ectoplasmic specialization, tubulobulbar complex and gap junctions between Sertoli-Sertoli cells, Sertoli-germ cells and testicular cells-extracellular matrix (6). Tight Sertoli cell junctions above the basal lamina of the seminiferous tubules in the testis act as a blood-testes barrier (BTB), which divides the seminiferous epithelium into basal and adluminal compartments and creates a selective, systemic-free environment for germ cell maturation. Being impermeable, it also restricts the access of biological substances such as nutrients, hormones and electrolytes into the seminiferous epithelium (7). The cytoskeletal network of Sertoli cells consisting of actin filaments, intermediate filaments and microtubules helps in the differentiation and migration of spermatocytes toward the adluminal compartment and the transport of spermatids (8,9). Several regulatory molecules such as cytokines, proteases, proteases inhibitors, GTPases, kinases and phosphatases play a pivotal role in the movement of germ cells (10).

The mitogen-activated protein kinases (MAPKs) are members of the serine/threonine family of protein kinases that regulate a wide variety of cellular programs by responding to extracellular signals (11). In the mammalian testes, MAPK plays an important role in the phosphorylation of key proteins to regulate the Sertoli-Sertoli and Sertoli–germ cell interface through modulation of the dynamics of ES junctions and BTB. Furthermore, these kinases are also important for sperm motility and fertilization and are key players for triggering apoptosis in germ cells, with the potential as targets for the development of male contraceptives (12,13). This chapter highlights the roles of three crucial MAPK members, namely, the extracellular signal-regulated kinase (ERK), the c-Jun N-terminal kinase (JNK) and the p38-MAPK, in modulating the dynamics of ES junctions, BTB and numerous male reproductive functions including cell-cycle progression, germ cell differentiation, apoptosis, Sertoli–germ cell interaction and sperm cell development.

10.2 MITOGEN-ACTIVATED PROTEIN KINASES: AN OVERVIEW

Mitogen-activated Ser/Thr protein kinases (MAPKs) are the most conserved classical pathways of signal transduction associated with an array of physiological activities such as proliferation, growth, migration, differentiation and cell survival (14–16). Mammalian cells express four MAPK families: the classical extracellular signal-regulated MAP

kinase (ERK1/2), the stress-activated protein kinase/c-Jun N-terminal protein kinases (SAPK-JNK), the p38 protein kinase (α, β, γ and δ) and the ERK5, which are activated by a specific MAPK kinase or MAPKK or MAP2K (17). All MAPKKs show redundancy for activation that adds up to the complexity and diversity in MAPK signaling cascades. Various signals from cell surface receptors are transduced directly or by means of small proteins, to a number of protein kinases that amplify these cues and lead to a physiological response in the cell (Table 10.1).

The pathway architecture involves a small G protein (RAS) and three protein kinases (RAF, MEK, ERK). The pathway commences with the binding of a ligand to the transmembrane receptor, which is a receptor tyrosine kinase (RTK). The signaling cascade finally results in the translocation of ERK to the nucleus where ERK transactivates different transcription factors that lead to the expression of specific genes to complete the cellular response (18). Furthermore, MAPKs orient with scaffold proteins to create a supportive environment to facilitate their interaction with specific proteins and substrates. Various protein phosphatases mediate the regulation of MAPK activity, the culmination of MAPK signaling. Such protein phosphatases dephosphorylate crucial proteins in the MAPK signaling and regulate the scale and extent of signaling (19,20).

In mammalian testes, MAPKs are involved in the maturation of spermatozoa in the epididymis, and MAPK isoforms regulate key cellular processes including cell-cycle progression and differentiation of germ cells, flagellar

Table 10.1 Mitogen-activated protein kinase (MAPKs) involved in spermatogenesis

Protein name	Protein family	Protein expression	Role in spermatogenesis
ERK			
ERK1	MAP kinase subfamily	Sertoli cells	Regulation of ectoplasmic specialization (ES) dynamics
ERK2	MAP kinase subfamily	Sertoli cells	Regulation of ES dynamics
ERK7	MAP kinase subfamily	Rat testis, Sertoli cells	Regulation of ES dynamics
JNK			
JNK1	MAP kinase	Tetraploid spermatocyte and spermatogonia	Spermatocyte loss through apoptosis
JNK2	MAP kinase	Tetraploid spermatocyte and spermatogonia	Spermatocyte loss through apoptosis
JNK3	MAP kinase	Mammalian testis	Spermatocyte loss through apoptosis
p38			
p38α	MAPkinase	Sertoli cells and elongated spermatids	Cell junction dynamics and apoptosis of germ cells
p38β	MAPkinase	Sertoli cells and elongated spermatids	Cell junction dynamics and apoptosis of germ cells
p38β2	MAPkinase	Sertoli cells and elongated spermatids	Cell junction dynamics and apoptosis of germ cells
p38δ	MAPkinase	Sertoli cells and elongated spermatids	Cell junction dynamics and apoptosis of germ cells

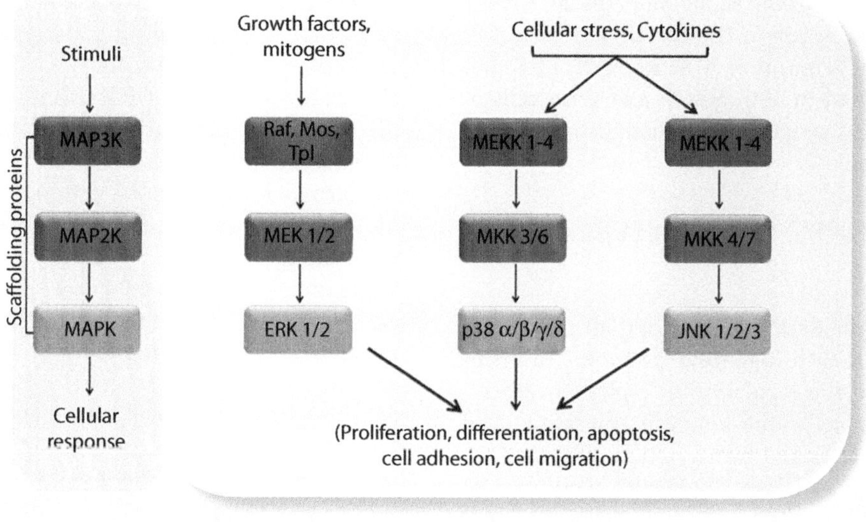

Figure 10.1 The core components of the MAPK signaling pathway. External stimuli mediate phosphorylation and activation of MAPKs which results in different cellular effects.

motility of spermatozoa, modulation of BTB dynamics, germ cell adhesion and acrosome reaction (21) (Figure 10.1).

10.3 JUNCTION DYNAMICS IN SPERMATOGENESIS AND ITS REGULATION

In mammalian testes, germ cells are anchored to the seminiferous epithelium through different types of anchoring junctions including cell-cell actin-based adhesion junctions, such as testis-specific ectoplasmic specializations and tubulobulbar complexes, cell-cell intermediate filament-based desmosome junctions (6). The testis-specific ectoplasmic specializations (ES) are basically found at the Sertoli-Sertoli and Sertoli–germ cell interface in the seminiferous epithelium and are classified as basal ES (at Sertoli-Sertoli cell interface restricted to BTB coexisting with TJs) and apical ES (at Sertoli-spermatid interface lacking TJs) with morphological similarity (22). The ES is a crucial anchoring device that is prominently involved in the movement of primary germ cells. It is known to provide an additional anchoring function to retain germ cells, specifically spermatids, in the epithelium until spermiation. Multiprotein complexes are found in the ES, namely, the cadherin/catenin, the afadin/nectin/ponsin and the integrin/laminin. Both cadherin/catenin and the nectin/afadin complexes are found at the apical and basal ES regions, though the integrin/laminin complex is restricted to the apical ES region (23). The cadherin/catenin, nectin-2/afadin and β1-integrin/FAK complexes, which are found at the apical ES, interact with cadherins, nectin 2/-3 and laminin-g3, present on the surface of spermatids (24). A group of molecules, including transmembrane adhesion proteins (e.g., adherins, integrins, laminins and nectins, etc.), adaptors

(e.g., α-, β- and γ-catenins, afadin, α-actinin, cortactin, fimbrin, paxillin, vinculin, zonula occludens-1 [ZO-1] etc.) and signaling molecules (e.g., protein/lipid kinases and phosphatases) constitute functional adhesion complexes that endow adhesiveness between the two cell types (25). These transmembrane adhesion proteins form a complex with different adaptor proteins in order to interact with the integral membrane protein in the cytoskeleton and facilitate the recruitment of other signaling molecules. Overall, this cytoskeletal complex of proteins supports cell-adhesion and germ cell movement (26,22). The complex dynamic architecture of ES allows it to make fine changes and restructure the ES complex in order to carry out the relay of an extracellular stimulus. Critical events such as the expression level of proteins, phosphorylation status, presence of essential proteins, adaptors, kinases, phosphatases and the actin cytoskeleton drive ES disassembly and reorganization (22).

Moreover, structural changes are required to be well coordinated by many intracellular factors to foster the adhesive ability of ES and the migration of germ cells. Hence, such coordinated movements at the ES permit external stimuli (e.g., environmental toxic substances, such as cadmium) to be transduced *via* Sertoli and germ cells. Sertoli and germ cells respond to the stimulus by secreting various cytokines such as TGF-β3 and TNF-α to exert the cellular response. An array of proteins involved in the concerted events related to ES dynamics is known as the MAPKs (10). Several *in vivo* or *in vitro* studies using the adult rat model and primary Sertoli/germ cell cocultures have demonstrated the essentiality and critical roles of MAPKs in junction restructuring events related to spermatogenesis by using hormones (e.g., FSH, testosterone, EGF), paracrine factors (e.g., TGF-β3, TNF-α) (27), chemical substances (cadmium, 1-[2,4-dichlorobenzyl]-1H-indazole-3carbohydrazide, nonylphenol, EDTA, EGTA, glycerol) and administration of adjudin (28),etc. Most of the signaling pathways invoke MAPKs to mediate adhesion at the Sertoli and germ cell interfaces. Almost all isoforms of MAPKs, JNK, ERK and p38, have been detected in both Sertoli and germ cells of mammalian testes and assigned key functions in the process of spermatogenesis.

10.3.1 MAPK-ERK1/2 signaling in junction dynamics

ERK1 and ERK2 are Ser/Thr kinases that participate in the Ras-Raf-MEK-ERK signaling pathway. This signaling is involved in the regulation of a plethora of cellular processes like cell adhesion, cell migration, cell growth, metabolic cycles and transcription of genes (29). Phosphorylation of ERK1/2 at Tyr204/187 and then at Thr202/185 is critical for their activation. While Raf and MEK have limited substrate specificity, ERK1/2 can catalyze the phosphorylation of a number of cytoplasmic and nuclear target proteins (30–32). ERK1/2 mediate the phosphorylation of a variety of substrates from the cytoplasmic and nuclear fractions of a cell including death-associated protein kinase (DAPK), tuberous sclerosis complex 2 (TSC2), RSK, MNK, NF-AT, Elk-1, myocyte enhancer factor 2 (MEF2), c-Fos, c-Myc, STAT3 and several other transcription factors and inhibitory molecules (11). Germ cells and Sertoli cells are known to express ERK1/2, which play a pivotal role in spermatogenesis, including germ cell survival, spermatocyte proliferation and meiotic divisions, as well as the acquisition of sperm motility (21).

ERK participates in maintaining the connection between Sertoli and germ cells, especially at the apical ES, where its activity is elevated through phosphorylation at the time of ES disassembly to facilitate spermiation (Figure 10.2). Hence, the phospho-ERK/ERK ratio is higher in the seminiferous epithelium during spermiation (3). Consequently, a reduction in intratesticular testosterone (T) levels by subdermal T and estradiol (E) implants in adult rats promoted loss of germ cells (step 8 spermatids and beyond) from the epithelium due to activation of ERK activity and abrogation of apical ES adhesion (33). Similarly, a dramatic activation of ERK and removal of germ cells was seen in rat epithelium after disruption of apical ES structure by adjudin (1-[2,4-dichlorobenzyl]-1H-indazole-3- carbohydrazide, formerly named AF-2364) (28), which could be inhibited by pretreatment with U0126, a specific inhibitor of upstream ERK kinase MEK (34).TNF-α, mostly secreted by germ cells, has been linked in the regulation of several cellular processes in spermatogenesis, including disruption of BTB through transient activation of ERK and p38MAPK (19), which implies that both ERK and p38MAPK play significant roles in the opening of BTB to aid migration of preleptotene and leptotene spermatocytes from the basal to the adluminal compartment (36). The ERK activation is primarily heralded by the activation of two focal adhesion components present at the apical ES, focal adhesion kinase (FAK) and c-Src, which supports the view that ERK serves as an important downstream signal transducer for the disorganization of the FA-like ES structure (37). The ERK plays critical roles via TGF-β3 in the regulation of adherens junctions of Sertoli cells (34).

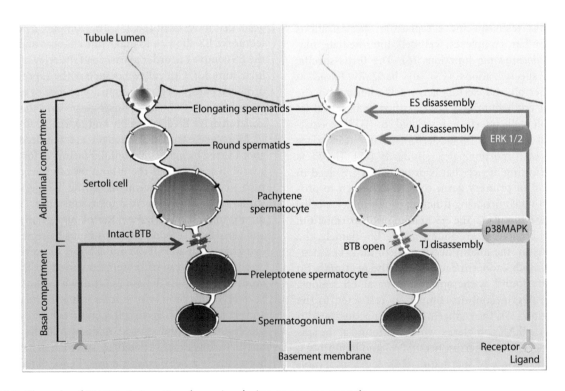

Figure 10.2 The role of MAPKs in junction dynamics during spermatogenesis.

10.3.2 MAPK-p38 in junction dynamics

The p38 mitogen-activated protein (MAP) kinases are serine-/threonine-based kinases composed of four members (p38α, p38β, p38γ and p38δ). These members show similarity in amino acid sequences, but their expression patterns are different (38). MAPK-p38 plays a key role in driving cellular activities in response to various extracellular stress stimuli. Interestingly, p38 MAPKs can also exert their function independent of its kinase activity, which it carries out by direct binding to its targets (39). Extracellular stress stimuli and inflammatory cytokines can also activate p38, which affects many biological activities downstream in the cell, such as inflammation, apoptosis, cell differentiation and the cell cycle (40). The upstream kinases MKK3 and MKK6 are responsible for p38 MAPK activation (41). Its activity is mainly controlled by phosphorylation-dephosphorylation mechanisms, and the duration of phosphorylation is pivotal in regulating cell fate (42). The MAP kinase-activated protein kinase 2 (MAPKAPK2 or MK2), the well-known substrate of MAPK p38, has been demonstrated to activate various transcription factors such as ATF1, c-Fos and c-Jun, which are reported to regulate steroid biosynthesis (43), and the molecular chaperone heat shock protein 27(Hsp27) that regulates actin dynamics to prevent its destabilization during stress (44). Besides MK2, Na^+/H^+ exchangers (NHE) are also reported as a substrate for p38MAPK, which ensures the spermatogenic event and the spermatozoal maturation by regulating pH and ionic balance (45,46).

It is well established that p38 regulates cell adhesion and motility by tempering actin organization *via* an actin-polymerizing factor, HSP27, or by changing the transcriptional expression of various adhesion molecules. All isoforms of p38 MAPK except p38-γ are found in the testes (13). TGF-β3 is involved in the activation of the p38 MAPK cascade, and when added to Sertoli cell cultures *in vitro*, it leads to the disruption of Sertoli cell TJ-barrier that can partially be reversed by a p38-specific inhibitor, SB202190 (47). It has been reported that epithelial TGF-β3 levels are increased during the cadmium-driven BTB restructuring, resulting in the BTB disassembly, which is accompanied by apical ES disintegration. The effect of this cytokine is partly mediated by the p38 MAPK, since an intratesticular injection of SB202190 before the cadmium application blocks the cadmium-mediated disruption of junction-associated proteins in the testes as well as impedes the expression of proteases at the cellular interface (48). Also, the inhibition of the p38 MAPK pathway averts the disruption of TJ-associated junction components, occludin and ZO-1, and apical ES-associated proteins such as catenins, cadherins, nectin-3 and afadin. These findings highlight the important role of MAPK signaling in sustaining both apical ES and the TJ dynamics (Figure 10.2).

10.3.3 JNK in junction dynamics

A stress-activated protein kinase (SAPK), c-Jun *N*-terminal kinase (JNK) plays diverse roles in a variety of cellular stress signals and is involved in different biological processes like programmed cell death and autophagy (49). In mammals, mainly three isoforms of JNK protein kinases are found, viz. JNK1, JNK2 and JNK3. Interestingly, JNK1 and JNK2 are ubiquitous in their expression, while JNK3 expression is mainly limited to the brain, cardiac smooth muscles and testes. In particular, the upstream kinases such as MKK4 and MKK7 mediate the stimulation of JNK by its double phosphorylation at the Thr-Pro-Tyr motif. The activated JNK is responsible for regulating an array of transcription factors including c-Jun, c-Fos, ATF-2, Elk, p53 and AP-1 (50). Also, JNK can activate cytoplasmic target molecules including cytoskeleton proteins and mitochondrial proteins, Bcl-2 and Bcl-xl. Collectively, the activation of JNK leads to cell growth, apoptosis, autophagy, cellular motility, metabolic shifts and DNA repair (51). Hence, JNKs are indispensable for cell proliferation, apoptosis and response to stresses. Several studies have indicated that JNK signaling is important for the formation and maintenance of adherens junctions (AJ), tight junctions (TJ) and gap junctions (GJ), as well as rapid and dynamic dissolution of adherens junctions (AJ) (52). JNK exists in three isoforms that are commonly present in the testes. JNK1 and JNK2 are localized in Sertoli and germ cells (53). The transcription factors activated by JNK, including c-jun, junB and junD, are also found in the testes. The function of Sertoli cell TJ-barrier is regulated by JNK cascade in the seminiferous tubules. Moreover, the JNK gets stimulated by TNF-α in Sertoli cell culture, and this cytokine disintegrates the Sertoli cell TJ-barrier, probably by stimulating the expression of a metalloproteinase, MMP-9 (54). Furthermore, it has also been demonstrated that cadmium-induced junction restructuring of epithelial layers augments the phosphorylation and enzymatic functions of JNK. Dimethylaminopurine (DMAP)-mediated specific inhibition of JNK activation results in BTB disruption and rapid depletion of germ cells from the epithelial tissues, as well as a regression of N-cadherin and h-catenin levels, suggesting its major role in maintaining rather than disintegrating the ES and TJ *in vivo*. Also, it has been demonstrated that JNK is involved in the upregulation of a protease inhibitor, α2-macroglobulin (α2 MG), that promotes the cellular adhesion between Sertoli and germ cells, *in vitro* (55). It is very clear from the available information that the activation of JNK in testes can either uphold or impede junction restructuring, depending on the type of external signal (Table 10.2) (10,24,56,57).

10.4 MAPK ROLE IN GERM CELL APOPTOSIS

Apoptosis is a precisely controlled and conspicuous process to maintain normal spermatogenesis, and deregulation of germ cell apoptosis can interrupt spermatogenesis, which leads to impaired fertility. For normal sperm output, this programmed germ cell death acts as a quality control system (58). Sertoli cells make a supporting framework and provide nutrition to facilitate germ cell development in the adult

Table 10.2 Classification of cell junctions found in the testis and their likely protein components

S.No.	Junction type	Cells participated	Locale	Components involved
1.	Occluding junction(tight junction)	Between Sertoli cells	BTB	**Integral membrane proteins**: Occludins, Claudin proteins, Junctional adhesion molecules **Adaptors or scaffolding proteins**: Zonula occludens, actin **Signaling proteins**: FAK, c-Src, p38MAPK, ERK1/2, JNK, PKB **Cytokines**: TNF, TGF-β3
2.	Anchoring (adhering) junction			
	a. Ectoplasmic specialization	Between Sertoli-Sertoli and Sertoli-germ cells	With actin filaments as an attachment site	**Integral membrane proteins**: Integrin, Laminin,N-cadherin, Nectin **Adaptors or scaffolding proteins**: Catenins, Afadin, vinculin, Paxillin, actin **Signaling proteins**: ERK1/2, Pi3-kinase, c-Src, FAK, PKB **Cytokines**: TNF, TGF-β3
	b. Tubulobulbar complex	Between Sertoli-Sertoli and Sertoli-germ cells	With actin filaments as an attachment site	**Tubulobulbar complex proteins**: MN7, actin, cofilin
	c. Focal contact	Between testicular cells and the extracellular matrix	With actin filaments as an attachment site	**Integral membrane proteins**: Integrins **Adaptors or scaffolding proteins**: Vinculin, paxillin, actin, **Signaling proteins**: FAK, c-Src, GSK
	d. Desmosome	Between Sertoli cells/ Sertoli cells-germ cells	With intermediate filaments as attachment sites	**Integral membrane proteins**: Desmoglein, Desmocollin **Adaptors or scaffolding proteins**: Plakoglobin, plakophilin, vimentin **Signaling proteins**: c-Src
	e. Hemidesmosome	Between testicular cells and the extracellular matrix	With intermediate filaments as attachment sites	**Integral membrane proteins**: Integrin, laminin **Adaptors or scaffolding proteins**: Paxillin
3.	Communicating junction		–	
	a. Gap junction	Between Sertoli cells,Sertoli-germ cells and Leydig cells	–	**Integral membrane proteins**: Connexins, connectin **Adaptors or scaffolding proteins**: Catenins **Signaling proteins**: c-Src

Source: Mruk DD, Cheng CY. *Endocr Rev.* 2004 Oct 1;25(5):747–806; Lui WY et al. *J Androl.* 2003 Jan 2;24(1):1–4; Cheng CY, Mruk DD. *Physiol Rev.* 2002 Jan 10;82(4):825–74; Cheng CY, Mruk DD. *Nat Rev Endocrinol.* 2010 Jul;6(7):380.
Note: This table includes information based on earlier reviews and reports.

testes. The number of Sertoli cells is fixed in adults, and each Sertoli cell can sustain ~30–50 developing germ cells (5). During spermatogenesis, up to 75% of germ cells are subjected to spontaneous apoptosis for maintaining the proper germ-Sertoli cell ratio. Besides spontaneous apoptosis, the environmental and pathological conditions (including intratesticular testosterone concentration, gonadotropins hormone deprivation or testicular hyperthermia) also affect germ cell apoptosis during spermatogenesis (59). Germ cell apoptosis involves a cascade of signals and pathways, among them mitogen-activated protein kinase (MAPK) family members are crucial in responding to various kinds of stimuli (60). The cytokine TNF-α predominantly secreted by the Sertoli cells also induces germ cell apoptosis via its downstream MAPK in a caspase-mediated process (61). The MAPK-p38 expression is found in Sertoli and germ cells, and its activation has a significant role in heat stress and hormone deprivation-mediated germ cell apoptosis (62,63). MAPK-p38 activation is mediated by the Fas ligand (FasL) binding to its receptor, which further phosphorylates

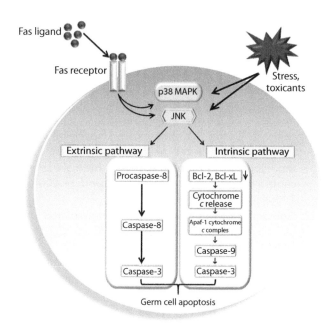

Figure 10.3 The role of MAPKs in germ cell apoptosis.

antiapoptotic molecules Bcl-x_L and Bcl-2 and prevents their accumulation within the mitochondria. Consequently, cytochrome *c* is released due to the loss of mitochondrial membrane potential, which results in caspase-3-mediated cell apoptosis. It is thus clear that activation of MAPK-p38 is a critical step for mitochondrial and FasL-mediated germ cell apoptosis (64) (Figure 10.3). Urriola-Muñoz reported that germ cell apoptosis induced by treatment of testes with endocrine disruptors, such as bisphenol-A (BPA) and non-ylphenol (NP), is mediated by MAPK-p38 signaling, which can be prevented by inhibiting MAPK-p38 activation (65). Similarly, MAPK-JNK also regulates germ cell apoptosis through both extrinsic and intrinsic pathways (51). MAPK-ERK-1/2 generally promotes cell survival, but under certain conditions, it may also exert proapoptotic action. Both ERK and PP2A can affect the antiapoptotic function of Bcl-2 by regulating its phosphorylation (66). A study has reported that the ERK-mediated activation of caspase-3 leads to apoptosis of malignant testicular germ cells (67). Long-term exposure to particulate matter 2.5 ($PM_{2.5}$) from automobile exhaust also impairs spermatogenesis and promotes germ cells apoptosis via activation of MAPKs (68).

10.5 MAPKs IN MALE INFERTILITY

Several studies have illustrated the importance of MAPKs in regulating spermatogenesis and fertility. Perturbation in this signaling leads to reproductive dysfunction, such as reduced sperm count and reduced semen quality (21). The phosphorylated levels of JNK/SAPK and p38-MAPK have been significantly correlated with sperm motility parameters, and the percentage of morphologically normal spermatozoa was positively correlated with the phosphorylated levels of p70 S6 kinase (69). In fact, MAPK-ERK1/2 stimulates and MAPK-p38 inhibits forward and hyperactivated motility of human sperm;

therefore, they can be used as markers of human sperm quality (70). In addition, junction dynamics play a significant role in the proper movement of germ cells, as its malfunction can disrupt the timely migration of preleptotene spermatocytes across the BTB. Also, the prolonged opening of these junctions can disrupt spermatogenesis, resulting in male infertility (24). Several *in vivo* or *in vitro* studies have demonstrated the critical roles of MAPKs in junction restructuring events related to spermatogenesis by using environmental toxicants (e.g., cadmium, bisphenol A) that damage germ-cell adhesions, which leads to germ-cell loss, reduced sperm count and male infertility or subfertility (8). Moreover, MAPK family members are crucial in responding to various kinds of stimuli for regulating germ cell apoptosis, which is an essential process for the production of healthy sperm and whose dysregulation can lead to male infertility (35).

10.6 CONCLUSION AND FUTURE DIRECTIONS

In summary, the MAPK signaling cascades participate in the concerted effort, plausibly under the influence of hormones and cytokines, to regulate restructuring events in the epithelium, which in turn facilitates germ cell movement during spermatogenesis. In addition, MAPK has been involved in the regulation of several critical processes of male germ cells, like differentiation and maturation. This chapter predominantly emphasizes the roles of three crucial MAPK members, namely, extracellular signal-regulated kinase (ERK), c-Jun N-terminal kinase (JNK) and p38 MAPK, in ES dynamics. Also, this review advocates and underscores the scope of targeting specific MAPK for the control and management of male reproductive abnormalities. Various kinases involved in the MAPK pathway hold the potential to become prime targets for developing male contraception and/or improving male fertility. A detailed understanding of the regulation of junction dynamics can contribute to the development of specific activators and inhibitors that can modulate the dynamics of BTB opening for controlling spermatogenesis at the testicular level. Further studies with specific knockout models may help in understanding the precise molecular mechanisms of MAPK signaling in controlling spermatogenesis and male fertility.

REFERENCES

1. Griswold MD. Spermatogenesis: The commitment to meiosis. *Physiol Rev.* 2015 Nov 4;96(1):1–7.
2. Ramaswamy S, Weinbauer GF. Endocrine control of spermatogenesis: Role of FSH and LH/testosterone. *Spermatogenesis.* 2014 Mar 4;4(2):e996025.
3. O'Donnell L, Nicholls PK, O'Bryan MK, McLachlan RI, Stanton PG. Spermiation: The process of sperm release. *Spermatogenesis.* 2011 Jan 1;1(1):14–35.
4. Petersen C, Söder O. The sertoli cell—A hormonal target and "super" nurse for germ cells that determines testicular size. *Horm Res Paediatr.* 2006;66(4):153–61.

5. Griswold MD. The central role of Sertoli cells in spermatogenesis. In: John Davey (Ed.), *Seminars in Cell andDevelopmental Biology*Aug 1 (Vol. 9, No. 4). Academic Press;1998, pp. 411–416.

6. Kopera IA, Bilinska B, Cheng CY, Mruk DD. Sertoligerm cell junctions in the testis: A review of recent data. *Philos Trans R Soc Lond B Biol Sci.* 2010 May 27;365(1546):1593–605.

7. Chen H, Lui WY, Mruk DD, Xiao X, Ge R, Lian Q, Lee WM, Silvestrini B, Cheng CY. Monitoring the integrity of the blood-testis barrier (BTB): An *in vivo* assay. In: Alves MG and Oliveira PF (Eds.), *Sertoli Cells.* New York, NY: Humana Press;2018, pp. 245–252

8. Cheng CY, Mruk DD. The blood-testis barrier and its implications for male contraception. *Pharmacol Rev.* 2012 Jan 1;64(1):16–64.

9. Mruk DD, Cheng CY. The mammalian blood-testis barrier: Its biology and regulation. *Endocr Rev.* 2015 Sep 10;36(5):564–91.

10. Mruk DD, Cheng CY. Sertoli-Sertoli and Sertoli-germ cell interactions and their significance in germ cell movement in the seminiferous epithelium during spermatogenesis. *Endocr Rev.* 2004 Oct 1;25(5):747–806.

11. Cargnello M, Roux PP. Activation and function of the MAPKs and their substrates, the MAPK-activated protein kinases. *Microbiol Mol Biol Rev.* 2011 Mar 1;75(1):50–83.

12. Almog T, Naor Z. Mitogen activated protein kinases (MAPKs) as regulators of spermatogenesis and spermatozoa functions. *Mol Cell Endocrinol.* 2008 Jan 30;282(1–2):39–44.

13. Wong CH, Cheng CY. Mitogen-activated protein kinases, adherens junction dynamics, and spermatogenesis: A review of recent data. *Dev Biol.* 2005 Oct 1;286(1):1–5.

14. Widmann C, Gibson S, Jarpe MB, Johnson GL. Mitogen-activated protein kinase: Conservation of a three-kinase module from yeast to human. *Physiol Rev.* 1999 Jan 1;79(1):143–80.

15. Sun Y, Liu WZ, Liu T, Feng X, Yang N, Zhou HF. Signaling pathway of MAPK/ERK in cell proliferation, differentiation, migration, senescence and apoptosis. *J Recept Signal Transduct Res.* 2015 Nov 2;35(6):600–4.

16. Johnson GL, Lapadat R. Mitogen-activated protein kinase pathways mediated by ERK, JNK, and p38 protein kinases. *Science.* 2002 Dec 6;298(5600):1911–2.

17. Zhang W, Liu HT. MAPK signal pathways in the regulation of cell proliferation in mammalian cells. *Cell Res.* 2002 Mar;12(1):9.

18. Daud A, Bastian BC. Beyond BRAF in melanoma. In: Mellinghoff K and Sawyers CL (Eds.), *Therapeutic Kinase Inhibitors.* Berlin, Heidelberg: Springer;2010, pp. 99–117.

19. Lie PP, Cheng CY, Mruk DD. Coordinating cellular events during spermatogenesis: A biochemical model. *Trends Biochem Sci.* 2009 Jul 1;34(7):366–73.

20. Karlsson M, Mandl M, Keyse SM. Spatio-temporal regulation of mitogen-activated protein kinase (MAPK) signalling by protein phosphatases.*Biochem Soc Trans.* 2006;34(Pt5):842–5.

21. Li MWM, Mruk DD, Cheng CY. Mitogen-activated protein kinases in male reproductive function. *Trends Mol Med.* 2009a Apr 1;15(4):159–68.

22. Lee NP, Cheng CY. Ectoplasmic specialization, a testis-specific cell–cell actin-based adherens junction type: Is this a potential target for male contraceptive development? *Hum Reprod Update.* 2004 Jul 1;10(4):349–69.

23. Goossens S, Van Roy F. Cadherin-mediated cell-cell adhesion in the testis. *Front Biosci.* 2005 Jan 1;10(51):398–419.

24. Lui WY, Mruk DD, Lee WM, Cheng CY. Adherens junction dynamics in the testis and spermatogenesis. *J Androl.* 2003 Jan 2;24(1):1–4.

25. Ogita H, Rikitake Y, Miyoshi J, Takai Y. Cell adhesion molecules nectins and associating proteins: Implications for physiology and pathology. *Proc Jpn Acad Ser B Phys Biol Sci.* 2010 Jun 11;86(6):621–9.

26. Wong EW, Mruk DD, Cheng CY. Biology and regulation of ectoplasmic specialization, an atypical adherens junction type, in the testis. *Biochim Biophys Acta.* 2008 Mar 1;1778(3):692–708.

27. Li MWM, Mruk DD, Lee WM, Cheng CY. Cytokines and junction restructuring events during spermatogenesis in the testis: An emerging concept of regulation. *Cytokine Growth Factor Rev.* 2009b Aug 1;20(4):329–38.

28. Siu MK, Wong CH, Lee WM, Cheng CY. Sertoli-germ cell anchoring junction dynamics in the testis are regulated by an interplay of lipid and protein kinases. *J Biol Chem.* 2005 Jul 1;280(26):25029–47.

29. Pouysségur J, Lenormand P. ERK1 and ERK2 map kinases: Specific roles or functional redundancy? *Front Cell Dev Biol.* 2016 Jun 8;4:53.

30. Rojas JM, Oliva JL, Santos E. Mammalian son of sevenless Guanine nucleotide exchange factors: Old concepts and new perspectives. *Genes Cancer.* 2011 Mar;2(3):298–305.

31. Nakamura Y, Hibino K, Yanagida T, Sako Y. Switching of the positive feedback for RAS activation by a concerted function of SOS membrane association domains. *Biophys Physicobiol.* 2016;13:1–1.

32. Wortzel I, Seger R. The ERK cascade: Distinct functions within various subcellular organelles. *Genes cancer.* 2011 Mar;2(3):195–209.

33. Beardsley A, O'Donnell L. Characterization of normal spermiation and spermiation failure induced by hormone suppression in adult rats. *Biol Reprod.* 2003 Apr 1;68(4):1299–307.

34. Xia W, Cheng CY. TGF-β3 regulates anchoring junction dynamics in the seminiferous epithelium of the rat testis via the Ras/ERK signaling pathway: An in vivo study. *Dev Biol.* 2005 Apr 15;280(2):321–43.

35. Shukla KK, Mahdi AA, Rajender S. Apoptosis, spermatogenesis and male infertility. *Front Biosci (Elite Ed)*. 2012 Jan 1;4:746–54.

36. Almog T, Naor Z. The role of mitogen activated protein kinase (MAPK) in sperm functions. *Mol Cell Endocrinol*. 2010 Jan 27;314(2):239–43.

37. Wong CH, Xia W, Lee NP, Mruk DD, Lee WM, Cheng CY. Regulation of ectoplasmic specialization dynamics in the seminiferous epithelium by focal adhesion-associated proteins in testosterone-suppressed rat testes. *Endocrinology*. 2005 Mar 1;146(3):1192–204.

38. Risco A, Cuenda A. New insights into the p38γ and p38δ MAPK pathways. *J Signal Transduct*. 2012;2012.

39. Gao J, Davidson MK, Wahls WP. Phosphorylation-independent regulation of Atf1-promoted meiotic recombination by stress-activated, p38 kinase Spc1 of fission yeast. *PLoS One*. 2009 May 14;4(5):e5533.

40. Cuenda A, Rousseau S. p38 MAP-kinases pathway regulation, function and role in human diseases. *Biochim Biophys Acta*. 2007 Aug 1;1773(8):1358–75.

41. Cuadrado A, Nebreda AR. Mechanisms and functions of p38 MAPK signalling. *Biochem J*. 2010 Aug 1;429(3):403–17.

42. Coulthard LR, White DE, Jones DL, McDermott MF, Burchill SA. p38MAPK: Stress responses from molecular mechanisms to therapeutics. *Trends Mol Med*. 2009 Aug 1;15(8):369–79.

43. Manna PR, Stocco DM. The role of specific mitogen-activated protein kinase signaling cascades in the regulation of steroidogenesis. *J Signal Transduct*. 2011;2011.

44. Roux PP, Blenis J. ERK and p38 MAPK-activated protein kinases: A family of protein kinases with diverse biological functions. *Microbiol Mol Biol Rev*. 2004 Jun 1;68(2):320–44.

45. Zarubin T, Jiahuai HA. Activation and signaling of the p38 MAP kinase pathway. *Cell Res*. 2005 Jan;15(1):11.

46. Martins AD, Bernardino RL, Neuhaus-Oliveira A, Sousa M, Sá R, Alves MG, Oliveira PF. Physiology of na$^+$/h$^+$ exchangers in the male reproductive tract: Relevance for male fertility. *Biol Reprod*. 2014 Jul 1;91(1):11.

47. Lui WY, Wong CH, Mruk DD, Cheng CY. TGF-β3 regulates the blood-testis barrier dynamics via the p38 mitogen activated protein (MAP) kinase pathway: An *in vivo* study. *Endocrinology*. 2003a Apr 1;144(4):1139–42.

48. Lui WY, Lee WM, Cheng CY. Transforming growth factor β3 regulates the dynamics of Sertoli cell tight junctions via the p38 mitogen-activated protein kinase pathway. *Biol Reprod*. 2003b May 1;68(5):1597–612.

49. Gkouveris I, Nikitakis NG. Role of JNK signaling in oral cancer: A mini review. *Tumor Biol*. 2017 Jun;39(6):1010428317711659.

50. Bode AM, Dong Z. The functional contrariety of JNK. *Mol Carcinog*. 2007 Aug;46(8):591–8.

51. Sui X, Kong N, Ye L, Han W, Zhou J, Zhang Q, He C, Pan H. p38 and JNK MAPK pathways control the balance of apoptosis and autophagy in response to chemotherapeutic agents. *Cancer Lett*. 2014 Mar 28;344(2):174–9.

52. You H, Lei P, Andreadis ST. JNK is a novel regulator of intercellular adhesion. *Tissue Barriers*. 2013 Dec 1;1(5):e26845.

53. Phelan DR, Loveland KL, Devereux L, Dorow DS. Expression of mixed lineage kinase 2 in germ cells of the testis. *Mol Reprod Dev*. 1999 Feb;52(2):135–40.

54. Siu MK, Lee WM, Cheng CY. The interplay of collagen IV, tumor necrosis factor-α, gelatinase B (matrix metalloprotease-9), and tissue inhibitor of metalloproteases-1 in the basal lamina regulates Sertoli cell-tight junction dynamics in the rat testis. *Endocrinology*. 2003 Jan 1;144(1):371–87.

55. Wong CH, Mruk DD, Siu MK, Cheng CY. Blood-testis barrier dynamics are regulated by α2-macroglobulin via the c-Jun N-terminal protein kinase pathway. *Endocrinology*. 2005 Apr 1;146(4):1893–908.

56. Cheng CY, Mruk DD. Cell junction dynamics in the testis: Sertoli-germ cell interactions and male contraceptive development. *Physiol Rev*. 2002 Jan 10;82(4):825–74.

57. Cheng CY, Mruk DD. A local autocrine axis in the testes that regulates spermatogenesis. *Nat Rev Endocrinol*. 2010 Jul;6(7):380.

58. Liu T, Wang L, Chen H, Huang Y, Yang P, Ahmed N, Wang T, Liu Y, Chen Q. Molecular and cellular mechanisms of apoptosis during dissociated spermatogenesis. *Front physiol*. 2017 Mar 29;8:188.

59. Boekelheide K, Fleming SL, Johnson KJ, Patel SR, Schoenfeld HA. Role of Sertoli cells in injury-associated testicular germ cell apoptosis (44558). *Proc Soc Exp Biol Med*. 2000 Nov;225(2):105–15.

60. Wada T, Penninger JM. Mitogen-activated protein kinases in apoptosis regulation. *Oncogene*. 2004 Apr;23(16):2838.

61. Lu Y, Luo B, Li J, Dai J. Perfluorooctanoic acid disrupts the blood–testis barrier and activates the TNFα/p38 MAPK signaling pathway *in vivo* and *in vitro*. *Arch Toxicol*. 2016 Apr 1;90(4):971–83.

62. Jia Y, Castellanos J, Wang C, Sinha-Hikim I, Lue Y, Swerdloff RS, Sinha-Hikim AP. Mitogen-activated protein kinase signaling in male germ cell apoptosis in the rat. *Biol Reprod*. 2009 Apr 1;80(4):771–80.

63. Vera Y, Erkkilä K, Wang C, Nunez C, Kyttänen S, Lue Y, Dunkel L, Swerdloff RS, Sinha Hikim AP. Involvement of p38 mitogen-activated protein kinase and inducible nitric oxide synthase in apoptotic signaling of murine and human male germ cells after hormone deprivation. *Mol Endocrinol*. 2006 Jul 1;20(7):1597–609.

64. Xu YR, Dong HS, Yang WX. Regulators in the apoptotic pathway during spermatogenesis: Killers or guards? *Gene*. 2016 May 15;582(2):97–111.

65. Urriola-Muñoz P, Lagos-Cabré R, Moreno RD. A mechanism of male germ cell apoptosis induced by bisphenol-A and nonylphenol involving ADAM17 and p38 MAPK activation. *PLOS ONE*. 2014 Dec 4;9(12):e113793.

66. Tamura Y, Simizu S, Osada H. The phosphorylation status and anti-apoptotic activity of Bcl-2 are regulated by ERK and protein phosphatase 2A on the mitochondria. *FEBS Lett*. 2004 Jul 2;569(1–3):249–55.

67. Schweyer S, Soruri A, Meschter O, Heintze A, Zschunke F, Miosge N, Thelen P, Schlott T, Radzun HJ, Fayyazi A. Cisplatin-induced apoptosis in human malignant testicular germ cell lines depends on MEK/ERK activation. *Br J Cancer*. 2004 Aug;91(3):589.

68. Liu B, Wu SD, Shen LJ, Zhao TX, Wei Y, Tang XL et al. Spermatogenesis dysfunction induced by PM2. 5 from automobile exhaust via the ROS-mediated MAPK signaling pathway. *Ecotoxicol Environ Saf*. 2019 Jan 15;167:161–8.

69. Silva JV, Freitas MJ, Correia BR, Korrodi-Gregório L, Patrício A, Pelech S, Fardilha M. Profiling signaling proteins in human spermatozoa: Biomarker identification for sperm quality evaluation. *Fertil Steril*. 2015 Oct;104(4):845–856.

70. Almog T, Lazar S, Reiss N, Etkovitz N, Milch E, Rahamim N et al. Identification of extracellular signal-regulated kinase 1/2 and p38 MAPK as regulators of human sperm motility and acrosome reaction and as predictors of poor spermatozoan quality. *J Biol Chem*. 2008 May 23;283(21):14479–89.

TGF-β signaling in testicular development, spermatogenesis, and infertility

POONAM MEHTA, MEGHALI JOSHI, AND RAJENDER SINGH

HIGHLIGHTS

- The TGF-β superfamily consists of a group of more than 40 ligands, which majorly includes activins, bone morphogenetic proteins (BMPs), Müllerian inhibiting substance (MIS), growth differentiation factors (GDFs) and glial cell–derived neurotrophic factors (GDNFs).
- These ligands in total regulate various developmental and testicular processes.
- Activin and inhibin signaling regulate gonadal development.
- GDNF signaling is required for the maintenance of spermatogonial stem cells (SSCs) pool.
- MIS signaling is required for Müllerian duct regression, an essential process in male sex differentiation.
- BMP signaling is required for primordial germ cell (PGC) specification, cell proliferation and differentiation.
- Abrogation of TGF-β signaling events is associated with testicular diseases, leading to male infertility.

11.1 INTRODUCTION

The transforming growth factor beta (TGF-β) field began in 1978 when De Larco and Todaro described the purification of sarcoma growth factor from fibroblasts transformed by Moloney sarcoma virus, an RNA virus (1). The identified growth factor has the ability to transform normal fibroblasts in soft agar colony-forming assay in *in vitro* conditions. Later, it became apparent that the growth of normal cells was largely controlled by several polypeptides, hormones and hormone-like growth factors that were secretions of the surrounding cells and acted in an autocrine or paracrine fashion. At present, TGF-β is a large family of secreted and functionally diverse growth factors and cytokines (2).

The TGF superfamily—a family of secreted differentiation factors—comprises a group of more than 40 ligands, which on receptor binding are capable of initiating a signaling cascade and regulating various developmental processes, such as gastrulation, axis patterning, lineage determination, specification and cellular processes including cell

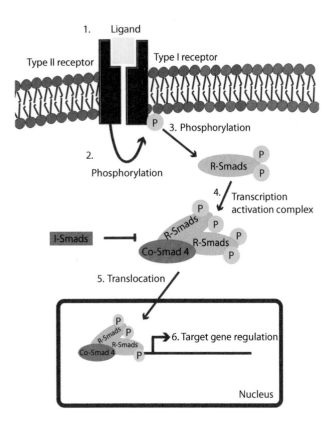

Figure 11.1 The TGF-β signaling. (1) Ligand-receptor interaction on the target cell. (2) Receptor dimerization and phosphorylation of type I subunit by type II receptor. (3) Phosphorylation of R-SMADs. (4) Formation of transcription activation complex. (5) Activated complex translocates to nucleus. (6) Target gene regulation.

proliferation, differentiation, adhesion and apoptosis from flies to humans (3–5). A TGF-β ligand initiates signaling by binding and bringing together two subunits of heteromeric complex of Ser/Thr Kinase receptor type I and type II, this receptor complex phosphorylates and activates another transcription regulator complex that consists of R-SMAD and Co-SMAD protein, which on translocation to the nucleus regulates transcription of the target genes (6). The general outline of the pathway is presented in Figure 11.1.

11.2 COMPONENTS OF TGF-β SIGNALING CASCADE

11.2.1 Ligands

Growth factors and other member proteins showing at least 25% homology to TGF-β were included in the TGF-β family. This family includes approximately 40 members, which share similar features, i.e., conserved cysteine residues (such as TGF-β 1–3 and inhibin β polypeptides that have nine characteristic cysteines, bone morphogenetic protein [BMPs] and growth differentiation factors [GDFs] that have seven and remaining BMP15A, GDF3, GDF9 that have six cysteines), which helps in intermolecular interaction for ligand dimerization and structural integrity. Ligands exist both as

homo- and heterodimers. The members of this superfamily include transforming growth factor β 1–3 (TGF-βs), inhibins and activins, BMPs, Müllerian inhibiting substance (MIS), also called anti-Müllerian hormone (AMH), GDFs and glial cell line-derived neurotrophic factor (GDNF) (7). These subfamilies have more members (Table 11.1), which have different cell functions depending upon their type, concentration, target tissue and developmental stage (8).

11.2.2 Receptors

All TGF-β ligands, on their binding to the receptor complex, transmit biological information to the cell. The receptor complex is heterotetrameric, consisting of two subunits of each receptor, i.e., type I and type II receptors. These receptors were classified on the basis of structural and functional properties—type I receptor shows higher sequence similarity in the kinase domain as compared to the type II receptor (8). These receptor molecules are characterized by their serine/threonine kinase activity and weaker tyrosine kinase activity (8). In mammals, there are seven type I receptors and five type II receptors. There is another receptor class called a type III receptor in mammals, which is known to regulate TGF-β signaling (8).

On ligand binding, the receptor subunits come together and type II phosphorylate the cytoplasmic domain of type I receptor, which further phosphorylates the downstream effector molecules, i.e., SMADs (9). Different ligands bind different receptor complexes, which are listed in Table 11.2.

11.2.3 SMAD proteins

For transmission of a signal from the cell surface to the intracellular compartments, transcription factors, i.e., SMADs, play important roles. Ligand receptor–mediated phosphorylation of SMAD proteins present in the cytosol translocate them to the nucleus for regulating target gene transcription (8,10). The term *SMAD* was coined after identification of human SMAD1, which shared sequence similarity with Sma and Mad proteins (11). There are eight SMAD proteins

Table 11.1 List of TGF-β superfamily ligands and their subtypes

Ligand	Subtypes
TGF-β	TGF-β1, TGF-β2, TGF-β3
BMP	BMP2, BMP4, BMP5, BMP6, BMP7, BMP8A, BMP8B, BMP9, BMP10
GDF	GDF1, GDF3, GDF5, GDF6, GDF8 (Myostatin), GDF7, GDF9, GDF9B, GDF10, GDF11, GDF15 (Macrophage inhibiting cytokine 1)
Activin and inhibin	Inhibin βA, Inhibin βB, Nodal
AMH	AMH (MIS)
GDNFs	—

Table 11.2 List of different types of receptors for various ligands

Ligands	Type I receptor	Type II receptor	Type III receptor (co-receptors)
TGF-βs	TβRI (ALK5), ALK1, ALK2, ALK3 (BMPRIA)	TβRII	TβRIII, Endoglin, Cripto3 (negative effect)
BMPs	BMPRIA (ALK3), BMPRIB (ALK6), ALK1, ALK2	BMPRII, ActRIIA, ActRIIB	RGMa, RGMb, RGMc
GDFs	BMPRIA (ALK3), BMPRIB (ALK6), ALK2, ActRIB (ALK4), ALK7, ALK5	BMPRII, ActRIIA, ActRIIB	Cripto 3
Activin and inhibin	ActRIB (ALK4), ALK7	ActRIIA, ActRIIB	Cripto 1, Cripto 3 (negative effect)
AMH	BMPRIA (ALK3), ALK2	AMHRII	Not known
GDNFs	GFRα 1–4		

encoded by the human genome, which are further classified into three classes, based on their function (8,10):

- *R-SMADs* (receptor-activated SMADs): Act as substrates for TGF-β receptors and include SMAD1, SMAD2, SMAD3, SMAD5, SMAD8. BMP ligands via its receptors activate SMADs 1, 5, 8, and activins, nodal and TGF-βs activate SMAD2 and SMAD3.
- *Co-SMADs* (common mediator SMADs): Partners for R-SMADs and make transcriptionally active complex. SMAD4 is the only Co-SMAD known.
- *I-SMADs* (inhibitory SMADs): Negative regulation of signaling and includes SMAD6 and SMAD7.

The structure of SMADs includes three domains: (a) an N-terminal Mad homology 1 domain that carries a nuclear localization signal and a DNA binding domain, (b) a linker domain-carries phosphorylatable serine and threonine and (c) a C-terminal Mad homology domain 2 for oligomerization of SMAD proteins (8).

11.3 KNOCKOUT MOUSE STUDIES

Mouse null for ligands, receptors and signaling proteins presented genetic evidence that these regulate multiple body functions from embryonic and extraembryonic development to defined body systems such as skeletal, renal, cardiac and reproductive (12). We filtered the knockout (KO) studies and present only those that are related to embryonic development and male infertility (Table 11.3). We also neglected those that were embryonically lethal and impaired other body functions. The KO studies have presented evidence for the involvement of BMP ligands in gonadal development, particularly primordial germ cell (PGC) number and

Table 11.3 Mouse knockout studies on TGF-β ligands, receptors and SMAD proteins

Knockout mouse model	Phenotype	References
TGF-β superfamily ligands		
Activin/inhibin βA	Lower Sertoli cell number; double the number of gonocytes	(13)
BMP-2	Embryonic lethal; reduced PGCs number, abnormal development of hindgut and allantois	(14,15)
BMP-4	Embryonic lethal; no mesoderm differentiation; lack an allantois; no PGCs	(16,17)
BMP-8A	Viable; epididymal integrity impaired; germ cell degeneration	(18)
BMP-8B	Male infertility because of germ cell depletion; defects in PGCs and allantois development	(19,20)
GDF-7	Male infertility because of abnormal seminal vesicle development	(21)
MIS	Male infertility; Leydig cell hyperplasia	(22)
GDNF+/−	Disrupted spermatogenesis; reduced SSCs population	(23)
TGF-β Receptors		
Activin receptor type IIA (ACVR2)	Delayed fertility in males	(24)
MIS type II receptor	Male infertility; Leydig cell hyperplasia	(25)
SMAD Proteins		
SMAD1	Defects in allantois development; dramatically reduced or absent PGCs	(26,27)
SMAD5	Extraembryonic defects; defective PGCs development	(28,29)
SMAD3	Delayed Sertoli cell maturation in testis	(30)

allantois development, activin ligands in regulating the proliferation of somatic and germ cell pool during development and GDNF in the maintenance of spermatogenesis.

From the above-mentioned KO studies, it is clear that TGF-β signaling plays an important role in regulating sexual differentiation, PGC development and specification, gonadal development and gastrulation (12).

11.4 TGF-β SUPERFAMILY ACTION IN TESTIS

TGF-β ligands play various roles in testicular development by influencing the proliferation, development and maturation from PGCs to spermatocytes and surrounding somatic cells (31). Various ligands come into play at different testicular developmental stages; for example, BMP signaling for PGCs specification (17,33), activin signaling for Sertoli cell proliferation and to expand testicular cords (13,34), TGF-β and activin signaling for negative regulation of gonocyte number and quiescence (13,35), GDNF signaling for SSC maintenance (23) and MIS-induced signaling for Müllerian

duct regression (36,37) (Figure 11.2 and Table 11.4). These signaling pathways are discussed in the following sections.

11.4.1 TGF-β signaling

The three isoforms of TGF-β, such as TGF-β1, TGF-β2 and TGFβ3, are expressed in mammalian testis (42) with their localization in different cellular pools, such as Leydig cells, Sertoli cells, germ cells and peritubular myoid cells (43). In Leydig cells, TGF-β1 along with its receptors ALK1, ALK5 and coreceptor endoglein have a role in Leydig cell proliferation (44).

In mammalian testis, the blood-testis barrier (BTB) segregates the seminiferous epithelium into basal and apical compartments (39), which undergo cyclic restructuring to allow the transition of preleptotene spermatocytes from basal to the apical compartment during the course of meiosis (39,45,49). The involvement of cytokines such as TGF-βs and testosterone facilitates the transit of spermatocytes across the BTB (46), and Cdc42 is the downstream effector of TGF-β3-induced BTB restructuring (47).

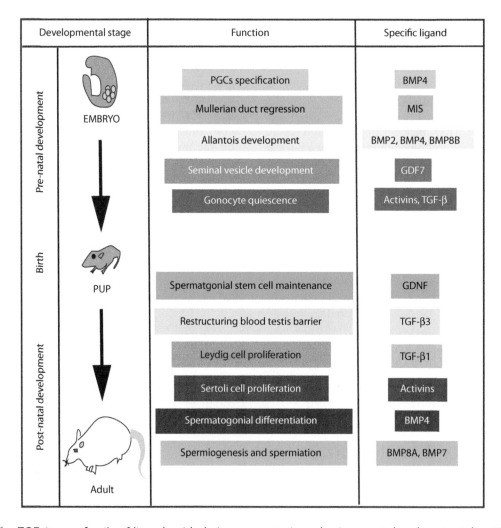

Figure 11.2 The TGF-β superfamily of ligands with their representative roles in prenatal and postnatal testicular development in the mouse.

Table 11.4 TGF-β superfamily with their representative functions in testis

TGF-β Superfamily	Function	References
TGF-β	Apoptosis and negative regulation of proliferation, blood testis barrier restructuring	(35,38,39)
BMP	Germline specification Spermatogonial differentiation	(17,33,40)
Activins and inhibins	Proliferation and apoptosis	(13,35)
GDFs	Seminal vesicle development	(21)
MIS	Regression of Müllerian duct	(36,37)
GDNFs	Spermatogonial stem cells maintenance	(23,41)

Beyond the testis, TGF-β1, TGF-β2 and TGF-β3 are also abundant in the seminal plasma, indicating their role in sperm fertility by direct or indirect mechanisms. The levels of these cytokines vary over time, though the exact causes and effects of this remain unknown (48). It has been suggested that the presence of these cytokines in seminal plasma helps in better receptivity and immune modulation in females to facilitate pregnancy (49).

11.4.2 Activin signaling

Activin, a TGF superfamily ligand, is known to regulate a plethora of developmental and reproductive functions in both males and females. Activins were initially identified and isolated for their capacity to induce FSH release (50,51). These are disulfide-linked dimers of inhibin β subunits (β_A, β_B, β_C), such as $\beta_A\beta_A$ (activin A) and $\beta_B\beta_B$ (activin B). Other activin units are also reported including activin C, activin D and activin E. Along with follicle-stimulating hormone (FSH) regulation, it has many other roles to play. Localization studies have identified the testis as the major site for activin production and activin action. In the murine testis, fetal Leydig cells are the source of activin A (34) and activin receptors ACVR2A and ACVR2B localized mainly in gonocytes, interstitial cells and Sertoli cells (13). KO studies have helped in understanding their specific functions, such as inhibin β A (Inhba$^{-/-}$) mice have lower Sertoli cell number and double the number of gonocytes, inhibin β B (Inhbb$^{-/-}$) or activin B deficient mice remain fertile (52) and abrogation of activin signaling results in testicular dysgenesis with reduced Sertoli cell number (34). These studies suggest activin A to be a regulator of Sertoli cell proliferation and differentiation, which decides testicular size and sperm production capacity.

The mechanism of action of activin involves its binding to one of the type II activin receptors (ACVR2A or ACVR2B) present on the target cell, ligand-receptor interaction, receptor dimerization which brings the type I receptor closer to the type II receptor. Binding of type I receptor to type II induces phosphorylation of the type I receptor, which in turn induces phosphorylation of intracellular and cytosolic proteins SMAD2 and SMAD3. These proteins along with Co-SMAD4 form a transcription activation complex, which on translocation to the nucleus regulates proliferation, differentiation and apoptotic genes (53).

11.4.3 Glial cell–derived neurotrophic factor signaling

GDNF, as the name suggests, was originally derived from glioma cell line cultures and is known for promoting survival and differentiation of dopaminergic neurons in mid brain (54). GDNF is a distant member of the TGF-β superfamily. It shares seven conserved cysteine residues with other members (53), but its signaling cascade is different from other ligands. It signals through a receptor complex composed of Gfrα1 (Gdnf family receptor alpha-1) and Ret (rearranged during transfection) tyrosine kinase transmembrane protein (55,56). GDNF is secreted by the Sertoli cells under the influence of FSH (57). Gdnf$^{-/-}$ mice died on the first day of birth due to renal and neuronal abnormalities (58), while Gdnf$^{+/-}$ mice survived to adulthood but with disturbed spermatogenesis evident through histological sections of the testis (23). In the case of Gdnf$^{+/-}$ 5-week-old mice, tubules lacked spermatogonia and by the eighth week, the SSC population was completely exhausted. Conversely, overexpression of GDNF in testis resulted in an overpopulation of undifferentiated spermatogonia. These studies suggest that GDNF is an essential factor for the maintenance of SSCs. Further, overexpression of GDNF in Sertoli cells via in vivo transfection using electroporation confirmed the proliferation increase and differentiation block in SSCs. Differentiation can be retrieved on their removal from the hyperstimulated environment. Thus, the level of GDNF secreted by Sertoli cells has an important role in regulating SSC proliferation and differentiation via the GDNF pathway (41).

Further exploration of the molecular mechanism of self-renewal revealed the involvement of other signaling pathways that are driven by GDNF. For example, Src family kinases, which activate P13 K/Akt signaling and ultimately N-myc expression, promote SSC proliferation. GDNF also activates Ras signaling, which further upregulates the transcription of cyclin A and cdk2, which are predominantly expressed during spermatogenesis. Thus, they are crucial for G1/S transition of Gfrα-1 positive spermatogonia (59). Microarray analysis of SSCs under the influence of GDNF helped in the identification of other target molecules such as Fgf2 (fibroblast growth factor receptor 2) and Bcl6b (B cell CLL/lymphoma 6, member B), which amplify the effect of GDNF and play roles in the maintenance of SSCs (60).

11.4.4 Müllerian inhibiting substance signaling

Sex determination is a complex process that involves multiple precisely regulated events. Before sexual determination, both Wolffian and Müllerian ducts are present. As the sexual differentiation proceeds, the Wolffian duct regresses in females and the Müllerian duct regresses in males (61). The Müllerian duct differentiates to form the uterus, the fallopian tubes, the uterine cervix and the superior portions of the vagina in females (61). MIS is a TGF-β family ligand secreted by the Sertoli cells of the fetal and adult testes. As the name suggests, MIS leads to the regression of the Müllerian duct in males (22). MIS KO male mice develop as pseudohermaphrodites with a complete male reproductive tract and retention of female ducts such as oviduct and uterus. This superimposed female tract due to the retention causes blockage of sperm transit, contributing to infertility (22,62).

The MIS ligand exerts its effect through receptor complexes I and II. The MIS type II receptor (AMHRII) is specific for the MIS ligand as the genetic analysis using KO studies produced a phenotype similar to the MIS KO (25,64). For type I receptor ALK2 and ALK3, ALK2 KO mice die at the gastrula stage (65,66), and tissue-specific ablation studies of ALK3 have shown the retention of oviduct and uteri (67). Further signals were carried from cytoplasm to nucleus via SMAD protein complexes such as SMAD5 and SMAD1 (68). The regulatory region upstream of the transcription start site has a binding site for SOX9 and SF-1. Further homozygous mutations in SOX9 and SF-9 binding site have shown blocked MIS transcription and pseudohermaphroditism only in case of SOX9 binding site mutation (69). Thus, SOX 9 and SF-1 are required for MIS transcription.

11.4.5 Bone morphogenetic protein signaling

Bone morphogenetic proteins were first identified in the mid-1960s as ectopic bone formation–inducing proteins (70). Since then, many studies have reported the ability of BMPs to induce mesenchymal stem cell differentiation into bone, suggesting their role in cartilage and bone formation. BMP signaling is involved in many processes, such as cell growth, apoptosis and differentiation (71–73). The role of BMP signaling in the development of male accessory sex organs was reported (21). In a study, the deletion of GDF7, a member of the BMP family, resulted in abnormal growth, branching and differentiation of seminal vesicle epithelium. It has been reported that ablation of BMP ligands, such as BMP4 (74) and their receptors, such as BMPR1A (75), leads to the lack of formation of PGCs, confirming their role in gonadal development. In testes, BMP4 signaling is involved in spermatogonial differentiation (40). Dorsomorphin (an inhibitor of BMP type I receptors) treatment to the spermatogonial culture system resulted in the inhibition of spermatogonial differentiation and promotion of proliferation (76). In another study, a mutation in the Zebrafish BMP

type I receptor resulted in impairment of spermatogonial differentiation *in vivo* (77), while the addition of BMP4 to mouse SSCs promoted differentiation and production of spermatids (40,78). It has been reported that BMP4 signaling along with retinoic acid signaling promote spermatogonial differentiation, suggesting a coordinated role of both of these pathways in spermatogonial differentiation (79). Similarly, other BMP ligands, BMP7 and BMP8a/b, are known to play important roles in male germ cell development (80,81). Their transcripts have been found in different stages of differentiation in male germ cells. Mutations in BMP8b in adult mice resulted in progressive germ cell apoptosis and degeneration, leading to small testes size (81). Mouse lacking BMP8a along with mutation in a single allele of BMP7 resulted in a similar phenotype as generated by BMP8b KO (80). BMP2 and BMP7 have been reported to be important for the proliferation of Sertoli and germ cells during early postnatal development in mice (82). In addition to BMP4, BMP7, BMP8a/b, growth-differentiation factor 9 (GDF9) expressed strongly in testes, specifically in the pachytene spermatocytes and early round spermatids (83). However, GDF9-deficient male mice were fertile (84), suggesting that the testicular GDF9 is not essential for normal spermatogenesis. Another member of the BMP family, GDF7, was seen in the seminal vesicle, and it was found that it is important for the development of seminal vesicle (21). Male mice deficient in GDF7 were found to be sterile and displayed defects in seminal vesicle development.

11.5 REPRODUCTIVE DISORDERS ASSOCIATED WITH ABERRANT TGF-β SIGNALING

The most well-studied members of TGF-β family in the male reproductive system are BMPs (BMP2, BMP4, BMP8), activins, MIS and GDNFs. The TGF-β superfamily exerts critical functions in the male reproductive tract by regulating development in prenatal to postnatal testicular events, like early postimplantation mouse embryonic and extraembryonic development (16,65,85,86,87), sexual differentiation (22,62), PGCs development (17,33), gonadal development (88) and maintenance of SSCs (23,41). Alterations in TGF-β signaling are also associated with various reproductive diseases, which increase the burden of male infertility. The associated reproductive diseases are discussed in the following sections.

11.5.1 Testicular cancer

Inhibin-α deficiency is associated with testicular tumors, because inhibin and FSH levels are inversely related and FSH regulates the gonadal cell proliferation (89). Recently, transcriptome analysis studies in seminomas and of TCam-2 seminoma model cell line revealed the potentially active pathways. Combined datasets from Affymetrix microarrays and RNAseq analysis revealed the presence of transcript levels of TGF-β signaling. GDF3, GDF11 and BMP7 transcripts were consistently detected in seminomas and TCam-2. Transcripts encoding receptor proteins such as ACVR1A and ACVR1B, ACVR2A and ACVR2B were also detected at high levels (90).

11.5.2 Disrupted spermatogenesis

Chronic activin signaling is associated with hypo-spermatogenesis with reduced testicular mass (91). In BMP signaling, BMP4 promotes SSC differentiation and production of spermatids, and its disruption results in impaired spermatogenesis (40,78).

11.5.3 Leydig cell hyperplasia

Leydig cell hyperplasia (LCH) is a benign condition, characterized by the presence of small, bilateral testicular nodules (92). Androgens are already known to stimulate the proliferation of Leydig cells (93–95). The involvement of TGF-β signaling components in Leydig cell hyperplasia is seen in various studies, such as with transgenic mice overexpressing hCG, and LCH showing increased levels of TGF-β1, ALK1 and co-receptor endoglein (96); increased levels of Smad 4 (97); increased levels of Smad 2/3 (98) and the fact that intratesticular injection of TGF-β1 plus progesterone increases Leydig cell volume (99).

11.5.4 Sertoli cell-only syndrome (germ cell aplasia)

Sertoli cell-only syndrome (SCOS), characterized by non-obstructive azoospermia, is a significant cause of male infertility. The involvement of activin signaling in SCOS is observed by Sun et al., where they have seen the increased levels of Smad 2 in testicular biopsies of SCOS patients (100).

11.5.5 Persistent Müllerian duct syndrome

MIS regresses the Müllerian duct in males. In the absence of MIS, the Müllerian duct will develop into a fallopian tube, uterus or superior portions of the vagina (101). Persistent Müllerian duct syndrome (PMDS) is associated with the levels of circulating MIS before puberty. In total, there are 38 mutations known to date, mostly missense, which are associated with PMDS. As described in Section 11.4.4, there is a specific type II receptor for the MIS ligand; accordingly, in PMDS patients with normal levels of MIS, mutations in its specific receptor AMHRII have been found. Still, there are PMDS patients who do not carry any ligand or receptor mutations, and the etiology remains unknown (102,103).

11.6 TGF-β CROSS TALK WITH OTHER PATHWAYS

In the complex molecular milieu, the TGF-β pathway engages in cross talk with other signaling pathways that are important for testicular development and spermatogenesis. SMAD proteins interlink the TGF-β pathway with other signaling pathways, including Wnt signaling (104), Hedgehog signaling (63) and Hippo signaling (32). Niche maintenance of SSCs is influenced by a number of signaling pathways discussed in this book. Identification of the whole network of extrinsic and intrinsic factors essential for SSCs would help in SSC proliferation in laboratory conditions and the scaling up of SSCs for clinical applications.

11.7 CONCLUSION AND FUTURE DIRECTIONS

The TGF-β field began in 1978 when De Larco and Todaro described the purification of sarcoma growth factor from fibroblasts transformed by Moloney sarcoma virus, an RNA virus. At present, TGF-β is a large family of secreted and functionally diverse growth factors and cytokines, which includes activins, BMPs, MIS, GDFs and GDNFs. A TGF-β ligand initiates signaling by binding and bringing together two subunits of a heteromeric complex of Ser/Thr Kinase receptor type I and type II; this receptor complex phosphorylates and activates another transcription regulator complex that consists of R-SMAD and Co-SMAD protein, which on translocation to the nucleus regulates the transcription of its target genes. The TGF-β family includes approximately 40 members, which share similar features, i.e., conserved cysteine residues. For transmission of a signal from the cell surface to the intracellular compartments, transcription factors, i.e., SMADs, play important roles.

In the testes, TGF-β ligands play various roles in testicular development by influencing the proliferation, development and maturation from PGCs to spermatocytes and surrounding somatic cells. It has been reported that the ablation of BMP ligands, such as BMP4 and their receptors, such as BMPR1A, leads to the lack of formation of PGCs, confirming their role in gonadal development. In the testes, BMP4 signaling is involved in spermatogonial differentiation, and BMP2 and BMP7 signaling is required for Sertoli cell proliferation. A number of disorders of the reproductive system, such as testicular cancer, hypospermatogenesis and Leydig cell hyperplasia are caused by aberrant TGF-β signaling. Investigations on the cross-linking of TGF-β signaling with other signaling pathways and the identification of new members of this family remain interesting subjects for further research.

ACKNOWLEDGMENTS

The authors would like to thank the University Grants Commission for fellowship, the Council of Scientific and Industrial Research (CSIR) for financial support and CSIR-CDRI for providing institutional support.

REFERENCES

1. De Larco JE, Todaro GJ. Growth factors from murine sarcoma virus-transformed cells. *Proc Natl Acad Sci USA*. 1978 Aug;75(8):4001.

2. Moses HL, Roberts AB, Derynck R. The discovery and early days of TGF-β: A historical perspective. *Cold Spring Harbor Perspect Biol*. 2016 Jul 1;8(7):a021865.

3. Massagué J. TGF-β signal transduction. *Annu Rev Biochem*. 1998;67:753–91.

4. Itman C, Mendis S, Barakat B, Loveland KL. All in the family: TGF-β family action in testis development. *Reproduction*. 2006 Aug 1;132(2):233–46.

5. Derynck R, Miyazono K (Eds). *The TGF-β Family*. Cold Spring Harbor, NY: CSHL Press; 2008.

6. Hata A, Chen YG. TGF-β signalling from receptors to Smads. *Cold Spring Harbor Perspect Biol*. 2016 Sep 1;8(9):a022061.

7. Sun PD, Davies DR. The cystine-knot growth-factor superfamily. *Annu Rev Biophys Biomol Struct*. 1995 Jun;24(1):269–92.

8. Moustakas A, Heldin CH. The regulation of TGFβ signal transduction. *Development*. 2009 Nov 15;136(22):3699–714.

9. Wrana JL, Ozdamar B, Le Roy C, Benchabane H. Signalling receptors of the TGF-β family. *Cold Spring Harbor Monogr Ser*. 2008;50:151.

10. Massagué J, Seoane J, Wotton D. Smad transcription factors. *Genes Dev*. 2005 Dec 1;19(23):2783–810.

11. Liu F, Hata A, Baker JC, Doody J, Cárcamo J, Harland RM, Massagué J. A human Mad protein acting as a BMP-regulated transcriptional activator. *Nature*. 1996 Jun;381(6583):620.

12. Chang H, Brown CW, Matzuk MM. Genetic analysis of the mammalian transforming growth factor-β superfamily. *Endocr Rev*. 2002 Dec 1;23(6):787–823.

13. Mendis SH, Meachem SJ, Sarraj MA, Loveland KL. Activin A balances Sertoli and germ cell proliferation in the fetal mouse testis. *Biol Reprod*. 2011 Feb 1;84(2):379–91.

14. Zhang H, Bradley A. Mice deficient for BMP2 are nonviable and have defects in amnion/chorion and cardiac development. *Development*. 1996 Oct 1;122(10):2977–86.

15. Ying Y, Zhao GQ. Cooperation of endoderm-derived BMP2 and extraembryonic ectoderm-derived BMP4 in primordial germ cell generation in the mouse. *Dev Biol*. 2001 Apr 15;232(2):484–92.

16. Winnier G, Blessing M, Labosky PA, Hogan BL. Bone morphogenetic protein-4 is required for mesoderm formation and patterning in the mouse. *Genes Dev*. 1995 Sep 1;9(17):2105–16.

17. Lawson KA, Dunn NR, Roelen BA, Zeinstra LM, Davis AM, Wright CV, Korving JP, Hogan BL. Bmp4 is required for the generation of primordial germ cells in the mouse embryo. *Genes Dev*. 1999 Feb 15;13(4):424–36.

18. Zhao GQ, Liaw L, Hogan BL. Bone morphogenetic protein 8A plays a role in the maintenance of spermatogenesis and the integrity of the epididymis. *Development*. 1998 Mar 15;125(6):1103–12.

19. Zhao GQ, Deng K, Labosky PA, Liaw L, Hogan BL. The gene encoding bone morphogenetic protein 8B is required for the initiation and maintenance of spermatogenesis in the mouse. *Genes Dev*. 1996 Jul 1;10(13):1657–69.

20. Ying Y, Liu XM, Marble A, Lawson KA, Zhao GQ. Requirement of Bmp8b for the generation of primordial germ cells in the mouse. *Mol Endocrinol*. 2000 Jul 1;14(7):1053–63.

21. Settle S, Marker P, Gurley K, Sinha A, Thacker A, Wang Y, Higgins K, Cunha G, Kingsley DM. The BMP family member Gdf7 is required for seminal vesicle growth, branching morphogenesis, and cytodifferentiation. *Dev Biol*. 2001 Jun 1;234(1):138–50.

22. Behringer RR, Finegold MJ, Cate RL. Müllerian-inhibiting substance function during mammalian sexual development. *Cell*. 1994 Nov 4;79(3):415–25.

23. Meng X, Lindahl M, Hyvönen ME, Parvinen M, de Rooij DG, Hess MW et al. Regulation of cell fate decision of undifferentiated spermatogonia by GDNF. *Science*. 2000 Feb 25;287(5457):1489–93.

24. Matzuk MM, Kumar TR, Bradley A. Different phenotypes for mice deficient in either activins or activin receptor type II. *Nature*. 1995 Mar;374(6520):356.

25. Mishina Y, Rey R, Finegold MJ, Matzuk MM, Josso N, Cate RL, Behringer RR. Genetic analysis of the Müllerian-inhibiting substance signal transduction pathway in mammalian sexual differentiation. *Genes Dev*. 1996 Oct 15;10(20):2577–87.

26. Lechleider RJ, Ryan JL, Garrett L, Deng CX, Wynshaw-Boris A, Roberts AB. Targeted mutagenesis of Smad1 reveals an essential role in chorioallantoic fusion. *Dev Biol*. 2001 Dec 1;240(1):157–67.

27. Tremblay KD, Dunn NR, Robertson EJ. Mouse embryos lacking Smad1 signals display defects in extra-embryonic tissues and germ cell formation. *Development*. 2001 Sep 15;128(18):3609–21.

28. Chang H, Huylebroeck D, Verschueren K, Guo Q, Matzuk MM, Zwijsen A. Smad5 knockout mice die at mid-gestation due to multiple embryonic and extraembryonic defects. *Development*. 1999 Apr 15;126(8):1631–42.

29. Chang H, Matzuk MM. Smad5 is required for mouse primordial germ cell development. *Mech Dev*. 2001 Jun 1;104(1–2):61–7.

30. Itman C, Wong C, Hunyadi B, Ernst M, Jans DA, Loveland KL. Smad3 dosage determines androgen responsiveness and sets the pace of postnatal testis development. *Endocrinology*. 2011 Mar 8;152(5):2076–89.

31. Loveland KL, Hime G. TGFβ superfamily members in spermatogenesis: Setting the stage for fertility in mouse and *Drosophila*. *Cell Tissue Res*. 2005 Oct 1;322(1):141–6.

32. Fujii M, Toyoda T, Nakanishi H, Yatabe Y, Sato A, Matsudaira Y et al. TGF-β synergizes with defects

in the Hippo pathway to stimulate human malignant mesothelioma growth. *J Exp Med.* 2012 Mar 12;209(3):479–94.

33. de Sousa Lopes SM, Roelen BA, Monteiro RM, Emmens R, Lin HY, Li E, Lawson KA, Mummery CL. BMP signalling mediated by ALK2 in the visceral endoderm is necessary for the generation of primordial germ cells in the mouse embryo. *Genes Dev.* 2004 Aug 1;18(15):1838–49.

34. Archambeault DR, Yao HH. Activin A, a product of fetal Leydig cells, is a unique paracrine regulator of Sertoli cell proliferation and fetal testis cord expansion. *Proc Natl Acad Sci USA.* 2010 Jun 8;107(23):10526–31.

35. Richards AJ, Enders GC, Resnick JL. Activin and TGFβ limit murine primordial germ cell proliferation. *Dev Biol.* 1999 Mar 15;207(2):470–5.

36. Donahoe PK, Cate RL, Maclaughlin DT, Epstein J, Fuller AF, Takahashi M, Oughlin JP, Ninfa EG, Taylor LA. Müllerian inhibiting substance: Gene structure and mechanism of action of a fetal regressor. In *Proceedings of the 1986 Laurentian Hormone Conference*, January 1. New York, NY: Academic Press; 1987:431–67.

37. Ross AJ, Tilman C, Yao H, MacLaughlin D, Capel B. AMH induces mesonephric cell migration in XX gonads. *Mol Cell Endocrinol.* 2003 Dec 15;211(1–2):1–7.

38. Olaso R, Pairault C, Boulogne B, Durand P, Habert R. Transforming growth factor β1 and β2 reduce the number of gonocytes by increasing apoptosis. *Endocrinology.* 1998 Feb 1;139(2):733.

39. Cheng CY, Mruk DD. An intracellular trafficking pathway in the seminiferous epithelium regulating spermatogenesis: A biochemical and molecular perspective. *Crit Rev Biochem Mol Biol.* 2009 Oct 1;44(5):245–63.

40. Pellegrini M, Grimaldi P, Rossi P, Geremia R, Dolci S. Developmental expression of BMP4/ALK3/SMAD5 signalling pathway in the mouse testis: A potential role of BMP4 in spermatogonia differentiation. *J Cell Sci.* 2003 Aug 15;116(16):3363–72.

41. Yomogida K, Yagura Y, Tadokoro Y, Nishimune Y. Dramatic expansion of germinal stem cells by ectopically expressed human glial cell line-derived neurotrophic factor in mouse Sertoli cells. *Biol Reprod.* 2003 Oct 1;69(4):1303–7.

42. Ingman WV, Robertson SA. Defining the actions of transforming growth factor beta in reproduction. *BioEssays.* 2002 Oct;24(10):904–14.

43. Zhang YQ, He XZ, Zhang JS, Wang RA, Zhou J, Xu RJ. Stage-specific localization of transforming growth factor β1 and β3 and their receptors during spermatogenesis in men. *Asian J Androl.* 2004 Jun;6(2):105–9.

44. Gonzalez CR, Calandra RS, Gonzalez Calvar SI. Testicular expression of the TGF-B1 system and the control of Leydig cell proliferation. *Adv in Biosci Biotech.* 2013;4(10):1–7.

45. Russell L. Movement of spermatocytes from the basal to the adluminal compartment of the rat testis. *Am J Anat.* 1977 Mar;148(3):313–28.

46. Yan HH, Mruk DD, Lee WM, Cheng CY. Blood-testis barrier dynamics are regulated by testosterone and cytokines via their differential effects on the kinetics of protein endocytosis and recycling in Sertoli cells. *FASEB J.* 2008 Jun;22(6):1945–59.

47. Wong EW, Mruk DD, Lee WM, Cheng CY. Regulation of blood–testis barrier dynamics by TGF-β3 is a Cdc42-dependent protein trafficking event. *Proc Natl Acad Sci USA.* 2010 Jun 22;107(25):11399–404.

48. Sharkey DJ, Tremellen KP, Briggs NE, Dekker GA, Robertson SA. Seminal plasma transforming growth factor-β, activin A and follistatin fluctuate within men over time. *Hum Reprod.* 2016 Sep 17;31(10):2183–91.

49. Robertson SA, Sharkey DJ. Seminal fluid and fertility in women. *Fertil Steril.* 2016 Sep 1;106(3):511–9.

50. Vale W, Rivier J, Vaughan J, McClintock R, Corrigan A, Woo W, Karr D, Spiess J. Purification and characterization of an FSH releasing protein from porcine ovarian follicular fluid. *Nature.* 1986 Jun;321(6072):776.

51. Ling N, Ying SY, Ueno N, Shimasaki S, Esch F, Hotta M, Guillemin R. Pituitary FSH is released by a heterodimer of the β-subunits from the two forms of inhibin. *Nature.* 1986 Jun;321(6072):779.

52. Vassalli A, Matzuk MM, Gardner HA, Lee KF, Jaenisch R. Activin/inhibin β B subunit gene disruption leads to defects in eyelid development and female reproduction. *Genes Dev.* 1994 Feb 15;8(4):414–27.

53. Wijayarathna RD, De Kretser DM. Activins in reproductive biology and beyond. *Hum Reprod Update.* 2016 Apr 1;22(3):342–57.

54. Lin LF, Doherty DH, Lile JD, Bektesh S, Collins F. GDNF: A glial cell line-derived neurotrophic factor for midbrain dopaminergic neurons. *Science.* 1993 May 21;260(5111):1130–2.

55. Treanor JJ, Goodman L, de Sauvage F, Stone DM, Poulsen KT, Beck CD, Gray C, Armanini MP, Pollock RA, Hefti F, Phillips HS. Characterization of a multicomponent receptor for GDNF. *Nature.* 1996 Jul;382(6586):80.

56. Jing S, Wen D, Yu Y, Holst PL, Luo Y, Fang M, Tamir R, Antonio L, Hu Z, Cupples R, Louis JC. GDNF–induced activation of the ret protein tyrosine kinase is mediated by GDNFR-α, a novel receptor for GDNF. *Cell.* 1996 Jun 28;85(7):1113–24.

57. Tadokoro Y, Yomogida K, Ohta H, Tohda A, Nishimune Y. Homeostatic regulation of germinal stem cell proliferation by the GDNF/FSH pathway. *Mech Dev.* 2002 Apr 1;113(1):29–39.

58. Moore MW, Klein RD, Fariñas I, Sauer H, Armanini M, Phillips H, Reichardt LF, Ryan AM, Carver-Moore K, Rosenthal A. Renal and neuronal abnormalities in mice lacking GDNF. *Nature.* 1996 Jul;382(6586):76.

59. Hofmann MC. GDNF signalling pathways within the mammalian spermatogonial stem cell niche. *Mol Cell Endocrinol.* 2008 Jun 25;288(1–2):95–103.

60. Hofmann MC, Braydich-Stolle L, Dym M. Isolation of male germ-line stem cells; influence of GDNF. *Dev Biol.* 2005 Mar 1;279(1):114–24.

61. Nef S, Parada LF. Hormones in male sexual development. *Genes Dev.* 2000 Dec 15;14(24):3075–86.

62. Behringer RR. The Müllerian inhibitor and mammalian sexual development. Philosophical Transactions of the Royal Society of London. *Series B: Biol Sci.* 1995 Nov 29;350(1333):285–9.

63. Dennler S, André J, Alexaki I, Li A, Magnaldo T, Ten Dijke P, Wang XJ, Verrecchia F, Mauviel A. Induction of sonic hedgehog mediators by transforming growth factor-β: Smad3-dependent activation of Gli2 and Gli1 expression *in vitro* and *in vivo*. *Cancer Res.* 2007 Jul 15;67(14):6981–6.

64. Mishina Y, Whitworth DJ, Racine C, Behringer RR. High specificity of Mullerian-inhibiting substance signalling *in vivo*. *Endocrinology.* 1999b May 1;140(5):2084–8.

65. Gu Z, Reynolds EM, Song J, Lei H, Feijen A, Yu L et al. The type I serine/threonine kinase receptor ActRIA (ALK2) is required for gastrulation of the mouse embryo. *Development.* 1999 Jun 1;126(11):2551–61.

66. Mishina Y, Crombie R, Bradley A, Behringer RR. Multiple roles for activin-like kinase-2 signalling during mouse embryogenesis. *Dev Biol.* 1999a Sep 15;213(2):314–26.

67. Jamin SP, Arango NA, Mishina Y, Hanks MC, Behringer RR. Requirement of Bmpr1a for Müllerian duct regression during male sexual development. *Nat Genet.* 2002 Oct 7;32(3):408.

68. Visser JA, Olaso R, Verhoef-Post M, Kramer P, Themmen AP, Ingraham HA. The serine/threonine transmembrane receptor ALK2 mediates Müllerian inhibiting substance signalling. *Mol Endocrinol.* 2001 Jun 1;15(6):936–45.

69. Arango NA, Lovell-Badge R, Behringer RR. Targeted mutagenesis of the endogenous mouse Mis gene promoter: *In vivo* definition of genetic pathways of vertebrate sexual development. *Cell.* 1999 Nov 12;99(4):409–19.

70. Urist MR. Bone: Formation by autoinduction. *Science.* 1965 Nov 12;150(3698):893–9.

71. Zou H, Niswander L. Requirement for BMP signalling in interdigital apoptosis and scale formation. *Science.* 1996 May 3;272(5262):738–41.

72. Kobayashi T, Lyons KM, McMahon AP, Kronenberg HM. BMP signalling stimulates cellular differentiation at multiple steps during cartilage development. *Proc Natl Acad Sci USA.* 2005 Dec 13;102(50):18023–7.

73. Stewart A, Guan H, Yang K. BMP-3 promotes mesenchymal stem cell proliferation through the TGF-β/activin signalling pathway. *J Cell Physiol.* 2010 Jun;223(3):658–66.

74. Wang RN, Green J, Wang Z, Deng Y, Qiao M, Peabody M et al. Bone morphogenetic protein (BMP) signalling in development and human diseases. *Genes Dis.* 2014 Sep 1;1(1):87–105.

75. Dudley B, Palumbo C, Nalepka J, Molyneaux K. BMP signalling controls formation of a primordial germ cell niche within the early genital ridges. *Dev Biol.* 2010 Jul 1;343(1–2):84–93.

76. Wong TT, Collodi P. Dorsomorphin promotes survival and germline competence of zebrafish spermatogonial stem cells in culture. *PLOS ONE.* 2013 Aug 1;8(8):e71332.

77. Neumann JC, Chandler GL, Damoulis VA, Fustino NJ, Lillard K, Looijenga L, Margraf L, Rakheja D, Amatruda JF. Mutation in the type IB bone morphogenetic protein receptor Alk6b impairs germ-cell differentiation and causes germ-cell tumors in zebrafish. *Proc Natl Acad Sci USA.* 2011 Aug 9;108(32):13153–8.

78. Nagano M, Ryu BY, Brinster CJ, Avarbock MR, Brinster RL. Maintenance of mouse male germ line stem cells in vitro. *Biol Reprod.* 2003 Jun 1;68(6):2207–14.

79. Yang Y, Feng Y, Feng X, Liao S, Wang X, Gan H, Wang L, Lin X, Han C. BMP4 cooperates with retinoic acid to induce the expression of differentiation markers in cultured mouse spermatogonia. *Stem Cells Int.* 2016;2016.

80. Zhao GQ, Chen YX, Liu XM, Xu Z, Qi X. Mutation in Bmp7 exacerbates the phenotype of Bmp8a mutants in spermatogenesis and epididymis. *Dev Biol.* 2001 Dec 1;240(1):212–22.

81. Zhao GQ, Hogan BL. Evidence that mouse Bmp8a (Op2) and Bmp8b are duplicated genes that play a role in spermatogenesis and placental development. *Mech Dev.* 1996 Jul 1;57(2):159–68.

82. Puglisi R, Montanari M, Chiarella P, Stefanini M, Boitani C. Regulatory role of BMP2 and BMP7 in spermatogonia and Sertoli cell proliferation in the immature mouse. *Eur J Endocrinol.* 2004 Oct 1;151(4):511–20.

83. Fitzpatrick SL, Sindoni DM, Shughrue PJ, Lane MV, Merchenthaler IJ, Frail DE. Expression of growth differentiation factor-9 messenger ribonucleic acid in ovarian and nonovarian rodent and human tissues. *Endocrinology.* 1998 May 1;139(5):2571–8.

84. Shimasaki S, Moore RK, Otsuka F, Erickson GF. The bone morphogenetic protein system in mammalian reproduction. *Endocr Rev.* 2004 Feb 1;25(1):72–101.

85. Nomura M, Li E. Smad2 role in mesoderm formation, left–right patterning and craniofacial development. *Nature.* 1998 Jun;393(6687):786.

86. Sirard C, De La Pompa JL, Elia A, Itie A, Mirtsos C, Cheung A et al. The tumor suppressor gene Smad4/Dpc4 is required for gastrulation and later for anterior development of the mouse embryo. *Genes Dev.* 1998 Jan 1;12(1):107–19.

87. Meno C, Gritsman K, Ohishi S, Ohfuji Y, Heckscher E, Mochida K et al. Mouse Lefty2 and zebrafish antivin are feedback inhibitors of nodal signalling during vertebrate gastrulation. *Mol Cell.* 1999 Sep 1;4(3):287–98.

88. Kumar TR, Varani S, Wreford NG, Telfer NM, de Kretser DM, Matzuk MM. Male reproductive phenotypes in double mutant mice lacking both FSHβ

and activin receptor IIA. *Endocrinology.* 2001 Aug 1;142(8):3512–8.

89. Matzuk MM, Finegold MJ, Su JG, Hsueh AJ, Bradley A. α-Inhibin is a tumour-suppressor gene with gonadal specificity in mice. *Nature.* 1992 Nov;360(6402):313.

90. Young JC, Wakitani S, Loveland KL. TGF-β superfamily signalling in testis formation and early male germline development. In: *Seminars in Cell and Developmental Biology* (Vol. 45). New York, NY: Academic Press; 2015 Sep 1, pp. 94–103.

91. Nicholls PK, Stanton PG, Chen JL, Olcorn JS, Haverfield JT, Qian H, Walton KL, Gregorevic P, Harrison CA. Activin signalling regulates Sertoli cell differentiation and function. *Endocrinology.* 2012 Dec 1;153(12):6065–77.

92. Carucci LR, Tirkes AT, Pretorius ES, Genega EM, Weinstein SP. Testicular Leydig's cell hyperplasia: MR imaging and sonographic findings. *Am J Roentgenol.* 2003 Feb;180(2):501–3.

93. Clegg ED, Cook JC, Chapin RE, Foster PM, Daston GP. Leydig cell hyperplasia and adenoma formation: Mechanisms and relevance to humans. *Reprod Toxicol.* 1997 Jan 1;11(1):107–21.

94. Ge RS, Hardy MP. Decreased cyclin A2 and increased cyclin G1 levels coincide with loss of proliferative capacity in rat Leydig cells during pubertal development. *Endocrinology.* 1997 Sep 1;138(9):3719–26.

95. Gould ML, Hurst PR, Nicholson HD. The effects of oestrogen receptors α and β on testicular cell number and steroidogenesis in mice. *Reproduction.* 2007 Aug 1;134(2):271–9.

96. Gonzalez CR, Gonzalez B, Rulli SB, Huhtaniemi I, Calandra RS, Gonzalez-Calvar SI. TGF-β1 system in Leydig cells. Part I: Effect of hCG and progesterone. *J Reprod Dev.* 2010b:1004150263.

97. Narula A, Kilen S, Ma E, Kroeger J, Goldberg E, Woodruff TK. Smad4 overexpression causes germ cell ablation and Leydig cell hyperplasia in transgenic mice. *Am J Pathol.* 2002 Nov 1;161(5):1723–34.

98. Gonzalez CR, Matzkin ME, Frungieri MB, Terradas C, Ponzio R, Puigdomenech E, Levalle O, Calandra RS, Gonzalez-Calvar SI. Expression of the TGF-β1 system in human testicular pathologies. *Reprod Biol Endocrinol.* 2010a Dec;8(1):148.

99. Gonzalez CR, Gonzalez B, Rulli SB, dos Santos ML, Costa GM, Franca LR, Calandra RS, Gonzalez-Calvar SI. TGF-β1 system in Leydig cells. Part II: TGF-β1 and progesterone, through Smad1/5, are involved in the hyperplasia/hypertrophy of Leydig cells. *J Reprod Dev.* 2010c:1004200265.

100. Sun T, Xin Z, Jin Z, Wu Y, Gong Y. Effect of TGF-β/Smad signalling on Sertoli cell and possible mechanism related to complete Sertoli cell-only syndrome. *Mol Cell Biochem.* 2008 Dec 1;319(1–2):1–7.

101. Teixeira J, Maheswaran S, Donahoe PK. Mullerian inhibiting substance: An instructive developmental hormone with diagnostic and possible therapeutic applications. *Endocr Rev.* 2001 Oct 1;22(5):657–74.

102. Belville C, Josso N, Picard JY. Persistence of Müllerian derivatives in males. *Am J Med Genet.* 1999 Dec 29;89(4):218–23.

103. Josso N, Belville C, Di Clemente N, Picard JY. AMH and AMH receptor defects in persistent Müllerian duct syndrome. *Hum Reprod Update.* 2005 May 5;11(4):351–6.

104. Charbonney E, Speight P, Masszi A, Nakano H, Kapus A. β-Catenin and Smad3 regulate the activity and stability of myocardin-related transcription factor during epithelial–myofibroblast transition. *Mol Biol Cell.* 2011 Dec 1;22(23):4472–85.

Notch signaling in spermatogenesis and male (in)fertility

MAHITHA SAHADEVAN AND PRADEEP G. KUMAR

HIGHLIGHTS

- Notch signaling is an evolutionarily conserved juxtacrine pathway that regulates stem cell renewal, cell proliferation, differentiation, cell fate determination and cell death.
- It consists of a bipartite protein receptor and a ligand.
- Four Notch receptors (NOTCH 1–4) and five ligands of the Delta-Serrate-Lag (DSL) family—jagged 1 (JAG1), jagged 2 (JAG2), delta-like 1 (DLL1), delta-like 3 (DLL3) and delta-like 4 (DLL4)—have been identified in mammals.
- Notch signaling is involved in spermatogenesis in worms, flies and mammals.

12.1 INTRODUCTION

Interaction between cells and their milieu is essential for retaining healthy cells in an organism. This is carried out with the aid of interconnections between various signaling pathways, through different routes like autocrine, paracrine, juxtracrine and endocrine. Disruption in any of these routes by either intrinsic or extrinsic factors can lead to germline and somatic cancers. Among various signaling pathways, the notch is a highly conserved pathway across species and has a versatile function in regulating cellular events like stem cell renewal, proliferation, differentiation and apoptosis. Recent studies have highlighted the dual function of the notch—as an oncogene as well as a tumor suppressor based on the cellular context and surroundings (1–5).

Spermatogenesis is the process of forming sperm from initially undifferentiated germ cells. Initially, these undifferentiated germ cells undergo a series of mitotic divisions to produce a clone of spermatogonial cells, followed by meiotic division and a final cytodifferentiation process, which results in the transformation of round spermatids into elongated spermatozoa. This entire process is tightly regulated at the cellular and hormonal levels to produce viable sperm for the existence of life in sexually reproducing organisms. The importance of notch in regulating spermatogenesis was reported in *Caenorhabditis elegans*, *Drosophila*, *Xenopus* and mammals (6–12). In *C. elegans*, it plays a critical role in germline stem cell renewal and differentiation. In the case of *Drosophila*, notch signaling plays an important role in deciding the fate of posterior somatic gonadal precursor cells to form hub cells. In mammals, constitutive activation of the notch receptor showed severe effects on the spermatogenic process, the formation of male gonads and accessory ducts (13). Hyperactivation of the notch signaling in both Sertoli and germ cells triggers apoptosis in germ cells, followed by a meiotic arrest. Sterility in male mice was also observed in cases of constitutive activation of the notch receptor (13). All these studies highlight the significance of notch signaling in regulating spermatogenesis across a wide range of organisms.

In this chapter, we focus on the role of notch signaling in regulating spermatogenesis, with special emphasis on *C. elegans*, *Drosophila melanogaster* and *Mus musculus*. This chapter is divided into three sections—the first section deals with the general concepts regarding the structure and function of the notch and the modulation of notch signaling. The second section focuses on how notch signaling regulates spermatogenesis and the cross talk between notch signaling and other pathways. The third section deals with how the dysfunction of notch signaling acts as a leading cause of male infertility. Finally, the future perspectives in this field are discussed.

12.2 NOTCH SIGNALING: GENERAL CONCEPTS

Notch signaling is a highly conserved juxtacrine signaling pathway, which was genetically identified 10 decades ago. This pathway plays a vital role in determining the fate of cells, based on spatiotemporal expression of its ligand and receptor. It regulates various cellular processes, like embryogenesis; maintenance of stem cell population, proliferation and differentiation; cell fate specification (by lateral inhibition/inductive signaling); pattern formation; and apoptosis (9,14–16). At the same time, dysfunction in any gear of this pathway, such as gain/loss of function, leads to various developmental blemishes and adult pathological conditions such as T-cell acute lymphoblastic leukemia, Alagille syndrome, spondylocostal dystoses and multiple sclerosis (2,15,17,18).

Notch signaling has a simple architecture in all metazoans, consisting of a bipartite protein receptor and ligands, without any amplifier molecules over and above like in other pathways, in between the signal transduction to the nucleus. Four notch receptors – NOTCH1, NOTCH2, NOTCH3 and NOTCH4 and five ligands of the DSL family – JAG1, JAG2, DLL1, DLL3 and DDL4 have been reported in mammals, a single notch receptor in *Drosophila* and LIN-12 and GLP-1 in *C. elegans*

(10,19–23). Typically, notch receptors consist of an extracellular domain having 36 epidermal growth factor (EGF)-like repeats, a subset of calcium binding sites within EGF-like repeats, three Notch-Lin12 (LN) repeats and a hydrophobic region, which helps in heterodimerization of the receptor. Simple Modular Architectural Research Tool (SMART) analysis of notch receptors in human is shown in Figure 12.1. Notch protein domain (NOD) and NODP represent a region present in many NOTCH proteins and NOTCH homologs in multiple species. The role of the NOD domain remains to be elucidated. DUF3454 also is a domain of unknown function.

The DSL family of notch ligands consists of an extracellular domain containing a conserved amino acid module at the N-terminus of notch ligands (MNNL domain, contains approximately 100 amino acids at *N*-terminal end). Following the MNNL domains, all DSL ligands contain a DSL (distinct cysteine-rich module) domain, a chain of iterated EGF-like repeats and a transmembrane segment. In addition to this region, serrate and jagged ligands contain a cysteine-rich domain between EGF-like repeats and a transmembrane region, unlike in the delta class of ligands, which lacks the same (9,19,20,22–24).

In the canonical notch pathway, the notch signal is initiated by the interaction of the single-pass transmembrane notch receptor with a notch ligand in the adjacent cell (*trans* activation). Different ligands can activate notch, and based on their combination, their fate differs. Recent studies report that DLL1 and DLL4 notch ligands can bind the same notch receptor, in which binding of the DLL1 ligand promotes myogenesis, whereas DLL4 binding inhibits it (9,22). Intriguingly, when both the receptor and ligand are expressed in the same cell, it results in *cis*-inhibitory action, which limits the activity of notch (25). Ligand binding to the notch receptor triggers a series of proteolytic cleavage called regulated intramembrane proteolysis (RIP), due to the exposure of the S2 site in the heterodimerization domain. This exposure is initiated as a result of mechanical pull generated by subsequent initiation of ligand endocytosis via ligand binding or conformational change in the negative regulatory region (NRR). The exposed S2 site is then cleaved by a-disintegrin- and metalloproteinases (ADAM)-type metalloprotease. Further, the membrane-tethered truncated fragment is sensitive to subsequent cleavage by γ-secretase at the S3 site of the receptor, resulting in the release of the intracellular domain

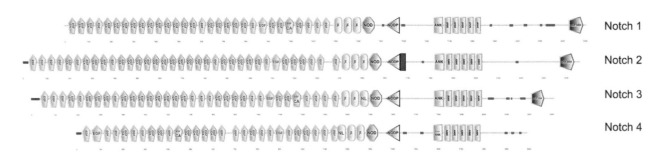

Figure 12.1 Simple Modular Architectural Research Tool (SMART; http://smart.embl-heidelberg.de/) analysis of the four NOTCH variants in human.

of the notch receptor from the membrane into the cytoplasm. The splitting of notch intracellular domain (NICD) from the membrane allows it to translocate to the nucleus and to assemble into a transcriptional activation complex. The main components of this complex include a DNA binding protein named CBF-1, Suppressor of Hairless, Lag-1 proteins family (CSL) (CBF1/RBP-J in mammals), Suppressor of hairless (in *D. melanogaster*), Lag1 (in *C. elegans*), NICD and a coactivator-Mastermind-like/Lag-3 family protein (19,20,26–30). In the transcriptional activation complex, CSL binds the DNA by recognizing the consensus sequence (C/T)GTGGGAA in the proximal promoter region of the notch target genes (31). The best characterized immediate downstream effectors/target genes of notch signaling are the basic hclix loop-helix (bHLH) group of transcriptional repressor—hes family bHLH transcription factor (HES) and HES-related genes, such as hairy/enhancer of split related with YRPW motif (HEY) (27,32–35). Upon activation of notch signaling, there is a competition between co-repressor molecules and NICD in cells to form the NICD-CSL complex,

which flips the cell from a transcriptional repressor stage to a transcriptionally active form by recruiting various coactivators like p300, which connect the general transcriptional machinery to core notch signaling (Figure 12.2). The turnover of notch signaling is highly modulated by several modulator molecules and cross talk between various signaling pathway components. Ligand responsiveness—epsin-dependent endocytosis of ligands and the stability and half-life of NICD—depends mainly on modifications like glycosylation, hydroxylation, ubiquitylation of receptor ectodomain (ECD), phosphorylation, acetylation and deacetylation of NICD (36).

Notch signaling has pleiotropic effects in regulating cellular functions based on the cellular context, microenvironment and activation dosage. Both lateral and inductive signaling of notch were first identified in invertebrates and later successively recognized in self-renewing organs of vertebrates (Figure 12.3). A plethora of studies has revealed the significance of notch signaling in self-renewal of stem cells, differentiation, apoptosis and in how its dysregulation promotes tumorigenesis (1–3,5,9,15,17,26,37,38).

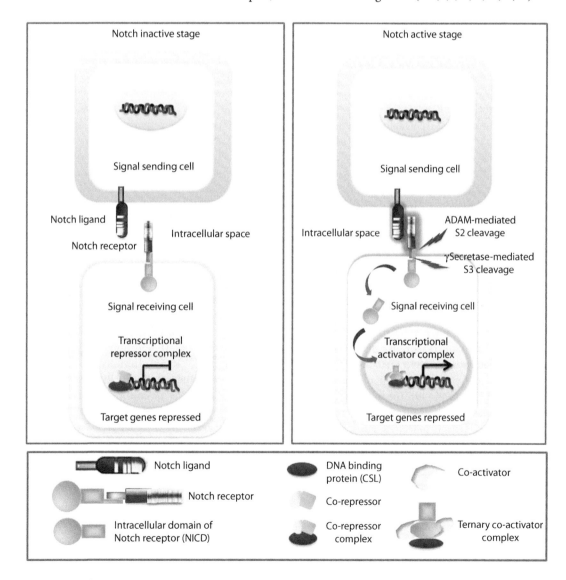

Figure 12.2 Notch signaling in inactive and active stages.

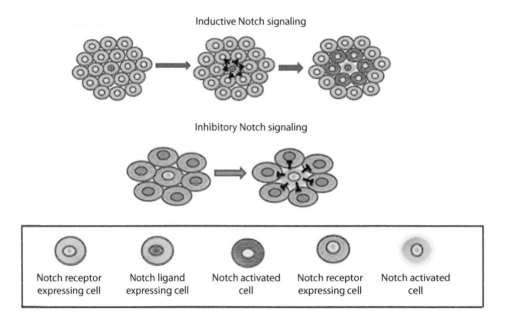

Figure 12.3 Functional aspects of the Notch signaling—Inductive Notch signaling and inhibitory Notch signaling.

12.3 HOW CRUCIAL IS NOTCH SIGNALING FOR SPERMATOGENETIC EVENTS?

Spermatogenesis is a tightly regulated process that results in the formation of the autonomous spermatozoa, which initially starts with syncytial clones of germ cells connected to specialized somatic cells. The formation of functional spermatozoa, which are capable of initiating the fundamental event of life (fertilization), is the result of well-harmonized and coordinated events carried out by many cells. The manufacturing of healthy sperm in testes is carried out with the assistance of three arms of cell signaling: juxtacrine, paracrine and endocrine signals. It has been reported that any error in the process of sperm formation in the testes, maturation journey of sperm in the epididymis, storage, as well as regulation at hormonal, transcriptional and translation levels may lead to male infertility (2,39–44). Although research in many fields has reached its summit, research on male infertility is still in its infancy, and many reasons for male infertility remain unknown. Various studies have verified that Notch signaling has a crucial role in the development of gonads and in sperm production (2,12,13,42,44–49). The role of notch signaling in the formation of spermatozoa from quiescent gonocytes in the adult testes and defects in this signaling pathway as a cause of male infertility need careful examination.

12.4 SPERMATOGENESIS IN CAENORHABDITIS ELEGANS AND NOTCH SIGNALING

Spermatogenesis exists in both sexes of *C. elegans*, males (genetically XO along with two sets of autosomes) and hermaphrodites (genetically XX along with two sets of

autosomes). In the case of male *C. elegans*, all germline cells differentiate into spermatozoa, whereas in hermaphrodites, switching of events takes place between spermatogenesis to oogenesis during the transition stage from larval form 4 (L4) to adult form. Hermaphrodites start life as male in the larval stage, produce spermatozoa and store the sperm in the proximal end and push it to spermatheca during the first time of ovulation (13,45,46,50–55).

C. elegans has a somatic gonadal niche consisting of two types of cells: a distal tip cell (DTC, single mesenchymal somatic cell with finger-like projection, which helps in the mitotic proliferation of germ cells) and germline cells. Thousands of germ cells in adult gonads are the result of continuous proliferation from a single primordial germ cell in the embryo, which initiates its division once it hatches (45,50,55–58). DTC crucial for germ cell proliferation and maintenance in the larval and adult stages. Studies have reported that aberration in DTC leads to the premature entry of germ cells into the meiosis stage. The opposite happens if additional DTC is placed in some other regions (7,45,58). Initially, in both sexes, germ cells undergo repeated miotic division before entering meiosis and form a large syncytium. Morphologically, there is no difference observed between immature germ cells in both sexes until reaching the pachytene stage of meiosis I. Later, shortly before the first meiotic division starts, germ cells bud off from the central cytoplasmic core of large syncytium called *rachis* (common cytoplasmic region shared by mitotic and progressively descent meiotic cell, connected by germ cell bridge). During the first meiotic division, primary spermatocytes (4N) divide and form two secondary spermatocytes (2N). Immediately thereafter, they undergo a second meiotic division, which results in budding of spermatids from a residual body (the anucleate body which contains many components of cytoplasm like a meiotic spindle, ribosomes, etc.), that results in the formation of four round sessile spermatids that lack all of these cellular components (59). Structurally, spermatids formed in the male are larger in size compared to those produced in hermaphrodites and are stored in the seminal vesicles (59–61). Intriguingly, these round sessile spermatids undergo drastic morphological changes during the process of spermiogenesis, which is initiated during copulation, resulting in the transformation of sessile spermatids to motile bipolar amoeboid spermatozoa (54,55,59–61).

The initial steps of spermatogenesis in *C. elegans* are tightly regulated by transcriptional and translational processes; later, it is carried over by various enzyme systems, which mainly include protein kinases (e.g., serine/threonine-protein kinase spe-6 (SPE-6) regulates the segregation of cell components during meiosis, sperm activation) and phosphatases (serine/threonine-protein phosphatase PP1-gamma (GSP-3) and serine/threonine-protein phosphatase PP1-delta (GSP4) which control the meiotic event during spermatogenesis and also help in dissembling the major sperm protein during movement) (54,55,59,61).

Also, spermatogenesis is regulated mainly by a sex-determination pathway, under the control of five main genes: two *Fog* genes (*Fog-1* and *Fog-3*) and three *Fem* genes (*Fem-1*, *Fem-2* and *Fem-3*). Genetic studies have reported that mutations in these genes misdirect the process of the spermatogenesis to oogenesis pathway (53,61–65). Feminization of germline (FOG-1) is a cytoplasmic polyadenylation binding protein, which is under the regulation of sex-determining transformer protein 1 (TRA-1), the latter belongs to the Gli family of protein, and functions as a transcription factor. In turn, the expression of TRA-1 expression is regulated by many other genes like-protein her-1 (Her-1), sex-determining transformer protein 2 (Tra-2), female germline-specific tumor suppressor gld-1 (Gld-1), feminization of germline (*Fog2*) and sex-determining protein fem (*Fem1/2/3*) (53,59,61,63,65–72).

Notch signaling plays an important role in two cell fate decisions in *C. elegans* such as the anchor cell (AC)/ventral uterine precursor cell (UV) decision and germ cell proliferation, along with the maintenance of the stem cell niche (73). It is observed that during the larval stage, the notch signal mainly regulates the proliferation of germline cells, whereas in adults it helps in proliferation as well as in self-renewal. The research on *C. elegans* has contributed a lot to the understanding of the structural, molecular and functional aspects of notch signaling. Most of the genetics and structural details of the notch and the role of γ-Secretase and its four components in notch signaling were first analyzed in *C. elegans* (45,51,56,57,59,74).

Two notch receptor proteins have been identified in *C. elegans*, encoded by the genes *lin-12* and *glp-1*, which were initially identified during genetic screening for developmental mutants (50,51,56,75). Mutations in the *lin-12* gene have been reported to result in defective early gonadogenesis and vulva formation (21,75). In the case of *glp-1*, both gain and loss of function of the gene exert an effect on gametogenesis.

The gain of function increases the mitotic proliferative rate of germline cells, which blocks their further differentiation; the loss of function forces the cell to enter premature meiosis (21,73,75). Any mutation in the NRR leads to constitutive activation of the notch receptor, leading to the dysfunction of this pathway.

The first notch ligand identified in *C. elegans* was *lag-2*, which showed the similarity between *Drosophila* Notch ligand Delta and Serrate (21,56,73,75). Later many other ligands were identified, such as *apx-1*, *arg-1* and *dsl-1* (76). Upon activation of the notch receptor, followed by binding of a ligand, intracellular domains cleave from an extracellular domain with the help of two sets of proteolytic enzymes, disintegrin and metalloproteinase domain-containing protein 10 homolog (SUP-17) and ADAM4, which cleave at site 2 of the receptor, followed by the cleavage of site 3 by SEL12/Presenilin (γ-Secretase) complex. The cleaved intracellular domain enters the nucleus and forms a transcriptional activation complex with the help of the LAG-1 protein, which is the CSL counterpart of *C. elegans*, instead of CBF1/RBP-J and Su (H) in mammals and *Drosophila*. The ternary transcriptional activation complex in *C. elegans* also contains another molecule called SER-8 (also called LAG-3). SER-8 is structurally (glutamine-rich region) and functionally similar to Mastermind in *Drosophila* and mammals (7,45,50,53,55,59,63,64,67,68,70,72,74,77–81). Thus, the transcriptional activation complex is formed by three components, intracellular region of the notch, LAG-1 and LAG-3/SER-8, which transforms the transcriptional repressor complex to an activator complex, which in turn activates the expression of target genes. Initially, the target genes were identified using computational approaches primarily based on the presence of the consensus binding site sequences, followed by experimental validation. Some such validated targets genes are protein lin-12 (*lin-12*), leukocyte specific transcript 1 (*lst-1*), lateral signaling target protein 2 (*lst-2*), *lst-3*, *lst-4*, dual specificity protein phosphatase lip-1 (*lip-1*), fem-3 mRNA-binding factor 1 (*fbf-1*) and fem-3 mRNA-binding factor 2 (*fbf-2*), which regulate the fate of vulva precursor and germline cells. The activity of notch signaling can be enhanced or suppressed by certain modulators such as putative neurobeachin homolog (*sel-2*), apoptosis linked gene 2-interacting protein X 1 (*alx-1*), enhancer of glp-one (glp-1) (*ego*), tetraspanin-12 (*tsp-12*) and tetraspanin-1 (*tsp-1*) (7,53,63,65,67,69,76,77,82,83). For instance, *ego* was identified as an enhancer of *glp-1*, which enhances the germline proliferation (84,85).

The DTC of the gonad regulates the mitotic and meiotic divisions in the germ cells through notch signaling with the help of certain ribonucleic acid regulators (like FBF-1, FBF-2, female germline-specific tumor suppressor gld-1 [GLD-1], poly(A) RNA polymerase gld-2 [GLD-2], defective in germ line development protein 3 [GLD-3] and nanOS related [NOS-3]). The proximity of the germ cells to the DTC is the main criteria for switching of the cell division from mitosis to meiosis due to signaling gradients generated among cells through diffusion barriers (21,58,76,86).

The whole region of gonads can be divided into three zones based on cell type—mitotic, transition and meiotic zones. A mitotic/progenitor zone (two progenitor zones in case of hermaphrodite at the distal end of gonadal arms and one in the male) is formed of the stem cell niche region, consisting of mitotically dividing cells, which have the capability of both self-renewal as well as production of differentiating gametes (Figure 12.4). DTC expresses protein lag-2 (LAG-2) notch ligand, whereas GLP-1/NOTCH receptor is expressed in the germ cells. The binding of LAG-2 to GLP-1 receptor in the germ cells triggers notch signaling and promotes mitotic division in the cells by inhibiting meiotic regulators. Although *glp-1* messenger RNA is present in all germ cells, its protein is expressed only in the germ cells near the distal

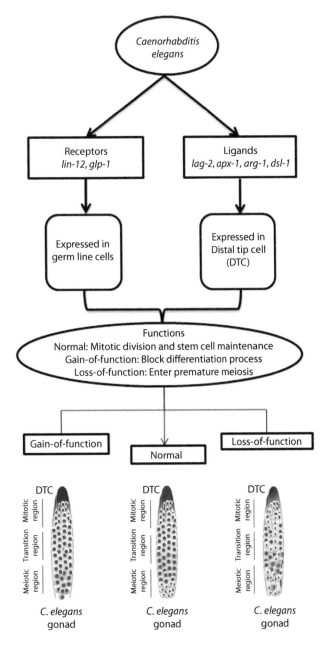

Figure 12.4 Summary of Notch signaling in the testes of *Caenorhabditis elegans*.

end. This gradient expression of GLP-1 protein is regulated by a translation repressor called GLD-1, which inhibits the translation of *glp-1* mRNA in the meiotic region germ cell by binding to their 3′UTR region (7,53,56,58,59,81,82). In addition to DTC, AC/VU precursor cells also regulate germline proliferation in larval form by the same mechanism, since it also expresses LAG-2 protein (73).

Notch signal activates the expression of the target genes, which regulate the decision-making of cells to follow either mitotic or meiotic division, with the help of a network of RNA regulatory molecules (GLD-1, GLD-2, GLD-3 and NOS-3). For instance, GLD-1 protein, which restricts the expression of the notch to the distal region, is in turn regulated by a protein called FBF (translation repressor of *gld-1*) (7,53,63,69,76,82,83). Initially, *fbf-2* and *fbf-1* were identified for their roles in regulating germline sex determination, and later it was found to be a direct target of notch signaling, enlightening how notch signaling regulates cell fate partially, since it is expressed only in the late larval stage and adult organism (63). Lee et al. recently identified two genes, *lst-1* (lateral signaling target) and *sygl-1* (synthetic Glp), as the direct targets of notch, which regulate the germline stem cells' renewal in larvae, since the *lst-1/sygl-1* double mutant produced a phenotype similar to that of the null mutant of GLP-1/NOTCH (7,75,88). They also identified that these genes were also expressed in the late larval and adult stages, which promotes FBF-2 function in retaining the germ stem cell population. Although a single mutant of *lst-1/sygl-1* did not show any severe defect, which represents its redundancy in function (75), tight regulation is identified to occur among *fbf-2, lst-1, sygl, gld-1, gld-2* and *gld-3* to maintain the balance of mitotic and meiotic cells. A recent study reported that LST-1 and SYG-1 form a repressive complex with FBF, which suppresses the expression of the signature target genes of FBF (50,63,76,88). At the same time, overexpression of LST-1 and SYGL-1 in the presence of FBF results in germline tumor. Hence, it is understood that its spatial restriction is crucial for "stemness" maintenance. Other notch target genes include *lip-1*, which promotes germ cell proliferation, but not self-renewal (50,66,76,88).

12.5 CROSS TALK BETWEEN NOTCH AND OTHER PATHWAYS IN REGULATING SPERMATOGENESIS IN *C. ELEGANS*

In a cellular context, mostly all cellular events are regulated by internetworking and intervening of various signaling pathways and by intrinsic mechanisms like epigenetic modifications. This regulation can be at the level of synthesis of the ligand/receptor or in the turnover number of signals. The two main axes through which notch regulate the spermatogenic events are direct regulation by activation of GLP-1/NOTCH through interaction between DTC niche and the germ cells and by the ribonucleic acid regulatory circuit formed by FBF/GLD/NOS within germline cells (50,51,53,57,63,66,68,69,72,76,78–80,83,89). The interaction of notch signaling with the Receptor Tyrosine Kinase/Ras/

Mitogen-activated protein kinase/transforming growth factor beta (TGF-β)/Wnt pathway is reported in vulva development and germline proliferation (7,30,45,52,55,68,82,90). Proper vulva development is the result of coordinated inductive signals from the epidermal growth factor receptor and the lateral signal from notch/LIN-12 (73). It has been reported that many of the target genes of the notch are repressed by PRC2 (polycomb repressor complex 2), by triggering the expression of H3K27 demethylase (71). In germline cells, PRC2 acts antagonistically to notch targets by an intrinsic mechanism, which enhances cellular reprogramming by enhancing the expression of genes like *cMyc* and *klf4* (71). It has been reported that dauer larva development regulatory growth factor daf-7 (DAF-7)/TGF-β regulates the expression of *lag-2* in DTC of the late larval stage by direct binding of DAF-3 to the promoter region of *lag-2* gene depending on milieu (91).

12.6 SPERMATOGENESIS IN *DROSOPHILA MELANOGASTER*

In *Drosophila*, the testes niche consists of three types of cell populations, which are interdependent: the hub (formed at apical end of testes), the somatic cyst stem cells (CySCs; connected to the hub and surrounding germline cells) and the germline stem cells (GSCs; attached to the hub) (47,91–93). During spermatogenesis, GSCs undergo asymmetric division and result in one self-renewing cell, which attaches to the hub, and a differentiating cell called gonialblast, which initiates spermatogenesis. Similarly, CySCs undergo asymmetric division resulting in two daughter quiescent cyst cells connected to the hub by a thin cytoplasmic bridge, which encapsulates each gonialblast, forming a microniche around it. Hub and cyst cells together form the niche in *Drosophila* for maintaining germ cell proliferation and differentiation, similar to the DTC in *C. elegans*. Gonialblast undergoes four rounds of transit mitotic amplifications resulting in a germ cell cyst containing 16 spermatogonia with incomplete cytokinesis, which further goes through two meiotic divisions resulting in 64 haploid spermatids (6,8,47,92–96).

The entire process is regulated by various signaling pathways, like janus kinase/signal transducers and activators of transcription (JAK-STAT), bone morphogenetic proteins (BMP), Hedgehog and epidermal growth factor (EGF/EGFR). The JAK-STAT pathway was the first signaling pathway reported to have a functional regulatory role in the maintenance of the CySCs and GSCs (8,47,97–99). The detailed mechanisms of the BMP and JAK-STAT signaling pathways in regulating spermatogenesis are discussed in greater detail in Chapters 11 and 15, respectively. In the case of notch signaling, it is reported to have a crucial role in Hub cell specification, as the mutant larvae of notch have complete abolition of hub cells in gonads, which is followed by early germ cell differentiation (8,23,37,100,101).

In *Drosophila*, notch signaling is initiated during the embryogenesis stage and proceeds onward, which is curial for hub cell specification among somatic gonadal precursor cells (SGPs), which in turn is necessary for proper maintenance and differentiation of CySCs and GSCs. Notch receptors were identified in hub cells a long time ago; however, the ligand that activates it was obscure until 2010 (8,47,96,99,100,102–104). Okegbe et al. identified that the notch ligand is presented to the SGPs by adjacent endodermal cells, which trigger the hub cell fate in them, and ablation of delta ligands reduces the number of hub cells in gonads (101). Although notch activation is observed in SGP cells in all regions of gonads, specifically hub cell fate is restricted to the anterior end by an antagonist mechanism played by the RTK pathway (105). The RTK pathway receptor sevenless (SEV) is expressed in the posterior SGPs, which is activated by Boss ligand exuded from the primordial germ cells (PGCs). Due to this activation of SEV, hub differentiation in the posterior SGPs is restricted. In addition to this, EGFR signaling is also activated in the posterior region of the gonads, which restricts hub differentiation by binding Spitz ligands secreted from PGCs to its receptor in the posterior SGPs (106,107). Thus, the interaction between SGPs and PGCs helps in proper formation of GSC in the anterior region and also helps in the continued production of sperm in male gonads by maintaining the germ line stem cell pool.

Notch ligands Delta and Serrate were identified in testes and its proximal tissues. Delta was highly expressed in the endodermal cells, which activate notch signaling in the hub cells. Although both ligands are present in the testes, Delta plays a prominent role with 70% of reductions in the hub cells being observed in Delta mutants, whereas only 30% were observed in Serrate mutants. Serrate was observed in the late anterior SGPs after gonad coalescence, which adds a small hub cell population to an already existing population of cells formed by Delta-Notch activation. Thus, in *Drosophila*, notch regulates the maintenance and differentiation of the hub cells in the testes, which in turn helps in the proliferation and differentiation of CySCs and GSC (Figure 12.5).

12.7 CROSS TALK BETWEEN NOTCH AND OTHER PATHWAYS IN *D. MELANOGASTER*

The hub cells act as the core niche in testes for promoting the self-renewal and differentiation of CySCs and GSCs through many signaling pathways like JAK-STAT, BMP and Hedgehog. Although the hub cells and cyst cells are derived from the SGPs, their fate is different due to the activation of notch signaling. Notch activation is reported in all SGPs, but still a few cells in the anterior region commit to form hub cells, which is due to antagonist mechanisms between the notch and EGFR signaling in the posterior region. Hub cell differentiation in the anterior region is also contributed by the synergetic effect of both RTK and EGFR signaling. Spitz (SPI) ligand is cleaved by a protease STET in the germ cells to activate the EGF signaling in cyst cells, which stimulates the differentiation of cyst cells from CySCs. Differentiated

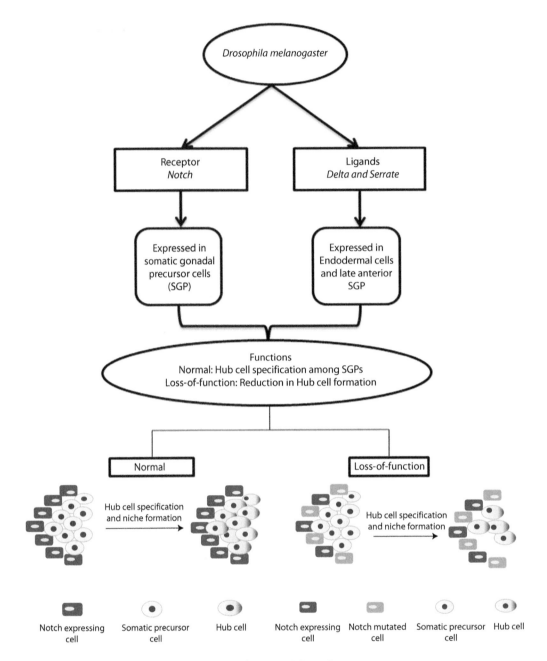

Figure 12.5 Summary of Notch signaling in the testes of *Drosophila melanogaster.*

cyst cells encapsulate germ cells, which in turn help in the differentiation of germ cells. Similarly, unpaired ligand secreted from the hub cells activates the JAK-STAT pathway in CySCs and GSC for their maintenance by downstream activation of the transcriptional factor Stat92E (23,98,100–102,105–110). Hence, there is major cross talk between signaling pathways, which leads to the development of defined embryonic gonads to adult gonads in *Drosophila.*

12.8 SPERMATOGENESIS IN *MUS MUSCULUS*

Mammalian spermatogenesis is a highly specialized and complex process occurring in the seminiferous tubule of the testes, which results in the formation of an array of germ cells at different developmental stages. In the mouse, spermatogenesis starts from 7.5 days postcoitum (dpc). The events start with the migration of PGCs from epiblast to the hind gut and finally colonizing the genital ridge, which is similar to gonad formation in *Drosophila* (41,44,102,111). The colonized PGCs undergo multiple mitotic divisions during their journey that result in the formation of gonocytes at 13.5 dpc, which are enclosed by peritubular myoid and Sertoli precursor cells. Gonocyte/prospermatogonia cells undergo further divisions until 16.5 dpc and enter G1/ G0 mitotic arrest in an unsynchronized manner until the time of birth (41,44,102,111). After birth, the mitotic arrest is released, and the gonocytes continue to proliferate to form postnatal spermatogonial stem cells (SSC). SSCs along the basal compartment of the seminiferous tubule form the stem cells niche in the testes, which help in balancing the self-renewal and differentiation processes (41,44,94,111). The time of resumption of mitotic proliferation in quiescent gonocytes varies among species in mammals. For instance, in mouse, it happens at around a week after birth, whereas in humans it may be prolonged until the time of puberty. SSCs undergo a self-renewal and differentiation process in the testes, thus forming the baseline cells for the formation of sperm. The spermatogenesis process can be divided into three phases: active mitotic proliferation, meiotic and cyto-differentiation. During the mitotic phase, spermatogonial mother cells (undifferentiated spermatogonia) undergo several series of mitotic divisions and form A1–A4, intermediate and B-type spermatogonia. The B-type spermatogonia, formed during the last mitotic division, get committed to undergo a differentiation process to form primary spermatocytes (41,44,94,111). The primary spermatocytes then undergo meiosis, which results in the formation of secondary spermatocytes and round spermatids. The round spermatids go through drastic morphological changes as a part of spermiogenesis (cytodifferentiation phase), resulting in elongated spermatozoon (44,112). The orchestration of these events occurring within the testes is assisted by the somatic cells, Sertoli cells (located inside seminiferous tubules) and Leydig cells (located in between tubules). The Sertoli cells provide an apt microenvironment for the nourishment of germ cells, which helps in their growth and survival, whereas the Leydig cells control the steroidogenic function in the testes (44,46,113). The elongated spermatozoa formed in the testes are immature, and their final maturation happens in the epididymis, where they undergo dramatic changes in the chemical and physical properties of their plasma membranes that make the sperm competent for fertilizing ovum (44,112,114–123).

Spermatogenesis is regulated by a precise expression of genes in a spatiotemporal manner, which is brought through regulations at hormonal, transcriptional, post-transcriptional, translational and epigenetic levels (41,44,94,113). A glut of transcription factors has been discovered in both somatic and germ cells, which play an important role in regulating the spermatogenesis progression. It can be generalized that transcriptional factors expressed in the germ cells mainly regulate a specific phase of germ cell progression, whereas those expressed in the Sertoli cells regulate all stages of spermatogenesis (41,42,44). The regulations at the post-transcriptional and epigenetic levels are pivotal for the late stage of spermatogenesis due to transcriptional arrest by chromatin compaction events. Recent studies have introduced new candidate microRNAs in the regulation of spermatogenesis at the post-transcriptional level (124–126).

The molecular level (transcriptional, post-transcriptional and translational) control is in turn exerted by various signaling pathways. It has been reported that various signaling pathways like Src, Ras and Notch are regulated by a molecule released by the Sertoli cells, called glial cell line-derived neurotrophic factor (GDNF) (33,46,127–130). Some recent studies have also reported the importance of BMP8A

in promoting self-renewal of SSC during the first round of spermatogenesis through activation of SMAD1/5/8 (130). In the case of mouse spermatogenesis, STAT3 regulates the differentiation of SSC colonies, which is contradictory to the function it plays in *Drosophila* (128,131,132). Notch signaling is reported to act as a trigger that facilitates the escape of gonocytes from the quiescent stage with the help of the Sertoli cells (33,129,133).

The scenario of Notch signaling in mammals is different from that of *C. elegans* and *Drosophila*. It regulates germline cell maintenance and development in mammals, whereas it helps in niche cell specification in fly and worm. However, there is controversy regarding whether notch is important for germ cell maintenance or differentiation in mammals (10,13,33,46,133–138). Spermatogenesis was normal in case of protein O-fucosyltransferase1 deletion in Sertoli cells, whereas *in vivo* blockage of notch severely affected spermatogenesis (139,140).

Although the expressions of all notch components in neonatal and adult mouse and human testes were first reported in 2001 by two groups concurrently, many questions regarding its function are still obscure (134,135). Lupien et al. developed a transgenic mouse constitutively expressing NICD of notch receptor 1 under the regulatory mechanism of mouse mammalian tumor virus. This led to the observation that notch expression outside the testes, including vas deferens and epididymis, resulted in hyperplasia of epithelial cells that led to the disruption in border formation and blockage of the efferent duct (13).

Sequential expressions of notch receptors, ligands and effectors were observed in both somatic (Sertoli and Leydig cells) and germ cells in the testes (10,134,137,138,141). All four notch receptors (NOTCH 1–4) and five ligands (DLLI, DLL3, DLL4, JAG1 and JAG2) were reported to have major roles in the development and maturation of the testes (33,46). The canonical notch pathway in them is activated by ligand engagement to the receptor, which finally results in the conversion of transcriptional repressor complex to activator complex. An activated notch signal mainly triggers the expression of target genes belonging to the HES and HEY families (33–35,46).

The expression of NOTCH receptors 1, 3 and 4 was reported in fetal and mature Sertoli cells, but its functional implications were only recently reported. Using reporter green fluorescence tag mice, it has been shown that notch signaling was active in fetal, neonatal and adult Sertoli cells. However, the loss of function of notch 1 receptor in the Sertoli cells did not implicate any functional defect, indicating the redundancy among receptors to balance their function (33,46). At the same time, the constitutive activation of the notch1 receptor from embryonic stage onward resulted in drastic changes in gonocyte behavior, although the morphology of Sertoli cells remained unaltered during the entire fetal and postnatal stage. Initially, premature differentiation and gonocyte apoptosis were observed followed by the complete absence of gonocytes after postnatal day 2. Further molecular analysis revealed that hyperactivation of

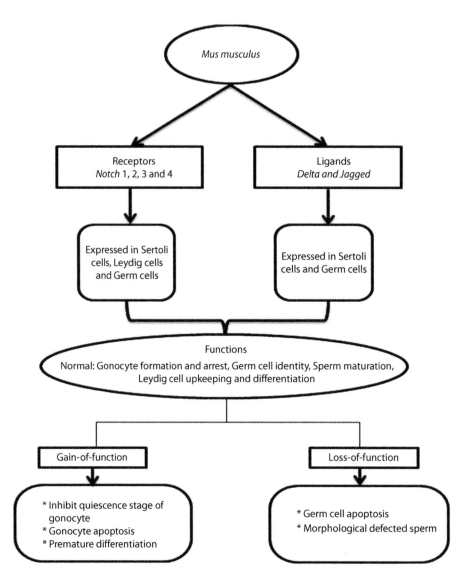

Figure 12.6 Summary of Notch signaling in the testes of *Mus musculus*.

the notch 1 intracellular domain dysregulated the expression of many Sertoli cell–specific genes crucial for germ cell maintenance, such as *Gdnf* and *Cyp26b1*. These genes were downregulated, whereas many meiosis-promoting genes like *Stra8*, *Sycp3* and *Rec8* were upregulated (46,129,133). It was thus revealed that tuning the timing of notch signaling is critical for maintaining gonocyte in the undifferentiated stage during fetal life. Otherwise, it jeopardizes the gonocyte development. Similarly *in vivo* blockage of the notch in adult mouse testes results in germ cell apoptosis, specifically zygotene spermatocytes, and also affects the morphology of mature sperm (142). The activation of notch signaling in germ cells is also time dependent. This was proved by the constitutive activation of NICD in the germ cells, since it did not show any effect immediately after birth, but drastic changes in the germ cells were observed with advancement of the age of the animal (33,46,133,136). In addition to this, it is also reported that notch signaling is critical for the maintenance of progenitor cells and for the differentiation

of Leydig cells during the fetal period (113,141,143). All these results indicate that notch signaling has an important role in regulating all events of spermatogenesis starting from gonocyte formation and arrest, germ cell identity, meiosis and finally in forming elongated mature sperm formation (Figure 12.6).

12.9 CROSS TALK BETWEEN NOTCH AND OTHER PATHWAYS

Notch signaling in mammals is reported to interact with other signaling pathways like GNDF, MAP kinase, TNF-α and fibroblast growth factor (16,90,100,127,128, 130,131,144,145). GDNF signaling is essential for the escape of gonocytes from mitotic arrest and for the maintenance of the SSC population in mammals (128,143). In AMH-NICDI (*Amh-cre*; *Rosa*$^{NICD/+}$) mice, downregulation of *Gdnf* resulted in an early exit of gonocytes from the quiescent stage, followed by gonocyte apoptosis and Sertoli cell–only phenotype after postnatal day 2 (46,128,133,143). So Notch acts as a negative regulator of GDNF and helps in balancing the proliferation and differentiation of spermatogonia. Currently, NFKB activating protein (*Nkap*) is reported as the transcriptional repressor of notch signaling specific to the germ cells as its deletion causes maturation arrest at pachytene spermatocyte (146).

In testes, the expression of notch receptor and ligands fluctuates between seminiferous epithelial cycles depending on extrinsic and intrinsic signals. Okada et al. reported that oscillation in the expression of jagged 1 in the Sertoli cells during the first wave of spermatogenesis is regulated by cross talk between cyclic adenosine monophosphate (cAMP) and tumor necrosis factor-α (TNF-α) signaling. The simultaneous addition of cAMP and TNF-α in an *in vitro* culture of Sertoli cells resulted in the suppression of jagged 1 ligand, indicating that cAMP has a dominating role over TNF-α in regulating this event (127,145,147). A recent study documented a new regulatory arm between notch signaling and aryl hydrocarbon receptor (AhR) in testes. Normally, AhR regulates various cellular events like cell proliferation and differentiation through interactions with other signaling pathways. In AhR$^{-/-}$ mice, a degenerative change occurred in the testes due to germ cell apoptosis that reduced the number of early spermatids, coinciding with downregulation of the notch receptor and its target genes (148). All of these studies provide strong evidence regarding the intertwining between major signaling pathways and notch.

12.10 MALE INFERTILITY DUE TO DYSREGULATION OF NOTCH SIGNALING

Fifty percent of infertility is caused by the male partner due to errors in spermatogenesis or inefficiency of the sperm to reach the ovum and fertilize it. The entire process of spermatogenesis is regulated by various signaling pathways, and its dysregulation may cause male infertility. As discussed in the previous sections, the evolutionarily conserved notch pathway regulates various steps in spermatogenesis, like stem cell renewal, niche specification, differentiation of germ cells, attachment of spermatids to the Sertoli cells, etc. Aberrant expression of notch components has been reported to cause male sterility in mice (13,133,136,137,148,149). Similar results were observed in rat testes when the notch signaling was suppressed (87,135). *In vivo* blockage of the notch in germ cell resulted in the significant loss of germ cell function and the formation of morphologically defective sperm (142). Studies using animal models have proven that notch signaling is crucial for the maintenance of the stem cell population in testes, and its dysregulation leads to an abrupt end to the progression of spermatogenesis (11,71,87,107,133,135,137,141,148,149). In humans, altered expression of the notch receptors was observed in infertile men when compared with fertile males (48,135).

12.11 CONCLUDING REMARKS AND FUTURE PERSPECTIVE

Notch signaling acts as the gatekeeper in regulating all events in spermatogenesis among various species. Functional versatility is observed among species, as in *C. elegans* it regulates maintenance and mitotic division of germ cells, whereas in *Drosophila* it regulates niche cell specification. However, in mammals, there are controversies in notch signal–mediated regulation of spermatogenic events. Recent studies related to the constitutive activation of notch receptor in both germ cells and somatic cells have highlighted the importance of notch signaling in regulating germ cell progression, meiotic events and maturation of sperm. Although a plethora of studies strongly invoke notch signaling in regulating spermatogenesis, very few direct targets have been reported so far. This is due to the huge amount of chaos that occurs during the cross talk between various signaling pathways. Similarly, there is less clarity regarding the upstream regulator of notch signaling in testicular biology. Novel experimental approaches blended with bioinformatics and computational biology would fill the gaps in the understanding of notch regulation in spermatogenesis in the near future and would come in handy in the development of new therapeutic targets to cure male infertility.

ACKNOWLEDGMENTS

The financial assistance received by MS (UGC Senior Research Fellowship No. 23/12/2012[i]EU-V) and PGK (BT/PR3600/MED/31/299/2017; RGCB Intramural Funds) is acknowledged. Rizwan R helped in file conversion during SMART analysis.

REFERENCES

1. Goriki A, Seiler R, Wyatt AW, Contreras-Sanz A, Bhat A, Matsubara A et al. Unravelling disparate roles of NOTCH in bladder cancer. *Nat Rev Urol*. 2018 Jun;15(6):345–57.
2. Miele L, Golde T, Osborne B. Notch signaling in cancer. *Curr Mol Med*. 2006 Dec;6(8):905–18.
3. Nowell CS, Radtke F. Notch as a tumour suppressor. *Nat Rev Cancer*. 2017 Mar;17(3):145–59.
4. Talora C, Campese AF, Bellavia D, Felli MP, Vacca A, Gulino A et al. Notch signaling and diseases: An evolutionary journey from a simple beginning to complex outcomes. *Biochim Biophys Acta*. 2008 Sep;1782(9):489–97.
5. Wilson A, Radtke F. Multiple functions of Notch signaling in self-renewing organs and cancer. *FEBS Lett*. 2006 May 22;580(12):2860–8.
6. Leatherman JL, DiNardo S. Germline self-renewal requires cyst stem cells and stat regulates niche adhesion in *Drosophila* testes. *Nat Cell Biol*. 2010 Aug;12(8):806–11.

7. Lee C, Sorensen EB, Lynch TR, Kimble JC. Elegans GLP-1/Notch activates transcription in a probability gradient across the germline stem cell pool. *Elife.* 2016 Oct 5;5.

8. Lim JG, Fuller MT. Somatic cell lineage is required for differentiation and not maintenance of germline stem cells in *Drosophila* testes. *Proc Natl Acad Sci USA.* 2012 Nov 6;109(45):18477–81.

9. Liu J, Sato C, Cerletti M, Wagers A. Notch signaling in the regulation of stem cell self-renewal and differentiation. *Curr Top Dev Biol.* 2010;92:367–409.

10. Mori S, Kadokawa Y, Hoshinaga K, Marunouchi T. Sequential activation of Notch family receptors during mouse spermatogenesis. *Dev Growth Differ.* 2003 Feb;45(1):7–13.

11. Morichika K, Kataoka K, Terayama K, Tazaki A, Kinoshita T, Watanabe K et al. Perturbation of Notch/suppressor of hairless pathway disturbs migration of primordial germ cells in *Xenopus* embryo. *Dev Growth Differ.* 2010 Feb;52(2):235–44.

12. Murta D, Batista M, Silva E, Trindade A, Henrique D, Duarte A et al. Dynamics of Notch pathway expression during mouse testis post-natal development and along the spermatogenic cycle. *PLOS ONE.* 2013;8(8):e72767.

13. Lupien M, Dievart A, Morales CR, Hermo L, Calvo E, Kay DG et al. Expression of constitutively active Notch1 in male genital tracts results in ectopic growth and blockage of efferent ducts, epididymal hyperplasia and sterility. *Dev Biol.* 2006 Dec 15;300(2):497–511.

14. Artavanis-Tsakonas S, Muskavitch MA. Notch: The past, the present, and the future. *Curr Top Dev Biol.* 2010;92:1–29.

15. Garg V. Chapter 53: Notch signaling in aortic valve development and disease. 2016. In: Nakanishi T, Markwald RR, Baldwin HS, Keller BB, Srivastava D, Yamagishi H (Eds.), *Etiology and Morphogenesis of Congenital Heart Disease: From Gene Function and Cellular Interaction to Morphology*, Tokyo: Springer. pp. 371–6.

16. Lucas TF, Nascimento AR, Pisolato R, Pimenta MT, Lazari MF, Porto CS. Receptors and signaling pathways involved in proliferation and differentiation of Sertoli cells. *Spermatogenesis.* 2014;4:e28138.

17. Lai EC. Notch signaling: Control of cell communication and cell fate. *Development.* 2004 Mar;131(5):965–73.

18. Weng AP, Ferrando AA, Lee W, Morris JP, Silverman LB, Sanchez-Irizarry C et al. Activating mutations of NOTCH1 in human T cell acute lymphoblastic leukemia. *Science.* 2004 Oct 8;306(5694):269–71.

19. D'Souza B, Miyamoto A, Weinmaster G. The many facets of Notch ligands. *Oncogene.* 2008 Sep 1;27(38):5148–67.

20. D'Souza B, Meloty-Kapella L, Weinmaster G. Canonical and non-canonical Notch ligands. *Curr Top Dev Biol.* 2010;92:73–129.

21. Lambie EJ, Kimble J. Two homologous regulatory genes, lin-12 and glp-1, have overlapping functions. *Development.* 1991 May;112(1):231–40.

22. Nandagopal N, Santat LA, LeBon L, Sprinzak D, Bronner ME, Elowitz MB. Dynamic ligand discrimination in the notch signaling pathway. *Cell.* 2018 Feb 8; 172(4):869–80.

23. Zeng C, Younger-Shepherd S, Jan LY, Jan YN. Delta and Serrate are redundant Notch ligands required for asymmetric cell divisions within the *Drosophila* sensory organ lineage. *Genes Dev.* 1998 Apr 15;12(8):1086–91.

24. Mitsiadis TA, Hirsinger E, Lendahl U, Goridis C. Delta-notch signaling in odontogenesis: Correlation with cytodifferentiation and evidence for feedback regulation. *Dev Biol.* 1998 Dec 15;204(2):420–31.

25. del AD, Rouault H, Schweisguth F. Mechanism and significance of *cis*-inhibition in Notch signalling. *Curr Biol.* 2011 Jan 11;21(1):R40–R47.

26. Baron M. An overview of the Notch signalling pathway. *Semin Cell Dev Biol.* 2003 Apr;14(2):113–9.

27. Bray S, Bernard F. Notch targets and their regulation. *Curr Top Dev Biol.* 2010;92:253–75.

28. Chillakuri CR, Sheppard D, Lea SM, Handford PA. Notch receptor-ligand binding and activation: Insights from molecular studies. *Semin Cell Dev Biol.* 2012 Jun;23(4):421–8.

29. Hori K, Sen A, Artavanis-Tsakonas S. Notch signaling at a glance. *J Cell Sci.* 2013 May 15;126(Pt 10):2135–40.

30. Poellinger L, Lendahl U. Modulating Notch signaling by pathway-intrinsic and pathway-extrinsic mechanisms. *Curr Opin Genet Dev.* 2008 Oct;18(5):449–54.

31. Tang Z, Kadesch T. Identification of a novel activation domain in the Notch-responsive transcription factor CSL. *Nucleic Acids Res.* 2001 Jun 1;29(11):2284–91.

32. Fischer A, Gessler M. Delta-Notch–and then? Protein interactions and proposed modes of repression by Hes and Hey bHLH factors. *Nucleic Acids Res.* 2007;35(14):4583–96.

33. Hasegawa K, Okamura Y, Saga Y. Notch signaling in Sertoli cells regulates cyclical gene expression of Hes1 but is dispensable for mouse spermatogenesis. *Mol Cell Biol.* 2012 Jan;32(1):206–15.

34. Zhou M, Yan J, Ma Z, Zhou Y, Abbood NN, Liu J et al. Comparative and evolutionary analysis of the HES/HEY gene family reveal exon/intron loss and teleost specific duplication events. *PLOS ONE.* 2012;7(7):e40649.

35. Iso T, Kedes L, Hamamori Y. HES and HERP families: Multiple effectors of the Notch signaling pathway. *J Cell Physiol.* 2003 Mar;194(3):237–55.

36. Andersson ER, Sandberg R, Lendahl U. Notch signaling: Simplicity in design, versatility in function. *Development.* 2011 Sep;138(17):3593–612.

37. Go MJ, Eastman DS, Artavanis-Tsakonas S. Cell proliferation control by Notch signaling in *Drosophila* development. *Development.* 1998 Jun;125(11):2031–40.

38. Leong KG, Karsan A. Recent insights into the role of Notch signaling in tumorigenesis. *Blood.* 2006 Mar 15;107(6):2223–33.

39. Aster JC, Pear WS, Blacklow SC. The varied roles of notch in cancer. *Annu Rev Pathol.* 2017 Jan 24;12:245–75.

40. Fan X, Mikolaenko I, Elhassan I, Ni X, Wang Y, Ball D et al. Notch1 and notch2 have opposite effects on embryonal brain tumor growth. *Cancer Res.* 2004 Nov 1;64(21):7787–93.

41. Jan SZ, Hamer G, Repping S, de Rooij DG, van Pelt AM, Vormer TL. Molecular control of rodent spermatogenesis. *Biochim Biophys Acta.* 2012 Dec;1822(12):1838–50.

42. Kostereva N, Hofmann MC. Regulation of the spermatogonial stem cell niche. *Reprod Domest Anim.* 2008 Jul;43 Suppl 2:386–92.

43. Lobry C, Oh P, Mansour MR, Look AT, Aifantis I. Notch signaling: Switching an oncogene to a tumor suppressor. *Blood.* 2014 Apr 17;123(16):2451–9.

44. Phillips BT, Gassei K, Orwig KE. Spermatogonial stem cell regulation and spermatogenesis. *Philos Trans R Soc Lond B Biol Sci.* 2010 May 27;365(1546):1663–78.

45. Crittenden SL, Eckmann CR, Wang L, Bernstein DS, Wickens M, Kimble J. Regulation of the mitosis/meiosis decision in the *Caenorhabditis elegans* germline. *Philos Trans R Soc Lond B Biol Sci.* 2003 Aug 29;358(1436):1359–62.

46. Garcia TX, Hofmann MC. NOTCH signaling in Sertoli cells regulates gonocyte fate. *Cell Cycle.* 2013 Aug 15;12(16):2538–45.

47. Gonczy P, DiNardo S. The germ line regulates somatic cyst cell proliferation and fate during *Drosophila* spermatogenesis. *Development.* 1996 Aug;122(8):2437–47.

48. Hayashi T, Yamada T, Kageyama Y, Negishi T, Kihara K. Expression failure of the Notch signaling system is associated with the pathogenesis of maturation arrest in male infertility patients. *Fertil Steril.* 2004 Mar;81(3):697–9.

49. Kiger AA, White-Cooper H, Fuller MT. Somatic support cells restrict germline stem cell self-renewal and promote differentiation. *Nature.* 2000 Oct 12;407(6805):750–4.

50. Kimble JE, White JG. On the control of germ cell development in *Caenorhabditis elegans. Dev Biol.* 1981 Jan 30;81(2):208–19.

51. Kipreos ET, Gohel SP, Hedgecock EM. The *C. elegans* F-box/WD-repeat protein LIN-23 functions to limit cell division during development. *Development.* 2000 Dec;127(23):5071–82.

52. Morgan CT, Noble D, Kimble J. Mitosis-meiosis and sperm-oocyte fate decisions are separable regulatory events. *Proc Natl Acad Sci USA.* 2013 Feb 26;110(9):3411–6.

53. Schvarzstein M, Spence AM. The *C. elegans* sex-determining GLI protein TRA-1A is regulated by sex-specific proteolysis. *Dev Cell.* 2006 Nov;11(5):733–40.

54. Shakes DC, Ward S. Initiation of spermiogenesis in *C. elegans*: A pharmacological and genetic analysis. *Dev Biol.* 1989 Jul;134(1):189–200.

55. Shakes DC, Wu JC, Sadler PL, Laprade K, Moore LL, Noritake A et al. Spermatogenesis-specific features of the meiotic program in *Caenorhabditis elegans. PLOS Genet.* 2009 Aug;5(8):e1000611.

56. Austin J, Kimble J. glp-1 is required in the germ line for regulation of the decision between mitosis and meiosis in *C. elegans. Cell.* 1987 Nov 20;51(4):589–99.

57. Chesney MA, Lam N, Morgan DE, Phillips BT, Kimble J. *C. elegans* HLH-2/E/Daughterless controls key regulatory cells during gonadogenesis. *Dev Biol.* 2009 Jul 1;331(1):14–25.

58. Cinquin A, Zheng L, Taylor PH, Paz A, Zhang L, Chiang M et al. Semi-permeable diffusion barriers enhance patterning robustness in the *C. elegans* germ line. *Dev Cell.* 2015 Nov 23;35(4):405–17.

59. Hansen D, Schedl T. The regulatory network controlling the proliferation-meiotic entry decision in the *Caenorhabditis elegans* germ line. *Curr Top Dev Biol.* 2006;76:185–215.

60. Ward S, Hogan E, Nelson GA. The initiation of spermiogenesis in the nematode *Caenorhabditis elegans. Dev Biol.* 1983 Jul;98(1):70–9.

61. Wu JC, Go AC, Samson M, Cintra T, Mirsoian S, Wu TF et al. Sperm development and motility are regulated by PP1 phosphatases in *Caenorhabditis elegans. Genetics.* 2012 Jan;190(1):143–57.

62. Guo Y, Chen X, Ellis RE. Evolutionary change within a bipotential switch shaped the sperm/oocyte decision in hermaphroditic nematodes. *PLOS Genet.* 2013;9(10):e1003850.

63. Lamont LB, Crittenden SL, Bernstein D, Wickens M, Kimble J. FBF-1 and FBF-2 regulate the size of the mitotic region in the *C. elegans* germ line. *Dev Cell.* 2004 Nov;7(5):697–707.

64. Shelton CA, Bowerman B. Time-dependent responses to glp-1-mediated inductions in early *C. elegans* embryos. *Development.* 1996 Jul;122(7):2043–50.

65. Varkey JP, Jansma PL, Minniti AN, Ward S. The *Caenorhabditis elegans* spe-6 gene is required for major sperm protein assembly and shows second site non-complementation with an unlinked deficiency. *Genetics.* 1993 Jan;133(1):79–86.

66. Barton MK, Kimble J. Fog-1, a regulatory gene required for specification of spermatogenesis in the germ line of *Caenorhabditis elegans. Genetics.* 1990 May;125(1):29–39.

67. Chen P, Ellis RE. TRA-1A regulates transcription of fog-3, which controls germ cell fate in *C. elegans. Development.* 2000 Jul;127(14):3119–29.

68. Jin SW, Kimble J, Ellis RE. Regulation of cell fate in *Caenorhabditis elegans* by a novel cytoplasmic polyadenylation element binding protein. *Dev Biol.* 2001 Jan 15;229(2):537–53.

69. Jin SW, Arno N, Cohen A, Shah A, Xu Q, Chen N et al. In *Caenorhabditis elegans*, the RNA-binding domains of the cytoplasmic polyadenylation element binding protein FOG-1 are needed to regulate germ cell fates. *Genetics*. 2001 Dec;159(4):1617–30.

70. Muhlrad PJ, Ward S. Spermiogenesis initiation in *Caenorhabditis elegans* involves a casein kinase 1 encoded by the spe-6 gene. *Genetics*. 2002 May;161(1):143–55.

71. Seelk S, Adrian-Kalchhauser I, Hargitai B, Hajduskova M, Gutnik S, Tursun B et al. Increasing Notch signaling antagonizes PRC2-mediated silencing to promote reprograming of germ cells into neurons. *Elife*. 2016 Sep 7;5.

72. Zarkower D, Hodgkin J. Molecular analysis of the *C. elegans* sex-determining gene tra-1: A gene encoding two zinc finger proteins. *Cell*. 1992 Jul 24;70(2):237–49.

73. Levitan D, Yu G, St George HP, Goutte C. APH-2/nicastrin functions in LIN-12/Notch signaling in the *Caenorhabditis elegans* somatic gonad. *Dev Biol*. 2001 Dec 15;240(2):654–61.

74. Kimble J, Crittenden SL. Controls of germline stem cells, entry into meiosis, and the sperm/oocyte decision in *Caenorhabditis elegans*. *Annu Rev Cell Dev Biol*. 2007;23:405–33.

75. Kershner AM, Shin H, Hansen TJ, Kimble J. Discovery of two GLP-1/Notch target genes that account for the role of GLP-1/Notch signaling in stem cell maintenance. *Proc Natl Acad Sci USA*. 2014 Mar 11; 111(10):3739–44.

76. Ellis RE, Stanfield GM. The regulation of spermatogenesis and sperm function in nematodes. *Semin Cell Dev Biol*. 2014 May;29:17–30.

77. Chen J, Li X, Greenwald I. sel-7, a positive regulator of lin-12 activity, encodes a novel nuclear protein in *Caenorhabditis elegans*. *Genetics*. 2004 Jan;166(1):151–60.

78. Crittenden SL, Bernstein DS, Bachorik JL, Thompson BE, Gallegos M, Petcherski AG et al. A conserved RNA-binding protein controls germline stem cells in *Caenorhabditis elegans*. *Nature*. 2002 Jun 6;417(6889):660–3.

79. Luitjens C, Gallegos M, Kraemer B, Kimble J, Wickens M. CPEB proteins control two key steps in spermatogenesis in *C. elegans*. *Genes Dev*. 2000 Oct 15;14(20):2596–609.

80. Mango SE, Thorpe CJ, Martin PR, Chamberlain SH, Bowerman B. Two maternal genes, apx-1 and pie-1, are required to distinguish the fates of equivalent blastomeres in the early *Caenorhabditis elegans* embryo. *Development*. 1994 Aug;120(8):2305–15.

81. Mello CC, Draper BW, Priess JR. The maternal genes apx-1 and glp-1 and establishment of dorsal-ventral polarity in the early *C. elegans* embryo. *Cell*. 1994 Apr 8;77(1):95–106.

82. Ellis RE, Kimble J. The fog-3 gene and regulation of cell fate in the germ line of *Caenorhabditis elegans*. *Genetics*. 1995 Feb;139(2):561–77.

83. Vaid S, Ariz M, Chaturbedi A, Kumar GA, Subramaniam K. PUF-8 negatively regulates RAS/MAPK signalling to promote differentiation of *C. elegans* germ cells. *Development*. 2013 Apr;140(8):1645–54.

84. Smardon A, Spoerke JM, Stacey SC, Klein ME, Mackin N, Maine EM. EGO-1 is related to RNA-directed RNA polymerase and functions in germ-line development and RNA interference in *C. elegans*. *Curr Biol*. 2000 Feb 24;10(4):169–78.

85. Qiao L, Lissemore JL, Shu P, Smardon A, Gelber MB, Maine EM. Enhancers of glp-1, a gene required for cell-signaling in *Caenorhabditis elegans*, define a set of genes required for germline development. *Genetics*. 1995 Oct;141(2):551–69.

86. Miller MA. Patterning with diffusion barriers. *Dev Cell*. 2015 Nov 23;35(4):395–6.

87. Sahin Z, Bayram Z, Celik-Ozenci C, Akkoyunlu G, Seval Y, Erdogru T et al. Effect of experimental varicocele on the expressions of Notch 1, 2, and 3 in rat testes: An immunohistochemical study. *Fertil Steril*. 2005 Jan;83(1):86–94.

88. Shin H, Haupt KA, Kershner AM, Kroll-Conner P, Wickens M, Kimble J. SYGL-1 and LST-1 link niche signaling to PUF RNA repression for stem cell maintenance in *Caenorhabditis elegans*. *PLOS Genet*. 2017 Dec;13(12):e1007121.

89. Kupinski AP, Muller-Reichert T, Eckmann CR. The *Caenorhabditis elegans* Ste20 kinase, GCK-3, is essential for postembryonic developmental timing and regulates meiotic chromosome segregation. *Dev Biol*. 2010 Aug 15;344(2):758–71.

90. Axelrod JD, Matsuno K, Artavanis-Tsakonas S, Perrimon N. Interaction between Wingless and Notch signaling pathways mediated by dishevelled. *Science*. 1996 Mar 29;271(5257):1826–32.

91. Pekar O, Ow MC, Hui KY, Noyes MB, Hall SE, Hubbard EJA. Linking the environment, DAF-7/TGFβ signaling and LAG-2/DSL ligand expression in the germline stem cell niche. *Development*. 2017 Aug 15;144(16):2896–906.

92. Demarco RS, Eikenes AH, Haglund K, Jones DL. Investigating spermatogenesis in *Drosophila melanogaster*. *Methods*. 2014 Jun 15;68(1):218–27.

93. Hardy RW, Tokuyasu KT, Lindsley DL, Garavito M. The germinal proliferation center in the testis of *Drosophila melanogaster*. *J Ultrastruct Res*. 1979 Nov;69(2):180–90.

94. Manku G, Culty M. Mammalian gonocyte and spermatogonia differentiation: Recent advances and remaining challenges. *Reproduction*. 2015 Mar;149(3):R139–R157.

95. Matunis EL, Stine RR, de CM. Recent advances in *Drosophila* male germline stem cell biology. *Spermatogenesis*. 2012 Jul 1;2(3):137–44.

96. Tran J, Brenner TJ, DiNardo S. Somatic control over the germline stem cell lineage during *Drosophila* spermatogenesis. *Nature*. 2000 Oct 12;407(6805):754–7.

97. Cheng J, Tiyaboonchai A, Yamashita YM, Hunt AJ. Asymmetric division of cyst stem cells in *Drosophila* testis is ensured by anaphase spindle repositioning. *Development*. 2011 Mar;138(5):831–7.

98. Issigonis M, Tulina N, de CM, Brawley C, Sandler L, Matunis E. JAK-STAT signal inhibition regulates competition in the *Drosophila* testis stem cell niche. *Science*. 2009 Oct 2;326(5949):153–6.

99. Tulina N, Matunis E. Control of stem cell self-renewal in *Drosophila* spermatogenesis by JAK-STAT signaling. *Science*. 2001 Dec 21;294(5551):2546–9.

100. Kiger AA, Jones DL, Schulz C, Rogers MB, Fuller MT. Stem cell self-renewal specified by JAK-STAT activation in response to a support cell cue. *Science*. 2001 Dec 21;294(5551):2542–5.

101. Okegbe TC, DiNardo S. The endoderm specifies the mesodermal niche for the germline in *Drosophila* via Delta-Notch signaling. *Development*. 2011 Apr;138(7):1259–67.

102. de Celis JF, Bray S. Feed-back mechanisms affecting Notch activation at the dorsoventral boundary in the *Drosophila* wing. *Development*. 1997 Sep;124(17):3241–51.

103. Leatherman JL, DiNardo S. Zfh-1 controls somatic stem cell self-renewal in the *Drosophila* testis and nonautonomously influences germline stem cell self-renewal. *Cell Stem Cell*. 2008 Jul 3;3(1):44–54.

104. Micchelli CA, Rulifson EJ, Blair SS. The function and regulation of cut expression on the wing margin of *Drosophila*: Notch, Wingless and a dominant negative role for Delta and Serrate. *Development*. 1997 Apr;124(8):1485–95.

105. Kitadate Y, Shigenobu S, Arita K, Kobayashi S. Boss/Sev signaling from germline to soma restricts germline-stem-cell-niche formation in the anterior region of *Drosophila* male gonads. *Dev Cell*. 2007 Jul;13(1):151–9.

106. Kitadate Y, Kobayashi S. Notch and Egfr signaling act antagonistically to regulate germ-line stem cell niche formation in *Drosophila* male embryonic gonads. *Proc Natl Acad Sci USA*. 2010 Aug 10;107(32):14241–6.

107. Xie T, Spradling AC. decapentaplegic is essential for the maintenance and division of germline stem cells in the *Drosophila* ovary. *Cell*. 1998 Jul 24;94(2):251–60.

108. Kawase E, Wong MD, Ding BC, Xie T. Gbb/Bmp signaling is essential for maintaining germline stem cells and for repressing bam transcription in the *Drosophila* testis. *Development*. 2004 Mar;131(6):1365–75.

109. Papagiannouli F, Lohmann I. Stage-specific control of stem cell niche architecture in the *Drosophila* testis by the posterior Hox gene Abd-B. *Comput Struct Biotechnol J*. 2015;13:122–30.

110. Schulz C, Wood CG, Jones DL, Tazuke SI, Fuller MT. Signaling from germ cells mediated by the rhomboid homolog stet organizes encapsulation by somatic support cells. *Development*. 2002 Oct;129(19):4523–34.

111. Yoshida S, Sukeno M, Nakagawa T, Ohbo K, Nagamatsu G, Suda T et al. The first round of mouse spermatogenesis is a distinctive program that lacks the self-renewing spermatogonia stage. *Development*. 2006 Apr;133(8):1495–505.

112. Lucas B, Fields C, Hofmann MC. Signaling pathways in spermatogonial stem cells and their disruption by toxicants. *Birth Defects Res C Embryo Today*. 2009 Mar;87(1):35–42.

113. Defalco T, Saraswathula A, Briot A, Iruela-Arispe ML, Capel B. Testosterone levels influence mouse fetal Leydig cell progenitors through notch signaling. *Biol Reprod*. 2013 Apr;88(4):91.

114. Casado ME, Huerta L, Ortiz AI, Perez-Crespo M, Gutierrez-Adan A, Kraemer FB et al. HSL-knockout mouse testis exhibits class B scavenger receptor upregulation and disrupted lipid raft microdomains. *J Lipid Res*. 2012 Dec;53(12):2586–97.

115. Fayomi AP, Orwig KE. Spermatogonial stem cells and spermatogenesis in mice, monkeys and men. *Stem Cell Res*. 2018 May;29:207–14.

116. Kierszenbaum AL. Intramanchette transport (IMT): Managing the making of the spermatid head, centrosome, and tail. *Mol Reprod Dev*. 2002 Sep;63(1):1–4.

117. O'Donnell L. Mechanisms of spermiogenesis and spermiation and how they are disturbed. *Spermatogenesis*. 2014 May;4(2):e979623.

118. Shadan S, James PS, Howes EA, Jones R. Cholesterol efflux alters lipid raft stability and distribution during capacitation of boar spermatozoa. *Biol Reprod*. 2004 Jul;71(1):253–65.

119. Taloni A, Font-Clos F, Guidetti L, Milan S, Ascagni M, Vasco C et al. Probing spermiogenesis: A digital strategy for mouse acrosome classification. *Sci Rep*. 2017 Jun 16;7(1):3748.

120. Shoeb M, Laloraya M, Kumar PG. Formation and dynamic alterations of horizontal microdomains in sperm membranes during progesterone-induced acrosome reaction. *Biochem Biophys Res Commun*. 2004 Mar 12;315(3):763–70.

121. Purohit SB, Laloraya M, Kumar GP. Role of ions and ion channels in capacitation and acrosome reaction of spermatozoa. *Asian J Androl*. 1999 Sep;1(3):95–107.

122. Kumar GP. Lipid phase transitions and a possible lipid-protein lattice structure as an activity regulator in maturing spermatozoa. *Biochem Mol Biol Int*. 1993 Apr;29(6):1029–38.

123. Singh A, Kumar P, Laloraya M, Verma S, Nivsarkar M. Superoxide dismutase activity regulation by spermine: A new dimension in spermine biochemistry and sperm development. *Biochem Biophys Res Commun*. 1991 May 31;177(1):420–6.

124. Bie B, Wang Y, Li L, Fang H, Liu L, Sun J. Noncoding RNAs: Potential players in the self-renewal of mammalian spermatogonial stem cells. *Mol Reprod Dev.* 2018 Aug;85(8–9):720–8.

125. Luo LF, Hou CC, Yang WX. Small non-coding RNAs and their associated proteins in spermatogenesis. *Gene.* 2016 Mar 10;578(2):141–57.

126. Royo H, Seitz H, Ellnati E, Peters AH, Stadler MB, Turner JM. Silencing of X-linked MicroRNAs by meiotic sex chromosome inactivation. *PLOS Genet.* 2015 Oct;11(10):e1005461.

127. Derynck R, Zhang YE. Smad-dependent and Smad-independent pathways in TGF-β family signalling. *Nature.* 2003 Oct 9;425(6958):577–84.

128. Hofmann MC. Gdnf signaling pathways within the mammalian spermatogonial stem cell niche. *Mol Cell Endocrinol.* 2008 Jun 25;288(1–2):95–103.

129. Li H, MacLean G, Cameron D, Clagett-Dame M, Petkovich M. Cyp26b1 expression in murine Sertoli cells is required to maintain male germ cells in an undifferentiated state during embryogenesis. *PLOS ONE.* 2009 Oct 19;4(10):e7501.

130. Wu FJ, Lin TY, Sung LY, Chang WF, Wu PC, Luo CW. BMP8A sustains spermatogenesis by activating both SMAD1/5/8 and SMAD2/3 in spermatogonia. *Sci Signal.* 2017 May 2;10(477).

131. Kamakura S, Oishi K, Yoshimatsu T, Nakafuku M, Masuyama N, Gotoh Y. Hes binding to STAT3 mediates crosstalk between Notch and JAK-STAT signalling. *Nat Cell Biol.* 2004 Jun;6(6):547–54.

132. Oatley JM, Kaucher AV, Avarbock MR, Brinster RL. Regulation of mouse spermatogonial stem cell differentiation by STAT3 signaling. *Biol Reprod.* 2010 Sep;83(3):427–33.

133. Garcia TX, Defalco T, Capel B, Hofmann MC. Constitutive activation of NOTCH1 signaling in Sertoli cells causes gonocyte exit from quiescence. *Dev Biol.* 2013 May 1;377(1):188–201.

134. Dirami G, Ravindranath N, Achi MV, Dym M. Expression of Notch pathway components in spermatogonia and Sertoli cells of neonatal mice. *J Androl.* 2001 Nov;22(6):944–52.

135. Hayashi T, Kageyama Y, Ishizaka K, Xia G, Kihara K, Oshima H. Requirement of Notch 1 and its ligand jagged 2 expressions for spermatogenesis in rat and human testes. *J Androl.* 2001 Nov;22(6):999–1011.

136. Huang Z, Rivas B, Agoulnik AI. NOTCH1 gain of function in germ cells causes failure of spermatogenesis in male mice. *PLOS ONE.* 2013;8(7):e71213.

137. Kitamoto T, Takahashi K, Takimoto H, Tomizuka K, Hayasaka M, Tabira T et al. Functional redundancy of the Notch gene family during mouse embryogenesis: Analysis of Notch gene expression in Notch3-deficient mice. *Biochem Biophys Res Commun.* 2005 Jun 17;331(4):1154–62.

138. Okada R, Fujimagari M, Koya E, Hirose Y, Sato T, Nishina Y. Expression profile of NOTCH3 in mouse spermatogonia. *Cells Tissues Organs.* 2017;204(5–6):283–92.

139. Shi S, Stanley P. Protein O-fucosyltransferase 1 is an essential component of Notch signaling pathways. *Proc Natl Acad Sci USA.* 2003 Apr 29;100(9):5234–9.

140. Stahl M, Uemura K, Ge C, Shi S, Tashima Y, Stanley P. Roles of Pofut1 and O-fucose in mammalian Notch signaling. *J Biol Chem.* 2008 May 16;283(20):13638–51.

141. Tang H, Brennan J, Karl J, Hamada Y, Raetzman L, Capel B. Notch signaling maintains Leydig progenitor cells in the mouse testis. *Development.* 2008 Nov;135(22):3745–53.

142. Murta D, Batista M, Trindade A, Silva E, Henrique D, Duarte A et al. In vivo notch signaling blockade induces abnormal spermatogenesis in the mouse. *PLOS ONE.* 2014;9(11):e113365.

143. von S, V, Wistuba J, Schlatt S. Notch-1, c-kit and GFRα-1 are developmentally regulated markers for premeiotic germ cells. *Cytogenet Genome Res.* 2004;105(2–4):235–9.

144. Estrach S, Ambler CA, Lo CC, Hozumi K, Watt FM. Jagged 1 is a β-catenin target gene required for ectopic hair follicle formation in adult epidermis. *Development.* 2006 Nov;133(22):4427–38.

145. Kluppel M, Wrana JL. Turning it up a Notch: Crosstalk between TGF-β and Notch signaling. *Bioessays.* 2005 Feb;27(2):115–8.

146. Okuda H, Kiuchi H, Takao T, Miyagawa Y, Tsujimura A, Nonomura N et al. A novel transcriptional factor Nkapl is a germ cell-specific suppressor of Notch signaling and is indispensable for spermatogenesis. *PLOS ONE.* 2015;10(4):e0124293.

147. Okada R, Hara T, Sato T, Kojima N, Nishina Y. The mechanism and control of Jagged1 expression in Sertoli cells. *Regenerative Therapy.* 2016;3:75–81.

148. Huang B, Butler R, Miao Y, Dai Y, Wu W, Su W et al. Dysregulation of Notch and ERα signaling in AhR-/- male mice. *Proc Natl Acad Sci USA.* 2016 Oct 18;113(42):11883–8.

149. Murta D, Batista M, Silva E, Trindade A, Henrique D, Duarte A et al. Notch signaling in the epididymal epithelium regulates sperm motility and is transferred at a distance within epididymosomes. *Andrology.* 2016 Mar;4(2):314–27.

13

Hedgehog signaling in spermatogenesis and male fertility

SANDEEP KUMAR BANSAL, MEGHALI JOSHI, AND RAJENDER SINGH

HIGHLIGHTS

- Hedgehog (hh) signaling plays a crucial role in testes development and maintenance.
- Desert hedgehog (Dhh) and Sonic hedgehog (Shh) are expressed in testes.
- Hedgehog signaling is important for the proliferation and differentiation of spermatogonial stem cells (SSCs).
- In Sertoli cells, hh signaling promotes the secretion of other signaling molecules like GDNF, BMP and SCF, which further helps in the proliferation of SSCs in an indirect way.
- Dhh produced by Sertoli cells promotes the maturation of Leydig cells, which in turn help in differentiation of SSCs.
- The expressions of hh signaling pathway components Hh, Gli1, Smo and ptc are detected in undifferentiated SSCs, showing an autocrine loop of hh signaling.

13.1 INTRODUCTION

Hedgehog (hh) signaling is one of the fundamental pathways having crucial roles in animal development and stem cell maintenance. This pathway has also been found to be involved in carcinogenesis. Recently, hedgehog signaling has been shown to have a role in adult organ homeostasis and repair (1). The hedgehog gene (*hh*) was first discovered in *Drosophila*, and since then many members of this gene family have been found in most metazoa. This signaling pathway is present in all bilaterians and got its name from its polypeptide ligand, an intercellular signaling molecule called hedgehog (hh). The signaling molecule hh got its name from the animal hedgehog, because of the resemblance of the fruit fly larva that lacks the *Hh* gene. In *Drosophila*, the *hh* gene is one of the segment polarity genes and is involved

in fly body plans. The lack of this gene results in small and spiny larvae, which look like an animal hedgehog. This gene is also important for the development of later stages of *Drosophila*, such as embryogenesis and metamorphosis.

13.2 HEDGEHOG MOLECULES

Hedgehog proteins are composed of two domains: the amino terminal "Hedge" domain (HhN) and the carboxy terminal "Hog" domain (HhC) (Figure 13.1). It was found that the carboxy-terminal domain of hh proteins is similar in sequence to the self-splicing inteins. Inteins are protein sequences that autocatalytically splice them out of the protein precursor and ligate the flanking regions into a functional protein. This region of similarity in hh proteins was named the "Hint" module.

133

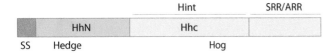

Figure 13.1 Basic structure of hedgehog proteins. (SS, signal peptide sequence [orange]; HhN, amino-terminal signaling domain [green]; HhC, the autocatalytic carboxy-terminal domain [blue] [Hint: this region shares similarities with self-splicing inteins]; and SRR, sterol recognition region, which binds with cholesterol. In hog proteins other than hh, the SRR region is termed as ARR [adduct recognition region].)

13.3 HEDGEHOG SIGNALING IN MAMMALS

Post-translation, HH proteins are extensively modified and released by the cell with the help of dispatched, a membrane transporter protein. Among hedgehog proteins, Shh is most widely expressed in vertebrates. Shh has its paracrine activity, which is the most common mode of signal transduction. However, HH also transduces signals in an autocrine manner. In the absence of HH ligand, patched 1(PTCH1) binds to smoothened (SMO) and represses it. In this situation, the GLI proteins (GLI2 and GLI3) are phosphorylated by casein kinase 1α (CK1), protein kinase A (PKA) and glycogen synthase kinase 3β (GSK3β), which leads to its partial proteolytic cleavage and removal of the C-terminal "activator" domain, resulting in the repressor forms (GLI2^R and GLI3^R), which in turn suppress the expression of HH target genes in the nucleus. In the presence of HH ligand, Hh binds to its receptor PTCH proteins and co-receptors CDO (cell adhesion molecule-related/downregulated by oncogenes), releasing ptch inhibition on smo. Now smo is phosphorylated by mainly CK1 and GRK2. Smo accumulates on the cell surface. Sufu is the major negative regulator of the pathway (kif7 is a minor one). In the presence of Hh, Sufu becomes destabilized and is degraded, which releases its repression on Gli. Gli proteins translocate to the nucleus and induce the expression of HH target genes. Hedgehog signaling is depicted in Figure 13.2.

13.4 HEDGEHOG SIGNALING IN SPERMATOGONIAL STEM CELL PROLIFERATION AND DIFFERENTIATION

Hedgehog signaling regulates the proliferation and differentiation of spermatogonial stem cells (SSCs) in direct and indirect ways. Earlier it was known that Hh signaling could regulate SSCs' proliferation and differentiation indirectly through the Sertoli cells. But recently, it was found that Hh ligands are also present on SSCs, thereby activating Hh signaling in SSCs directly.

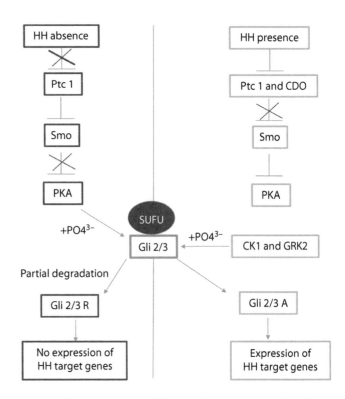

Figure 13.2 Hedgehog (hh) signaling pathway. Red highlights show the signaling pathway in the absence of the Hedgehog molecule; green highlights show the signaling pathway in the presence of the Hedgehog molecule.

13.5 INDIRECT HEDGEHOG SIGNALING IN SSCs

In adult mice, the expression of Dhh has been reported in the Sertoli cells (SCs). After Sertoli cells start expressing Dhh, it initiates Hh signaling, which further promotes the expression of other signaling molecules like glial cell–derived neurotrophic factor (GDNF), bone morphogenetic protein (BMP) and stem cell factor (SCF). Most of these molecules have receptors on SSCs, which upon binding activates signaling pathways such as BMP, Src, RAS/ERK1/2 and PI3K-Akt. On activation of these signaling pathways, SSCs restore their self-renewal capacity while inhibiting their differentiation (2,3). Leydig cells (LCs) and their precursor stem cells are located beneath the basement membrane of the seminiferous tubules, and Ptc and Smo are on the surface of the precursor stem cells. Dhh secreted by the SCs promotes differentiation of Leydig lineage cells into mature Leydig cells, which in turn helps in the growth and development of SSCs (4,5). It has been reported that Dhh secreted by the SCs is important for the maturation of Leydig cells, which is ultimately important for SSCs differentiation (6). Therefore, in order to maintain a balance between SSCs proliferation and differentiation, there should be a balance between Sertoli cells and Leydig cells regulated by Hh signaling (7).

13.6 DIRECT HEDGEHOG SIGNALING IN SSCs

The expression of Hh signaling pathway components Hh, Gli1, Smo and ptc was detected in undifferentiated SSCs, suggesting an autocrine loop of Hh signaling, where it only promotes SSCs' proliferation and inhibits their differentiation (8). In addition to this, a negative regulator of the Hh pathway, SuFu (suppressor of fused) expression was undetected in the proliferating SSCs, while its expression constantly increases, inhibiting Gli transcription and suppressing Dhh signaling during the differentiation process when SSCs develop into mature spermatids (9–11). Hence, Hh signaling negatively regulates the differentiation of SSCs.

13.7 HEDGEHOG SIGNALING IN SPERMATOGENESIS

Sperm production or spermatogenesis is a complex process that is regulated by various signaling pathways. These pathways are controlled at many checkpoints. There is a fine-tuning between germ cell proliferation and differentiation for successful sperm production, which is coordinated by regulated cross talk between various signaling pathways. Dysregulation of these pathways could lead to abnormal spermatogenesis. Hedgehog (hh) signaling is one of the fundamental pathways whose crucial roles have been found in the development and maintenance. Recently, this signaling pathway was found to play an important role in bone formation. Moreover, a few studies have shown the presence of this signaling pathway in mouse testis (12,13). To date, three members of this gene family are known: Dhh (Desert hedgehog), Shh (Sonic hedgehog) and Ihh (Indian hedgehog).

13.7.1 Desert hedgehog

Desert hedgehog protein is encoded by the DHH gene and has a role in hedgehog signaling. The human homolog (DHH) of this gene is located on chromosome band 12q13.1. The expression of the Dhh gene is widely reported in mouse testis. Bitgood et al. (12) revealed that *Dhh* expression starts in mouse Sertoli cell precursors after activation of the *Sry* gene and is maintained in the testis to adulthood. They also found that male mice homozygous for a Dhh-null mutation were viable, but infertile (12). Umehara et al. reported that in humans, mutations in the *DHH* gene may cause 46, *XY PGD* (partial gonadal dysgenesis) (13). They reported that a homozygous missense mutation (ATG→ACG) at the initiating codon in exon 1 of the desert hedgehog (*DHH*) gene leads to the failure of translation of this gene. Clark et al. reported that the Dhh gene is required in mouse testis for the formation of adult-type Leydig cells and normal development of peritubular cells and seminiferous tubules (14).

13.7.2 Sonic hedgehog (Shh)

Sonic hedgehog protein in humans is encoded by the *SHH* gene. This gene has been found to have the most critical roles in development via patterning many systems, such as limbs, brain, spinal cord, lungs, thalamus and teeth. The expression of this gene has also been linked to some specific cancerous tumors, such as embryonic cerebellar tumors, medulloblastoma and the progression of prostate cancer tumors. A few studies have been conducted on the role of the shh gene in spermatogenesis; however, the significance of the Shh gene in spermatogenesis is not clear. Recently, Zou et al. studied a case report of a cryptorchid man and checked Shh signaling in mice and patient with obstructive azoospermia and a patient with prostate cancer (15). They reported Shh immunostaining in spermatocytes of juvenile and adult mouse testis and in patients with obstructive azoospermia and prostate cancer. Earlier, Turner et al. revealed that Shh signaling genes are expressed and transcribed in adult mouse epididymis (16). From these studies, it is clear that the shh gene is expressed in human and mouse testis; however, their expression and roles at different stages of spermatogenesis remain unclear. Earlier, Yuasa et al. found that sonic hedgehog is involved in osteoblast differentiation by cooperating with BMP-2 (17). Similarly, the expression of Shh in mouse and human spermatocytes may be associated with germ cell differentiation. Moreover, Amankulor et al. revealed that acute brain injury activates sonic hedgehog signaling (18). Chen et al. reported that sonic hedgehog signaling has a protective role in endotoxin-induced acute lung injury in a mouse model (19). Shh signaling has been found in the adult immune system, participating in CD[4+] T-lymphocyte activation. Shh expression is also upregulated in acute lung injury (20). These studies indicate that sonic hedgehog may have some crucial roles in the testis, like repairing testicular injuries.

13.7.3 Indian hedgehog

The role of Indian hedgehog has been shown in bone formation. St-Jacques et al. revealed that Indian hedgehog signaling regulates proliferation and differentiation of chondrocytes and is required for bone formation (21). Its expression in testis has not been well studied and documented.

13.8 CONCLUSION

In conclusion, it is worth stating that hedgehog signaling is crucial for testis development and maintenance. There are three members of the hedgehog gene family, i.e., Desert hedgehog (Dhh), Sonic hedgehog (Shh) and Indian hedgehog (Ihh). Out of the three members, two (Dhh and Shh) are expressed in the testes. Dhh is expressed in the Sertoli cell precursors, which are maintained in the adult testes as well. Mutations in the Dhh gene are known to cause infertility in male mice, whereas in humans, mutations in this gene cause partial gonadal dysgenesis. Shh is expressed in the spermatocytes of juvenile and adult mouse testes, suggesting its possible role in germ cell differentiation. Hedgehog signaling is important for the proliferation and differentiation of the SSCs. Hh signaling regulates SSC proliferation and differentiation in direct and indirect ways. Hh signaling initiates in the Sertoli cells to regulate the proliferation of SSCs by producing other signaling molecules like GDNF, BMP and SCF. Indirectly, the Sertoli cells help in the maturation of the Leydig cells by secreting Dhh. Ultimately, these mature Leydig cells help in the differentiation of SSCs. An autocrine loop of Hh signaling as an expression of the components of Hh signaling (Hh, Gli1, Smo and Ptc) is seen in undifferentiated SSCs. Though the hedgehog signaling works via cell-cell communication and cross talk, the full mechanism and all members of this signaling pathway in the testis are yet to be discovered. To date, many studies have been published on this pathway; however, this pathway has not been well elucidated in human testis. A better understanding, exploration of unknown molecules and connections of this pathway to other known signaling pathways could help in the understanding of the etiology of infertility and pave the way to its treatment.

REFERENCES

1. Petrova R, Joyner AL. Roles for Hedgehog signaling in adult organ homeostasis and repair. *Development.* 2014 Sep 15;141(18):3445–57.

2. Meng X, Lindahl M, Hyvönen ME, Parvinen M, de Rooij DG, Hess MW, Raatikainen-Ahokas A, Sainio K, Rauvala H, Lakso M, Pichel JG. Regulation of cell fate decision of undifferentiated spermatogonia by GDNF. *Science.* 2000 Feb 25;287(5457):1489–93.

3. Inaba M, Yamashita YM, Buszczak M. Keeping stem cells under control: New insights into the mechanisms that limit niche-stem cell signaling within the reproductive system. *Mol Reprod Dev.* 2016 Aug;83(8):675–83.

4. Hazra R, Jimenez M, Desai R, Handelsman DJ, Allan CM. Sertoli cell androgen receptor expression regulates temporal fetal and adult Leydig cell differentiation, function, and population size. *Endocrinology.* 2013 Jun 13;154(9):3410–22.

5. Martin LJ. Cell interactions and genetic regulation that contribute to testicular Leydig cell development and differentiation. *Mol Reprod Dev.* 2016 Jun;83(6):470–87.

6. Franco HL, Yao HH. Sex and hedgehog: Roles of genes in the hedgehog signaling pathway in mammalian sexual differentiation. *Chromosome Res.* 2012 Jan 1;20(1):247–58.

7. Shetty GU, Zhou W, Weng CC, Shao SH, Meistrich ML. Leydig cells contribute to the inhibition of spermatogonial differentiation after irradiation of the rat. *Andrology.* 2016 May;4(3):412–24.

8. Sahin Z, Szczepny A, McLaughlin EA, Meistrich ML, Zhou W, Ustunel I, Loveland KL. Dynamic Hedgehog signalling pathway activity in germline stem cells. *Andrology.* 2014 Mar;2(2):267–74.

9. Kroft TL, Patterson J, Won Yoon J, Doglio L, Walterhouse DO, Iannaccone PM, Goldberg E. GLI1 localization in the germinal epithelial cells alternates between cytoplasm and nucleus: Upregulation in transgenic mice blocks spermatogenesis in pachytene. *Biol Reprod.* 2001 Dec 1;65(6):1663–71.

10. Szczepny A, Hime GR, Loveland KL. Expression of hedgehog signalling components in adult mouse testis. *Dev Dyn.* 2006 Nov;235(11):3063–70.

11. Mäkelä JA, Saario V, Bourguiba-Hachemi S, Nurmio M, Jahnukainen K, Parvinen M, Toppari J. Hedgehog signalling promotes germ cell survival in the rat testis. *Reproduction.* 2011 Nov 1;142(5):711–21.

12. Bitgood MJ, Shen L, McMahon AP. Sertoli cell signaling by Desert hedgehog regulates the male germline. *Curr Biol.* 1996 Mar 1;6(3):298–304.

13. Umehara F, Tate G, Itoh K, Yamaguchi N, Douchi T, Mitsuya T, Osame M. A novel mutation of desert hedgehog in a patient with 46,XY partial gonadal dysgenesis accompanied by minifascicular neuropathy. *Am J Hum Genet.* 2000 Nov 1;67(5):1302–5.

14. Clark AM, Garland KK, Russell LD. Desert hedgehog (Dhh) gene is required in the mouse testis for formation of adult-type Leydig cells and normal development of peritubular cells and seminiferous tubules. *Biol Reprod.* 2000 Dec 1;63(6):1825–38.

15. Zou S, Wang Y, Chen T, Song P, Xin D, Ping P, Huang Y, Li Z, Hu H. Ectopic expression of sonic hedgehog in a cryptorchid man with azoospermia: A case report. *J Int Med Res.* 2014 Apr;42(2):589–97.

16. Turner TT, Bomgardner D, Jacobs JP. Sonic hedgehog pathway genes are expressed and transcribed in the adult mouse epididymis. *J Androl.* 2004 Jul 8;25(4):514–22.

17. Yuasa T, Kataoka H, Kinto N, Iwamoto M, Enomoto-Iwamoto M, Iemura SI, Ueno N, Shibata Y, Kurosawa H, Yamaguchi A. Sonic hedgehog is involved in osteoblast differentiation by cooperating with BMP-2. *J Cell Physiol.* 2002 Nov 1;193(2):225–32.

18. Amankulor NM, Hambardzumyan D, Pyonteck SM, Becher OJ, Joyce JA, Holland EC. Sonic hedgehog pathway activation is induced by acute brain injury and regulated by injury-related inflammation. *J Neurosci.* 2009 Aug 19;29(33):10299–308.

19. Chen X, Jin Y, Hou X, Liu F, Wang Y. Sonic hedgehog signaling: Evidence for its protective role in endotoxin induced acute lung injury in mouse model. *PLOS ONE.* 2015 Nov 6;10(11):e0140886.

20. Smelkinson M. The Hedgehog signaling pathway emerges as a pathogenic target. *J Dev Biol.* 2017 Dec;5(4):14.

21. St-Jacques B, Hammerschmidt M, McMahon AP. Indian hedgehog signaling regulates proliferation and differentiation of chondrocytes and is essential for bone formation. *Genes Dev.* 1999 Aug 15;13(16):2072–86.

mTOR signaling in spermatogenesis and male infertility

ARCHANA DEVI AND GOPAL GUPTA

HIGHLIGHTS

- mTOR signaling ensures the continuance of male fertility by regulating spermatogonial stem cell (SSC) self-renewal and differentiation.
- Signaling through mTORC1 promotes SSC differentiation.
- Sertoli cell polarity, necessary for the framework of microenvironment for developing germ cells, is maintained by mTOR signaling.
- mTORC1 signaling disorganizes the blood-testis barrier (BTB) for entry of primary spermatocytes into the immunoprotected adluminal compartment.
- mTORC2 signaling regulates the restructuring of BTB to shield the advanced germ cells from systemic circulation.
- Treatment with rapamycin causes infertility in men.

14.1 INTRODUCTION

Spermatogenesis is a continuous and critical process of maintaining male fertility. The undifferentiated diploid spermatogonium proliferates and differentiates to ultimately give rise to mature haploid male gametes, called *spermatozoa* (1). Within the seminiferous tubules, the spermatogonia lie along the basement membrane in a highly ordered manner. The process begins with the mitotic cell division of spermatogonial stem cells (SSCs), which either self-renew or differentiate. The differentiated spermatogonium gets separated from the basement membrane and after a series of mitotic divisions enters meiosis to produce preleptotene primary spermatocytes. These primary spermatocytes divide meiotically into secondary spermatocytes that further divide meiotically to form round, haploid

spermatids. Thereafter, the process of spermiogenesis further differentiates spermatids into spermatozoa. This final process of cell differentiation produces a highly specialized germ cell (spermatozoon), which is structurally and functionally programmed to carry the paternal DNA to the oocyte. Spermiogenesis involves tail elongation, maturation, acrosome formation and nuclear changes to produce elongated spermatids (2).

Self-renewal or differentiation of spermatogonium is precisely regulated not only to maintain normal spermatogenesis but also to sustain the reproductive health of the male, as excessive or insufficient differentiation can result in testicular cancer or decreased (or lost) sperm production leading to infertility. Emerging evidence suggests that mTOR signaling plays a significant role in balancing this self-renewal and in the differentiation of spermatogonia (3).

The seminiferous epithelium consists of Sertoli cells that provide structural, functional and metabolic support to the developing germ cells. These cells are well ordered according to the developmental stages of germ cells and extend from the basement membrane to the lumen of the seminiferous tubule. Adjacent Sertoli cells form tight junctions or a blood-testis barrier (BTB) to divide the seminiferous tubule lumen into basal and adluminal compartments. During spermatogenesis, preleptotene spermatocytes are actively transported through this barrier to reach the adluminal compartment. The process of preleptotene spermatocyte transport is strictly coordinated and regulated through multiple signaling pathways without compromising the functional integrity of BTB. Several studies have reported that mTOR signaling regulates the dynamics of BTB remodeling, which facilitates the transport of preleptotene spermatocyte across the BTB (4,5). During spermatogenesis, the balance between self-renewal and differentiation of SSCs and the maintenance of BTB are two crucial events that are critically regulated by mTOR signaling. Any alteration in these events may lead to male infertility.

14.2 mTOR-SIGNALING PATHWAY AND mTOR COMPLEXES

The mammalian Target of Rapamycin (mTOR) is a Ser/Thr kinase that belongs to the phosphoinositide-3-kinase (PI3 K)–related kinase family (6). Depending on its binding partner Raptor or Rictor, mTOR forms two structurally and functionally distinct multiprotein complexes known as mTOR complex1 (mTORC1) and mTOR complex2 (mTORC2) (7). In addition to mTOR (the catalytic subunit of the complex), mTORC1 contains Raptor (regulatory-associated protein of mammalian target of rapamycin), PRAS40 (proline-rich AKT/PKB substrate of 40 kDa), mLST8 (mammalian lethal with SEC13 protein 8, also known as GβL) and Deptor (DEP domain containing mTOR-interacting protein) (Figure 14.1). Raptor is important for stable association of PRAS40 with mTORC1, since PRAS40 interacts with mTORC1 through the substrate-binding site of raptor (6). PRAS40 and Deptor both are considered as repressors of mTORC1 in the dephosphorylated state. Upon activation, mTOR (catalytic component of the mTORC1 complex) directly phosphorylates both PRAS40 and Deptor, which results in weakening of their interaction with the rest of mTORC1 components and consequently the activation of mTORC1 signaling (8–10). The role of mLST8 in mTORC1 function is not very clear (6).

The subunits of the mTORC2 are mTOR, Rictor (Rapamycin-insensitive companion of mammalian target of rapamycin), mLST8/GβL, DEPTOR and mSIN1 (Stress-activated MAP kinase-interacting protein 1) (10). Rictor and SIN1 subunits maintain the stability and integrity of mTORC2 and are supposed to carry the regulatory functions of this complex. DEPTOR interacts specifically with mTOR in both mTORC1 and mTORC2 and is believed to be an endogenous inhibitor of both the complexes (11). The

mTORC2 assembles by forming a complex between the heterodimers rictor/SIN1 and mTOR/mLST8, which is the first step in the assembly of mTORC2 (Figure 14.1). The core subunits Rictor and Sin1 determine the integrity and stability of the mTORC2 complex. The mLST8 is a small adaptor protein, which is essential for maintaining the interaction between rictor-mTOR but not between raptor-mTOR. It regulates the kinase activity of mTOR by binding to the kinase domain of mTOR. A study reported that mTOR without mLST8 failed to bind to the rictor/SIN1 heterodimer, and knockout of mLST8 only disrupted the mTORC2 assembly (12). The two mTOR complexes show different sensitivity toward rapamycin (or Sirolimus, a macrocyclic lactone produced by *Streptomyces hygroscopicus*): mTORC1 is highly sensitive to rapamycin, whereas mTORC2 is relatively less sensitive (13,14).

Cumulative evidence indicates that this versatile kinase regulates cellular growth, proliferation, autophagy, protein synthesis, motility and survival, and is itself regulated through a number of signals including stress conditions and nutrients (15,16). Both the complexes show a difference in sensitivity toward rapamycin in upstream signals and the downstream processes they regulate (17).

14.3 ROLE OF mTOR SIGNALING IN SPERMATOGENESIS

14.3.1 mTOR signaling in spermatogonial proliferation and Sertoli cell polarity

Incessant spermatogenesis is dependent on the proliferation and differentiation of spermatogonia. The decision of SSCs to self-renew (to maintain its own population) or to differentiate into sperm cells is critical for maintaining tissue homeostasis, as imbalances (insufficient or excessive differentiation) can lead to male infertility or testicular cancer (18). Of the several signaling pathways controlling the appropriate balance between spermatogonial self-renewal and differentiation, mTOR signaling is the most important pathway. It acts as an important regulator of spermatogonial proliferation and differentiation in the developing testes (19). In the seminiferous tubules, spermatogonia reside at the base surrounded by the Sertoli cells. The Sertoli cells secrete the glial cell line–derived neurotrophic factor (GDNF), which is supposed to activate the mTOR pathway in spermatogonia. GDNF activity is crucial in balancing spermatogonial self-renewal and differentiation, and its overexpression results in the accumulation of spermatogonia (3). In C57Balb-c adult male mice, the spermatogonial stem cells and preleptotene spermatocytes express mTOR, phospho-mTOR, p70S6 K, phospho-p70S6 K and p-4EBP1. Rapamycin treatment causes a significant decrease in the expression level of p-p70S6 K, p-4EBP1, which indicates that mTOR signaling plays a prominent role in the proliferation and stimulation of spermatogonial stem cells for the initiation of meiosis (20). Injecting mTOR inhibitor rapamycin in SD rats results in decreased

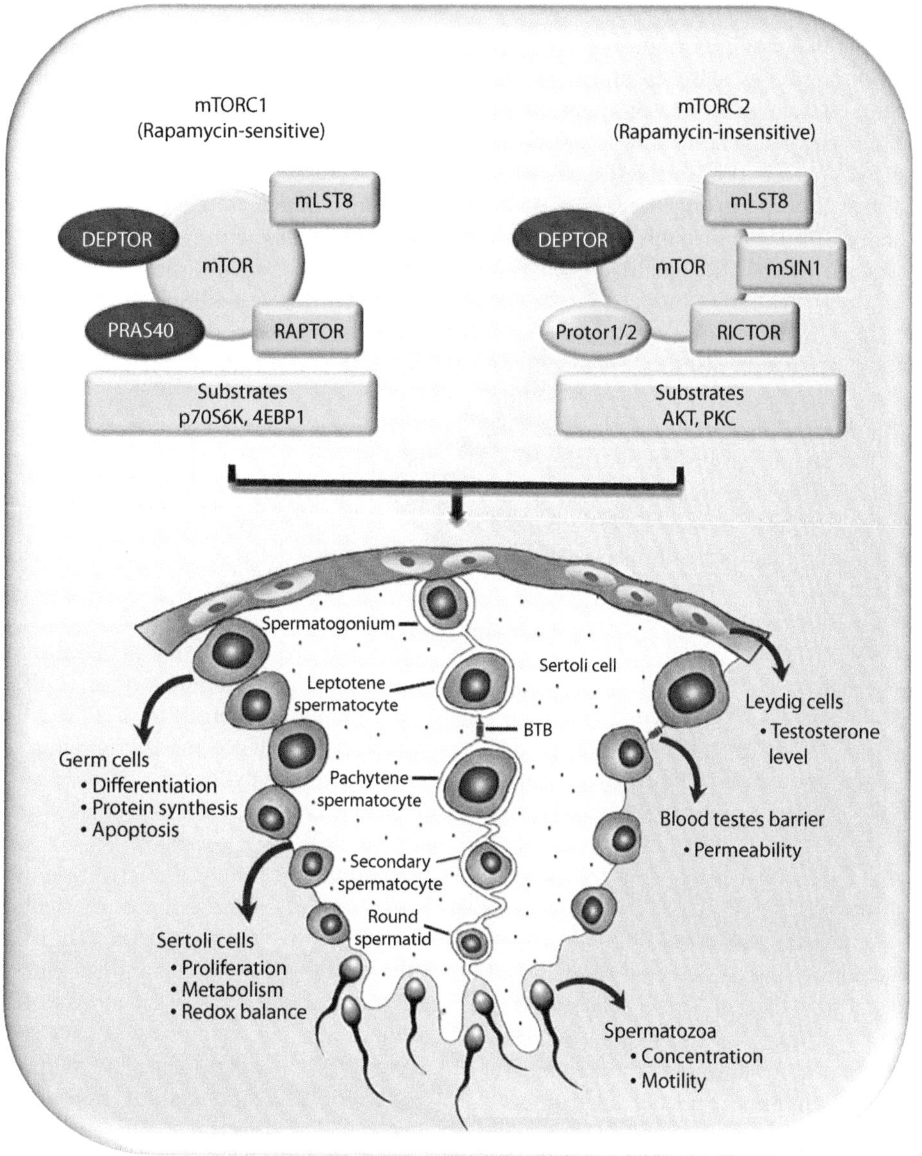

Figure 14.1 mTORC1 and mTORC2 subunits and the key steps of spermatogenesis regulated by mTOR signaling.

phosphorylation of mTOR downstream targets p70S6 K and rps6, but the phosphorylation level of 4e-bp1 remains unchanged (21). Furthermore, the inactivation of mTOR by rapamycin reduces the sperm count by inhibiting spermatogonial proliferation (21). Also, treating spermatogonia with specific PI3 K inhibitor LY294002 decreased the level of phosphorylated p70S6 K, rps6 and 4ebp1 and decreased the expression of mTOR (21). During postnatal testicular development, the undifferentiated spermatogonia display low mTORC1 activity, while the differentiated spermatogonia show high activity. In mutant mice with conditional deletion of spermatogonium-specific TSC1 (tuberous sclerosis 1, which negatively regulates mTORC1 activity), the hyperactivation of mTORC1 in undifferentiated spermatogonia accelerated their differentiation at the cost of germline maintenance and led to early germ cell depletion and impairment of spermatogenesis (18). P70S6 K is recognized as a downstream target of mTOR, phosphorylation

of which can facilitate the translation of mRNA and promotion of cell proliferation. In rapamycin-treated rats, p-p70S6 K and the ratio of p-p70S6 K/p70S6 K were much lower as compared with controls, resulting in the arrest of spermatogonial proliferation. However, the interruption of rapamycin treatment was able to induce recovery of spermatogenesis in the low-dose group (22). Retinoic acid is also shown to signal through the mTOR pathway for regulating the spermatogonial differentiation and stimulating the initiation of meiosis by controlling STRA8 (retinoic acid-stimulated gene 8) expression. Treatment with rapamycin inhibited the mTOR pathway that reduced retinoic acid-stimulated STRA8 expression and caused an accumulation of undifferentiated spermatogonia (19,23). In fact, mutant mice with Raptor (a component of mTORC1) knockout spermatogonia have accelerated differentiation of spermatogonia without self-renewing, resulting in total loss of germline by adulthood and complete infertility (24).

The Sertoli cell number plays an important role in deciding the sperm production capacity and in determining adult testicular size. Abnormal development and proliferation of Sertoli cells can impair spermatogenesis and/or cause the development of testicular cancer. Within the testes, estrogen regulates several aspects of spermatogenesis, like proliferation and differentiation, plausibly through the regulation of Sertoli cell proliferation via mTOR signaling. On treatment with rapamycin, the 17β-estradiol-induced Sertoli cell proliferation is decreased (25).

The vital involvement of Sertoli cells in spermatogenesis is also through the supply of nutrition to the developing germ cells and maintenance of the BTB for protection of advanced germ cells. The Sertoli cell polarity is also essential for the maintenance of normal spermatogenesis. It is believed that the cytoskeletal network maintains the Sertoli cells' polarity in the seminiferous epithelium. Several studies have established that the *in vitro* function of mTORC2 is in the regulation of actin dynamics. Sertoli cell–specific deletion of rictor (a component of mTORC2) in mice results in perturbed actin dynamics, leading to disrupted Sertoli cells polarity and spermatogenic arrest, accompanied with excessive germ cell loss (26,27). Thus, it can be concluded that altered mTOR signaling also results in disruption of Sertoli cell polarity and impaired spermatogenesis.

14.3.2 Role of mTOR signaling in blood-testes barrier

The Sertoli cells provide the essential microenvironment and signals for spermatogenesis. Adjacent Sertoli cells establish a BTB by specialized tight junctions and divide the seminiferous tubule into basal and adluminal compartments, which provides a unique immunoregulated environment to the developing germ cells. They also provide a structural framework for the differentiating germ cells to move from the basal to the adluminal compartment (28). Morphological segregation created by the BTB is crucial for spermatogenesis. Spermatogonia and preleptotene spermatocytes reside in the basal compartment and have unrestricted access to hormones, nutrients and biomolecules from the blood supply, unlike the more developed germ cells, which reside in the adluminal compartment across the BTB, that is sequestered from the systemic circulation (4). The BTB is composed of several integral membrane proteins that include tight junction (TJ) proteins (claudins, occludin, junctional adhesion molecules [JAMs], etc.), basal ectoplasmic specialization (basal ES, a testis-specific adherens junction or AJ), gap junction (GJ) and desmosome (DS), and is considered as one of the tightest BTBs. One of the TJ proteins, claudin-11, is precisely expressed in the Sertoli cells, and its knockdown leads to male infertility in mice due to the lack of BTB formation caused by inhibition of TJ strand formation between Sertoli cells (28–30). Despite the atypical tightness, the BTB go through extensive remodeling at the time of transit of preleptotene spermatocytes from the basal to the adluminal compartment. A new BTB is assembled behind the transiting

spermatocytes, and the old BTB (above the transiting spermatocyte) gets disassembled in a temporal fashion to avoid entry of harmful material into the adluminal compartment. The different types of junctions of BTB are connected with actin cytoskeleton, and the cyclic reorganization of the F-actin filament is regulated by different actin-regulating proteins such as actin-related protein 3 (Arp3) and epidermal growth factor pathway substrate 8 (Eps8). Studies have demonstrated that in addition to the actin-regulating proteins, several signaling pathways also play a crucial role in modulating the BTB function. A number of studies have identified that mTOR signaling is one among them, which plays a crucial role in the extensive reorganization of the F-actin network to assist BTB restructuring during spermatogenesis (30). A study has reported that mTOR is highly expressed in the seminiferous epithelium at the BTB to regulate the precisely coordinated events of BTB disassembly and assembly during the transport of preleptotene spermatocytes across the immunological barrier (4). Both the complexes of mTOR signaling, mTORC1 and mTORC2, possess antagonistic effects on BTB function, with mTORC1 exerting a disruptive function in contrast to mTORC2, which promotes BTB assembly (31). Hence, mTOR signaling complexes play a crucial role in BTB dynamics.

14.3.2.1 mTORC1 IN BTB

Several factors lead to the activation of mTORC1 signaling, such as cellular energy status, nutrients and growth factors, which involve PI3 K and Akt as upstream regulators and ribosomal protein S6 kinase (also known as p70 S6 K) as an activator of downstream effector molecule rpS6 (ribosomal protein S6) (30). Some studies have reported a crucial role of mTORC1 in spermatogenesis by promoting the restructuring of BTB and making it leaky (32). rps6 is highly expressed at all stages of the epithelial cycle during spermatogenesis in adult rat testes, and its expression is found to be consistent with its localization at the BTB. Phospho-rps6 (activated form of rps6) is highly expressed at the BTB and co-localized with BTB proteins ZO-1, N-cadherin and Arp3. Phosphorylation of rps6 was confined at the time of BTB restructuring to facilitate the transit of preleptotene spermatocytes and was restricted to late stages VIII–IX of the epithelial cycle. This stage-specific upregulation of activated rps6 (p-rps6) at the BTB suggests that p-rps6 induces the opening of BTB to transit preleptotene spermatocytes into the adluminal compartment. Knockdown of rpS6 by RNAi (using either rpS6-specific siRNA or shRNA), *in vitro* or *in vivo*, promoted the formation of BTB by making it tighter. Conversely, rpS6 phosphomimetic mutant p-rpS6 overexpression in cultured Sertoli cells with an established TJ barrier (mimicking the BTB *in vivo*) made the BTB leaky. The possible mechanisms explained were that the mutant p-rpS6 in Sertoli cells downregulates Akt1/2, which induces matrix metalloproteinase 9 (MMP-9) production by the Sertoli cells causing proteolysis of TJ and/or basal adhesion protein complexes, making the BTB leaky (32). Another mechanism explained (33,31) was through upregulation of p-rps6 causing downregulation of p-Akt1/2, which in turn increased association of Arp3 and its upstream activator N-WASP (neuronal Wiskott-Aldrich syndrome protein), resulting in actin nucleation at the barbed ends of a linear actin microfilament (i.e., branched actin polymerization). This reorganizes the actin filaments from a bundled to a branched/un-bundled network, thereby destabilizing cell adhesion protein complexes at the BTB (e.g., occluding, ZO-1, N-cadherin, α-catenin which utilize F-actin for attachment at the basal ES/BTB), making the BTB leaky (31,33). These studies are further supported by the study of Wen et al. on Sertoli cells with an established TJ-permeability barrier that mimicked the BTB. On treating these cells with Rapamycin, the mTORC1 complex function was blocked causing the barrier to become tighter (30). These studies highlighted that the mTORC1 signaling exerts its disruptive effects on BTB dynamics during spermatogenesis (Figure 14.2).

14.3.2.2 mTORC2 IN BTB

During the spermatogenic cycle, the expression of rictor (key binding partner of mTORC2) is higher at the BTB from stage I to stage VI. However, it gets downregulated from late-stage VII and becomes hardly detectable at stage IX. This stage-specific expression of rictor suggests that mTORC2 signaling plays a role in maintaining the BTB integrity during all stages of the epithelial cycle of spermatogenesis, excluding stages VIII–IX, when it is downregulated at the time of BTB restructuring. Several studies were performed to confirm the role of the mTORC2 complex in maintaining the integrity of the BTB. Rictor knockdown *in vivo* and *in vitro* disrupted the TJ barrier. Rictor knockdown with

RNAi *in vivo* disrupted the organization of F-actin at the ES and made the BTB leaky, while in Sertoli cells with established TJ-permeability barrier *in vitro*, rictor knockdown disrupted the N-cadherin–α-catenin and occludin-ZO-1 association (4). Furthermore, mice with Sertoli cell-specific deletion of Rictor showed infertility with defects in the cytoskeletal organization of Sertoli cells across the seminiferous epithelium. Lost cytoskeletal organization compromised the polarity of Sertoli cells and BTB function, resulting in spermatogenic arrest (34). Rictor knockdown obstructed the Sertoli cell junction-based channel communication suggesting that mTORC2 promotes BTB dynamics by exerting its effect through gap junctions or GJs (26). Germ cell apoptosis and infertility are also reported on conditional knockout of mTOR (Mtor[flox/flox]; Amhr2[cre/+]) in mice causing disorganization of seminiferous epithelium, redistribution of BTB gap junction protein-1 (GJA1) and Sertoli cell polarity loss (35). During spermatogenesis, the testes express almost a dozen GJ proteins, one of them is Connexin 43 (Cx43), also known as GJA1 (gap junction α-1 protein). Its expression in Sertoli cells is important for normal testicular development, spermatogenesis and fertility. Downregulated rictor, at the time of BTB remodelling, promotes endocytosis of TJ proteins and downregulation of GJ proteins to destabilize BTB for the transit of spermatocytes into the adluminal compartment (30). Further, in Sertoli cell–specific Cx43 (Connexin-43) knockout mice, spermatogonia fail to differentiate into spermatocytes to enter into meiosis, whereas the Sertoli cells fail to terminally differentiate to form functional BTB, thus hampering spermatogenesis (36). The role of mTORC2 in BTB dynamics is briefly highlighted in Figure 14.2.

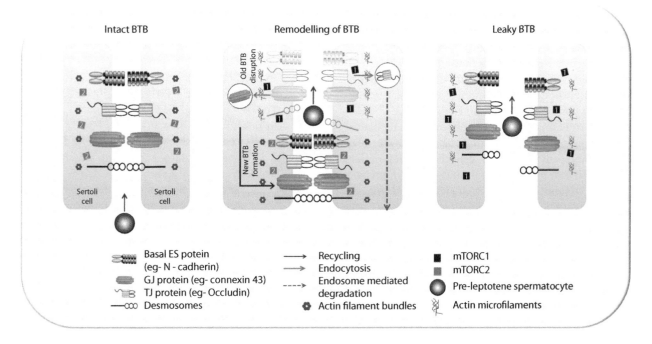

Figure 14.2 Two complexes mTORC1 and mTORC2 show antagonistic effects in disassembly and assembly (leaky and intact) of blood-testes barrier during transit of preleptotene spermatocyte.

14.4 CLINICAL EVIDENCE OF THE ROLE OF mTOR IN MALE FERTILITY

The role of the mTOR pathway in male reproductive function emerged when several clinical reports suggested that treatment with mTOR inhibitor sirolimus (also known as Rapamycin) is related to changes in sex hormone levels (lower testosterone, increased levels of luteinizing and follicle-stimulating hormones LH and FSH) and male infertility (37). Further studies also reported low sperm count (oligozoospermia), decreased sperm motility (asthenozoospermia), loss of sperm vitality and reduced percentage of normal sperm (38). A case study reporting sirolimus-associated infertility in a young male after heart-lung transplant provided the potential mechanism of sirolimus effects on spermatogenesis through mTOR and p70S6 kinase-mediated signaling pathways causing sexual hormone dysfunction, seminiferous tubule dystrophy and spermatogenesis blockade (39). Fortunately, the cessation of sirolimus treatment showed complete normalization of the sex hormones and sperm quality parameters (38–40).

14.5 CONCLUSION

The evidence presented in this chapter provides enough support to conclude that in the developing testes, mTOR signaling is an important molecular regulator of spermatogenesis. Essentially, mTOR signaling regulates three key processes of spermatogenesis, viz. SSC proliferation and differentiation, maintenance of Sertoli cell polarity and BTB dynamics. One of the primary functions of mTOR signaling is maintaining a balance between the SSCs' self-renewal and differentiation. This is an important step for the maintenance of male fertility and an endless supply of spermatozoa throughout the reproductive life. Aberrations in mTOR signaling may cause depletion of SSCs or their uncontrolled proliferation leading to testicular cancer. Highly polarized Sertoli cells that lie along the basement membrane and extend up to the lumen of the seminiferous tubule are dependent on their cytoskeletal network for maintaining the cell-polarity. Loss of Sertoli cell polarity has been shown to cause male infertility. mTOR signaling plays an important role in regulating actin organization for maintaining the Sertoli cell polarity. Furthermore, adjacent Sertoli cells form tight junctions called the BTB that provide an immunoprotective environment for the advanced germ cells, shielding them from the systemic circulation. Temporal opening and closing of the BTB ensures the safe passage of meiotic germ cells across the BTB, whose dynamics is regulated by contrasting effects of the two mTOR multiprotein complexes mTORC1 and mTORC2 that help in the disorganization and restructuring of the BTB, respectively. Future investigations of the mTOR pathway in testis may facilitate the development of improved treatments for male infertility, as well as pave the way for the development of novel male contraceptives, through pharmacological targeting of mTOR complexes using designed molecules.

REFERENCES

1. Sharma R, Agarwal A. Spermatogenesis: An overview. In: Zini A and Agarwal A (Eds.), *Sperm Chromatin.* New York, NY: Springer; 2011, pp. 19–44.
2. Sharma RK. Physiology of male gametogenesis. In: Falcone T and Hurd WW (Eds.), *Clinical Reproductive Medicine and Surgery.* 2007, pp73–83, Elsvier.
3. Carnevalli LS, Trumpp A. Tuning mTORC1 activity for balanced self-renewal and differentiation. *Dev Cell.* 2010 Aug 17;19(2):187–8.
4. Mok KW, Mruk DD, Cheng CY. Regulation of blood–testis barrier (BTB) dynamics during spermatogenesis via the "Yin" and "Yang" effects of mammalian target of rapamycin complex 1 (mTORC1) and mTORC2. *Int Rev Cell Mol Biol.* 2013a;301:291–358.
5. Jesus TT, Oliveira PF, Sousa M, Cheng CY, Alves MG. Mammalian target of rapamycin (mTOR): A central regulator of male fertility? 2017 May 4;52(3):235–53.
6. Zhou H, Huang S. The complexes of mammalian target of rapamycin. *Curr Protein Pept Sci.* 2010 Sep 1;11(6):409–24.
7. Watanabe R, Wei L, Huang J. mTOR signaling, function, novel inhibitors, and therapeutic targets. *J Nucl Med.* 2011 Apr 1;52(4):497–500.
8. Rahman A, Haugh JM. Kinetic modeling and analysis of the Akt/Mechanistic Target of Rapamycin Complex 1 (mTORC1) signaling axis reveals cooperative, feedforward regulation. *J Biol Chem.* 2017 Feb 17;292(7):2866–72.
9. Wiza C, Nascimento EB, Ouwens DM. Role of PRAS40 in Akt and mTOR signaling in health and disease. *Am J Physiol Endocrinol Metab.* 2012 Feb 21;302(12):E1453–60.
10. Wang Z, Zhong J, Inuzuka H, Gao D, Shaik S, Sarkar FH, Wei W. An evolving role for DEPTOR in tumor development and progression. *Neoplasia.* 2012 May 1;14(5):368–75.
11. Oh WJ, Jacinto E. mTOR complex 2 signaling and functions. *Cell cycle.* 2011 Jul 15;10(14):2305–16.
12. Yao CA, Ortiz-Vega S, Sun YY, Chien CT, Chuang JH, Lin Y. Association of mSin1 with mTORC2 Ras and Akt reveals a crucial domain on mSin1 involved in Akt phosphorylation. *Oncotarget.* 2017 Sep 8;8(38):63392.
13. Jacinto E, Loewith R, Schmidt A, Lin S, Rüegg MA, Hall A, Hall MN. Mammalian TOR complex 2 controls the actin cytoskeleton and is rapamycin insensitive. *Nat Cell Biol.* 2004 Nov;6(11):1122.
14. Blenis J. TOR, the gateway to cellular metabolism, cell growth, and disease. *Cell.* 2017 Sep 21;171(1):10–3.
15. Oliveira PF, Cheng CY, Alves MG. Emerging role for mammalian target of rapamycin in male fertility. *Trends Endocrinol Metab.* 2017 Mar 1;28(3):165–7.
16. Su KH, Dai C. mTORC1 senses stresses: Coupling stress to proteostasis. *BioEssays.* 2017 May;39(5):1600268.
17. Zarogoulidis P, Lampaki S, Turner JF, Huang H, Kakolyris S, Syrigos K. mTOR pathway: A current,

up-to-date mini-review (Review). *Oncol Lett.* 2014, 8: 2367–2370.

18. Wang C, Wang Z, Xiong E, Dai H, Zou Z, Jia C, Bai X, Chen Z. mTORC1 activation promotes spermatogonial differentiation and causes subfertility in mice. *Biol Reprod.* 2016 Nov 1;95(5).

19. Serra ND, Velte EK, Niedenberger BA, Kirsanov O, Geyer CB. Cell-autonomous requirement for mammalian target of rapamycin (Mtor) in spermatogonial proliferation and differentiation in the mouse. *Biol Reprod.* 2017 Apr 1;96(4):816–28.

20. Sahin P, Sahin Z, Gungor-Ordueri NE, Donmez BO, Celik-Ozenci C. Inhibition of mammalian target of rapamycin signaling pathway decreases retinoic acid stimulated gene 8 expression in adult mouse testis. *Fertil Steril.* 2014 Nov 1;102(5):1482–90.

21. Xu H, Shen L, Chen X, Ding Y, He J, Zhu J, Wang Y, Liu X. mTOR/P70S6 K promotes spermatogonia proliferation and spermatogenesis in Sprague Dawley rats. *Reprod Biomed Online.* 2016 Feb 1;32(2):207–17.

22. Liu S, Huang L, Geng Y, He J, Chen X, Xu H, Li R, Wang Y, Ding Y, Liu X. Rapamycin inhibits spermatogenesis by changing the autophagy status through suppressing mechanistic target of rapamycin-p70S6 kinase in male rats. *Mol Med Rep.* 2017 Oct 1;16(4):4029–37.

23. Busada JT, Niedenberger BA, Velte EK, Keiper BD, Geyer CB. Mammalian target of rapamycin complex 1 (mTORC1) Is required for mouse spermatogonial differentiation *in vivo. Dev Biol.* 2015 Nov 1;407(1):90–102.

24. Serra N, Velte EK, Niedenberger BA, Kirsanov O, Geyer CB. The mTORC1 component RPTOR is required for maintenance of the foundational spermatogonial stem cell pool in mice. *Biol Reprod.* 2018 Sep 10. doi: 10.1093/biolre/ioy198.

25. Yang WR, Wang Y, Wang Y, Zhang JJ, Zhang JH, Lu C, Wang XZ. mTOR is involved in 17β-estradiol-induced, cultured immature boar Sertoli cell proliferation via regulating the expression of SKP2, CCND1, and CCNE1. *Mol Reprod Dev.* 2015 Apr;82(4):305–14.

26. Dong H, Chen Z, Wang C, Xiong Z, Zhao W, Jia C, Lin J, Lin Y, Yuan W, Zhao AZ, Bai X. Rictor regulates spermatogenesis by controlling Sertoli cell cytoskeletal organization and cell polarity in the mouse testis. *Endocrinology.* 2015 Sep 11;156(11):4244–56.

27. Tanwar PS, Kaneko-Tarui T, Zhang L, Teixeira JM. Altered LKB1 /AMPK /TSC1 /TSC2 /mTOR signaling causes disruption of Sertoli cell polarity and spermatogenesis. *Hum Mol Genet.* 2012 Jul 12;21(20): 4394–405.

28. Mruk DD, Cheng CY. The mammalian blood-testis barrier: Its biology and regulation. *Endocr Rev.* 2015 Sep 10;36(5):564–91.

29. Cheng CY, Mruk DD. The blood-testis barrier and its implications for male contraception. *Pharmacol Rev.* 2012 Jan 1;64(1):16–64.

30. Wen Q, Tang EI, Gao Y, Jesus TT, Chu DS, Lee WM, Wong CK, Liu YX, Xiao X, Silvestrini B, Cheng CY. Signaling pathways regulating blood–tissue barriers—Lesson from the testis. *Biochim Biophys Acta Biomembr.* 2018 Jan;1860(1):141–53.

31. Mok KW, Chen H, Lee WM, Cheng CY. rpS6 regulates blood-testis barrier dynamics through Arp3-mediated actin microfilament organization in rat Sertoli cells. An *in vitro* study. *Endocrinology.* 2015 Feb 25;156(5):1900–13.

32. Mok KW, Mruk DD, Silvestrini B, Cheng CY. rpS6 regulates blood-testis barrier dynamics by affecting F-actin organization and protein recruitment. *Endocrinology.* 2012 Oct 1;153(10):5036–48.

33. Mok KW, Mruk DD, Cheng CY. rpS6 regulates blood–testis barrier dynamics through Akt-mediated effects on MMP-9. *J Cell Sci.* 2014 Nov 15;127(22):4870–82.

34. Mok KW, Mruk DD, Lee WM, Cheng CY. Rictor/mTORC2 regulates blood-testis barrier dynamics via its effects on gap junction communications and actin filament network. *FASEB J.* 2013b Mar;27(3):1137–52.

35. Boyer A, Girard M, Thimmanahalli DS, Levasseur A, Céleste C, Paquet M, Duggavathi R, Boerboom D. mTOR regulates gap junction α-1 protein trafficking in Sertoli cells and is required for the maintenance of spermatogenesis in mice. *Biol Reprod.* 2016 Jul 1;95(1):13.

36. Li N, Cheng CY. Mammalian target of rapamycin complex (mTOR) pathway modulates blood-testis barrier (BTB) function through F-actin organization and gap junction. *Histol Histopathol.* 2016 Sep;31(9):961.

37. Huyghe E, Zairi A, Nohra J, Kamar N, Plante P, Rostaing L. Gonadal impact of target of rapamycin inhibitors (sirolimus and everolimus) in male patients: An overview. *Transpl Int.* 2007 Apr;20(4):305–11.

38. Bererhi L, Flamant M, Martinez F, Karras A, Thervet E, Legendre C. Rapamycin-induced oligospermia. *Transplantation.* 2003 Sep 15;76(5):885–6.

39. Deutsch MA, Kaczmarek I, Huber S, Schmauss D, Beiras-Fernandez A, Schmoeckel M, Ochsenkuehn R, Meiser B, Mueller-Hoecker J, Bruno Reichart B. Sirolimus-associated infertility: Case report and literature review of possible mechanisms. *Am J Transplant.* 2007 Oct;7(10):2414–21.

40. Rovira J, Diekmann F, Ramírez-Bajo MJ, Banón-Maneus E, Moya-Rull D, Campistol JM. Sirolimus-associated testicular toxicity: Detrimental but reversible. *Transplantation.* 2012 May 15;93(9):874–9.

JAK-STAT pathway: Testicular development, spermatogenesis and fertility

POONAM MEHTA AND RAJENDER SINGH

HIGHLIGHTS

- The JAK-STAT pathway is an intracellular cell signaling cascade activated in response to the extracellular ligands and cell surface receptor interaction.
- Components of the JAK-STAT pathway have been identified in *Drosophila melanogaster*, *Caenorhabditis elegans*, slime molds and mammals.
- In mammals, it is known to regulate cellular development, proliferation, differentiation and apoptosis.
- In *Drosophila*, it is known to regulate segmentation, blood cell development, eye development, wing development, sex determination, spermatogenesis and oogenesis.
- During sexual development in *Drosophila*, Upd (Unpaired) acts as an X-linked signal element and regulates Sxl expression in females and also regulates male-specific cell division in germ cells through somatic support.
- For sustained spermatogenesis throughout the reproductive life, the germ stem cell population is maintained by JAK-STAT signaling.
- Sperm motility and the process of sperm capacitation are regulated by the levels of JAK-STAT pathway mediators, i.e., cytokines, in the human reproductive tract.

15.1 INTRODUCTION

JAK-STAT is a signal transduction cascade involving various intracellular, extracellular and intercellular key molecules regulating the process of transcription. This pathway is an excellent example of intercellular communication and

transcriptional control in eukaryotes, through which it regulates various biological responses. The JAK-STAT pathway is activated in response to a diverse range of ligands and signal progression through different classes of mediators, suggesting multiple functions of this pathway. Identification of a complete set of JAK-STAT in *Drosophila melanogaster* has facilitated functional studies. Murine knockout models, loss and gain of function mutations and overactivation studies defined the role of the JAK-STAT pathway in immune functions, cellular development, proliferation, differentiation, polarization and apoptosis (1–3). The various complex biological processes from embryonic development to aging are regulated by JAK-STAT signaling. Today, JAK-STAT is known to play a role in segmentation, blood cell development, eye development, wing development, sex determination, spermatogenesis and oogenesis (4,5). Irregularities in these processes are associated with disease development, including multiple myeloma, mycosis fungoides, myelogenous leukemia, SCID (severe combined immunodeficiency), myocardial hypertrophy and bronchial asthma (1).

The following are the sequential events of the cascade, also described schematically in Figure 15.1 (6):

1. Recognition of the extracellular or intercellular signaling molecule by the receptor complex
2. Dimerization of the receptor
3. Association of the JAK to the intracellular domain of the receptor
4. Autophosphorylation or transphosphorylation of JAK and phosphorylation of tyrosine residues of the intracellular domain of the receptor

5. Recognition of receptor's phosphorylated motifs by STAT (signal transducer and activator of transcription)
6. Phosphorylation of cytoplasmic STAT by JAK, resulting in homo- and heterodimerization of STATs
7. Translocation of STAT dimer to the nucleus
8. Action of STAT dimer as a transcription regulator

15.2 MODEL ORGANISMS FOR STUDYING THE JAK-STAT PATHWAY

The JAK-STAT pathway has been extensively studied in a wide range of organisms from slime molds to mammals. In mammals, it was originally identified through cytokine (IFNα, IFNγ) and growth factor–induced signaling (7) by which it regulates various cellular events such as cell proliferation, differentiation and apoptosis (1). The components of the JAK-STAT pathway have been identified in a wide range of organisms including *Drosophila melanogaster*, *Caenorhabditis elegans* and mammals. In mammals, there are more than 50 cytokine-like molecules that mediate JAK-STAT signaling. The diverse functions of this pathway in different cells are regulated by four JAK family members, i.e., JAK1, JAK2, JAK3 and TYK2, and seven STAT family members, i.e., STAT1, STAT2, STAT3. STAT4, STAT5a, STAT5b and STAT6 (8) (Table 15.1). Because of the

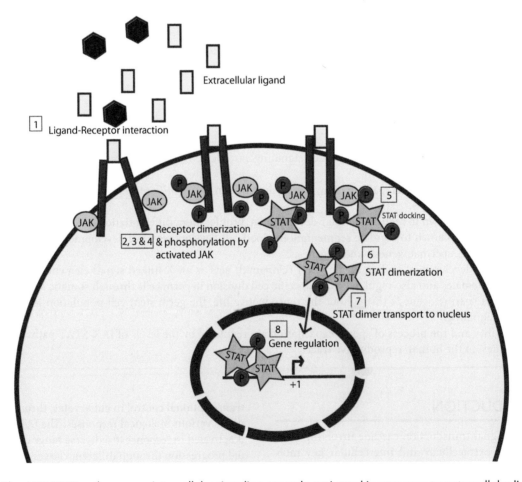

Figure 15.1 The JAK-STAT pathway—an intracellular signaling cascade activated in response to extracellular ligand.

Table 15.1 List of JAK-STAT pathway components known in mammals

Components	Members in mammals	References
Ligand	Interferons (IFNα, IFNγ), interleukins (IL-2, IL-4, IL-6, IL-7, IL-11, IL-9, IL-11, IL-15, etc.), Growth factors (IGFs), prolactin, erythropoietin, etc.	(10)
Receptor	gp130 receptor, gp140 receptor, growth hormone family receptor, IL-2 family receptor	(10,11)
JAK	JAK1, JAK2, JAK3, TYK2	(12)
STAT	STAT1, STAT2, STAT3, STAT4, STAT5a, STAT5b, STAT6	(13)
Negative regulators	SOCS, PIAS, PTPs	(14)

Abbreviations: IGF, insulin-like growth factor; PIAS, protein inhibitors of activated STAT; PTP, protein tyrosine phosphatase; SOCS, suppressors of cytokine signaling.

Table 15.2 List of JAK-STAT pathway components known in *Drosophila melanogaster*

Basic components	Known components in *D. melanogaster*	References
Ligand	Unpaired (upd), upd2, upd3	(16,17,18,19)
Receptor	Domeless	(20,21)
JAK	Hopscotch	(22)
STAT	STAT92E	(23,24)

numerous JAK and STAT homologues, study of the system is more complex (3,9).

Luckily, the *D. melanogaster* model system offers a simple system due to the ease of genetic manipulation. The downstream signaling molecules associated with the JAK-STAT pathway are present in a single copy and offer an easy understanding of the pathway. The complete system includes three ligands, a receptor, a JAK and a STAT (15) (Table 15.2).

15.3 COMPONENTS OF THE JAK-STAT PATHWAY

The key molecules involved are an extracellular ligand, a receptor molecule, Janus kinase (JAK), signal transducer and activator of transcription (STAT) and target regulatory sequence (25).

15.3.1 Ligand molecules

Ligand molecules are the extracellular molecules that cannot cross the membrane but through ligand-receptor interaction have the potential to activate an intracellular cell signaling

Table 15.3 List of known extracellular ligand molecules involved in the JAK-STAT pathway activation

Ligand family	Members
IFN family	IFNα, IFNγ, IL-10
gp130 family	IL-6, IL-11, IL-12, CNTF LIF, leptin
IL-2 family	IL-2, IL-4, IL-7, IL-9, IL-13, IL-15
gp140 family	IL-3, IL-5, GM-CSF
Growth hormone family	Erythropoietin, growth hormone, prolactin, thrombopoietin

Abbreviations: CNTF, ciliary neurotrophic factor; GM-CSF, granulocyte-macrophage colony stimulating factor; IFN, interferon; IL, interleukin; LIF, leukemia inhibitory factor.

cascade. Initially, the JAK-STAT pathway was discovered by interferon (IFN)-induced intracellular signaling. But later, a large number of cytokines, interferons and growth hormones were known to induce JAK-STAT signaling. In mammals, these ligand molecules are classified into various families depending on their structural and functional characteristics (10) (Table 15.3). In *Drosophila*, Upd is the only known ligand molecule for inducing JAK-STAT signaling. The unpaired gene encodes a 47 kDa secretory glycoprotein, localized to an extracellular matrix (ECM) (16). While curating a *Drosophila* database, other *Upd*-like genes have also been identified, such as *Upd2* (19) and *Upd3* (17).

15.3.2 Receptors

For transcending signal to the cell, a receptor complex interacts with an extracellular ligand. Cytokine signaling is known to be mediated by three receptor families: protein tyrosine kinase, nonreceptor protein tyrosine kinase and G-protein-coupled receptors (GPCRs) (10).

In JAK-STAT signaling, nonreceptor tyrosine kinase is the main class of receptors. These are single-membrane receptors with no intrinsic tyrosine kinase activity. Their intracellular cytoplasmic tails are associated with JAK, which gets phosphorylated on ligand binding and recruits STAT for further extending pathway function. In mammals, the subfamilies are gp130 family receptor, IL-2 family receptors, gp140 family receptors and growth hormone family receptors (10,11). In *Drosophila*, Domeless is the only known receptor that is encoded by the *Dome* gene (20) and also named as Master of Marelle (MOM) by another group (21). These nonreceptor tyrosine kinase receptors have a cytoplasmic membrane proximal domain through which they associate with tyrosine kinase-JAK (26). Domeless is a membrane-associated protein. Its extracellular domain consists of five fibronectin type III domains (FNIII). Out of these, two show similarity to the cytokine binding module of vertebrate cytokine receptor family I, which includes four conserved cysteine residues in the N-terminal domain and an incomplete WSXWS motif in the C-terminal domain (20) (Figure 15.2).

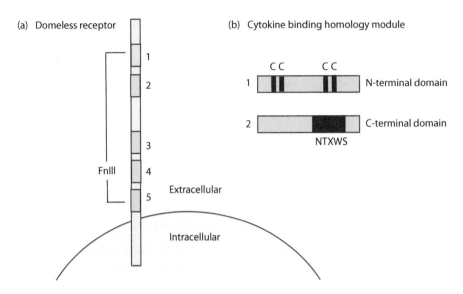

Figure 15.2 Domain structure of domeless receptor. **(a)** Extracellular domain consists of five fibronectin type III domains. **(b)** Cytokine binding module (CBM) consists of two fibronectin type III domains: an *N*-terminal consists of two pairs of cysteines and *C*-terminal has NTXWS motif.

15.3.3 Janus kinases

JAKs are a family of nonreceptor tyrosine kinase, with four homologues in mammals such as JAK1 (135 kDa), JAK2 (130 kDa), JAK3 (120 kDa) and TYK2 (140 kDa) (10,13), and only one homologue, i.e., hopscotch in *D. melanogaster* (22). In mammals, three members JAK1, JAK2 and JAK3 are present ubiquitously, and TYK2 has a restricted expression in hematopoietic cells only (12). In *D. melanogaster*, JAK was originally identified as a hopscotch locus, which plays an important role in embryonic segmentation. After identification of its domain structures, it is related to mammalian JAKs. It shows 27% homology to mammalian JAK2. Hopscotch encodes a protein of 1,177 amino acids, and similar to mammalian JAK, it is subdivided into FERN (band4.1/ezrin/radixin/moiesin) domain (JH4-JH7), SH2 (Src homology) domain (JH3) and protein kinase domains (JH1 and JH2) (Figure 15.3) (4,5,22). JAKs are associated with the intracellular cytoplasmic tail of the receptor through their FERN domain, but the exact binding interaction mechanism is not known. Different family members of JAK associate with different intracellular receptors (13) (Table 15.4).

Table 15.4 List of known Janus kinase family members along with associated receptor complex

Janus kinase	Receptor
JAK1	IFNα, IFNγ, IL-2 and IL-6 receptors
JAK2	Growth hormone receptor, erythropoietin receptor, prolactin receptor, IL-3 receptor, IL-5 receptor, granulocyte-macrophage colony stimulating factor receptor (GM-CSFR)
JAK3	IL-4, IL-7, IL-15, IL-21
TYK2	IFNα, IL-6, IL-10, IL-12, IL-23

Abbreviations: GM-CSFR, granulocyte-macrophage colony stimulating factor receptor; IFN, interferon; IL, interleukin.

15.3.4 Signal transducer for activation of transcription

STAT molecules are the transcription factors, which reside in the cytoplasm in an inactive form, and on activation, they dimerize and translocate to the nucleus (27, 28). In mammals, there are seven STAT family members, i.e., STAT1, STAT2,

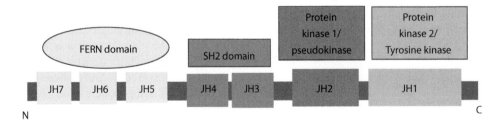

Figure 15.3 The domain structure of Janus kinase-hopscotch.

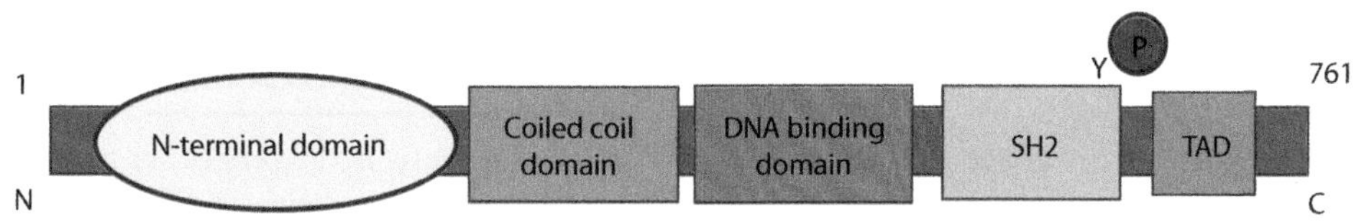

Figure 15.4 The domain structure of transcription factor-STAT92E.

Table 15.5 List of known mammalian STAT molecules along with their ligands

Mammalian STAT molecules	STAT activator
STAT1	IFN type I and IFN type II
STAT2	IFN type I
STAT3	IL-6, IL-11, IL-31, LIF, CNTF, IL-10, IL-19, IL-20, IL-21, IL-22, IL-24, IL-26, leptin, GCSF
STAT4	IL-12, IL-23
STAT5a, STAT5b	IL-3, IL-5, GM-CSF, GH, EPO, prolactin
STAT6	IL-4, IL-13

Abbreviations: CNTF, ciliary neurotrophic factor; EPO, Erythropoietin; GCSF, granulocyte colony stimulating factor; GH, Growth hormone; GM-CSF, granulocyte-macrophage colony stimulating factor; IFN, interferon; IL, interleukin; LIF, leukemia inhibitory factor.

STAT3, STAT4, STAT5a, STAT5b and STAT6. The STATs are known to include several domains—amino-terminal domain, coiled-coil domain, DNA binding domain, linker, SH2 domain, tyrosine activation domain and transcriptional activation domain (Figure 15.4) (4,13,15). This conserved SH2 domain mediates the interaction of STAT with phosphotyrosyl residue of JAK and receptor dimerization (29). The N-terminal domain is important for dimer-dimer interaction or tetramerization of STAT complex, which provides a stable complex for DNA binding (30). These different STAT molecules are known to be activated by different ligand molecules (Table 15.5), thus regulating different cellular functions (13).

In *Drosophila*, STAT homolog was identified and named as D-STAT with 33% identity to STAT5 and STAT6 and 25%–29% identity to other mammalian stats. D-STAT is also called as STAT92E because of its localization on salivary gland chromosome band 92E. The identified DNA binding sequence for STAT92E is TTCNNNGAA (24). Another group at the same time reported the same receptor molecule and called it marelle. They reported that marelle show 37% identity to mammalian STAT5 and is involved in regulating two developmental pathways in *Drosophila*, i.e., pair rule gene regulation and cell proliferation (23).

15.3.5 Regulators of the JAK-STAT pathway

For fine-tuning of the pathway, there are positive and negative regulators that exist in the vertebrate and invertebrate systems. Positive regulation involves the ligand molecules

(15), and negative regulation involves three basic mechanisms: dephosphorylation by protein tyrosine phosphatase (PTPs), STAT inhibition by protein inhibitors of activated STAT (PIAS) and negative feedback by suppressors of the cytokine signaling (SOCS) (14). As tyrosine phosphorylation is a central event in the pathway and activates the major players such as JAK and STAT, dephosphorylation of these positive regulators will have a negative effect on the pathway. The enzymes that are involved in dephosphorylation are called phosphatases. In mammals, the known tyrosine phosphatases are SHP1 (SH2 domain containing phosphatase), SHP2, protein tyrosine phosphatase B1 (PTPB1) and T-cell protein tyrosine phosphatase (TC-PTPs) (31). PIAS, as the name suggests, are the inhibitors of phosphorylated STAT. They constitute an E3 sumo ligase family and have four members present in mammals: PIAS1, PIASx, PIAS3 and PIASy (32). SOCS proteins suppress the JAK-STAT signaling pathway and generate a negative feedback loop in both mammals and *Drosophila* (33).

15.4 JAK-STAT SIGNALING IN GONAD DEVELOPMENT

Gonad development is an integrated process that involves a variety of signaling pathways, i.e., hedgehog, delta-notch, bone morphogenetic protein (BMP), platelet-derived growth factor (PDGF) and JAK-STAT signaling (4,34–37). In male gonads, from gonad formation and sexual identification to continuous sperm production and maturation, JAK-STAT signaling is involved (5,38–41). The functions of the JAK-STAT pathway in the male reproductive system studied in different model organisms are discussed in the following sections.

15.4.1 Germline sexual development in *Drosophila melanogaster*

There are two existing cell populations in *Drosophila* that include germline and somatic cells. How do these cells achieve sexual identity? In *Drosophila* somatic cells, male and female identity is defined by counting the ratio of X chromosome to an autosome, where an X/A ratio of 1 indicates normal female and X/A ratio of 0.5 indicates normal male (42). There is a double copy of X-linked signal elements (XSEs) in females as compared to males. These X-linked elements include sisterless-a (sis-a), scute (sis-b), runt (run) which encodes transcription factor and unpaired (sisterless-c) which encodes a secretory ligand (16,42). These double copies of XSEs are important for regulating the transcription

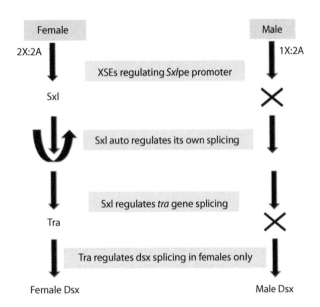

Figure 15.5 Representation of the hierarchy of splicing regulators in sexual development in *Drosophila melanogaster*.

of *Sxl* (sex-lethal) from Sxl-pe (promoter for the establishment) in females. The resultant protein from Sxl-pe regulates its own synthesis from Sxl-pm promoter (promoter for maintenance). Thus, Sex-lethal is turned on only in females. Sxl acts through a transformer (tra) and regulates splicing of doublesex RNA (dsx) in females. But in males, because Sxl is not present, default Splicing of dsx results in males (Figure 15.5). Another ligand, Upd, is considered to be a weak XSE because Upd and other downstream components, such as Hop and STAT92E, in mutational studies had little effect on Sxl expression in females (43–46).

Another role of Upd was identified through germline sex-determination studies. Wawersik et al. showed that the sex of the germline is dependent on the sex of the surrounding somatic tissue (38). Their experimental observations of the upregulation of STAT92E in male germ cells at the time of gonad formation and expression of Upd in the male somatic gonad indicates the male-specific activation of the JAK-STAT pathway. They also observed the upregulation of STAT92E in germ cells surrounding masculine soma (expressing dsx)—i.e., if XX germ cells are surrounded by masculine soma, they express STAT92E but if XY germ cells surround feminized soma, there was no expression of STAT92E. To address the masculine soma and germline association, they performed deletion studies of zygotic STAT92E and Upd mutant studies, resulting in the reduction of germ cell proliferation. This showed that JAK-STAT is required for male-specific cell division in the gonad (38). Thus, JAK-STAT expression is male specific, and female germ cells can be induced with Upd, resulting in male-specific gene expression in female germ cells. The JAK-STAT pathway is also known to maintain mgm1 (male germline marker 1) in male germ cells (38).

15.5 JAK-STAT PATHWAY AND SPERMATOGENESIS

Spermatogenesis is the process of production of spermatozoa from germline stem cells (46). Stem cells have a long-term capacity to divide and self-renew (47). For sustained spermatogenesis throughout the reproductive life, there should be regular maintenance and division of the stem cell population. In the testis, germline stem cells reside in a specialized microenvironment called niche that regulates the behavior of the stem cell population (48). Germline stem cells in the testis divide asymmetrically to produce two daughter cells: one retains stem cell characteristics and another differentiates and undergoes proliferation and development into mature sperm (48,49). To understand the importance of niche in the process of spermatogenesis, let us first understand the *Drosophila* stem cell niche.

15.5.1 *Drosophila* testis stem cell niche

Adult male *Drosophila* has two pairs of testis, each is tube-like, coiled and blunt ended. The testis is a production house for spermatozoa, and it contains all the developmental stages from stem cell to mature sperm. The existing population of stem cells includes germline stem cells (GSCs) and cyst stem cells (CysSCs), which are in close contact with compactly packed nondividing cells called hub (48). There are ~10–15 cells which constitute hub, located at the apical tip, both GSCs and CysSCs are anchored to hub cells in a 2:1 ratio, because two cyst cells surround one GSC. The process of spermatogenesis starts from germline stem cells, which divide asymmetrically resulting in two daughter cells. One daughter cell that remains in close proximity to the hub cells retains the characteristics of the germline stem cell, i.e., self-renews, and another daughter cell, which displaces away from the hub, differentiates and is called gonialblast (GB). The gonialblast undergoes four mitotic divisions and results in 16 primary spermatocytes that are interconnected through intercellular bridges. Further growth and two meiotic divisions result in 64 spermatids, which in the final stages of spermatogenesis undergo elongation and maturation and get stored in seminal vesicle (50, 51) (Figure 15.6). Each gonialblast is enveloped by the cyst cells, which only grow and do not divide and encase gonialblast throughout spermatogenesis (48). These cyst cells are the differentiated daughters of the cyst stem cell, which like GSCs can also self-renew (52–54). Is this self-renewal signal in both the populations coming from the niche environment, or do they coordinate and regulate each other for their renewal? These questions can be answered only if one understands the intercellular communication signals.

15.5.2 Intercellular communications

Cellular junctions and physical distance between the cells are important for intercellular communications or receiving signals. In *Drosophila* testis, three different populations

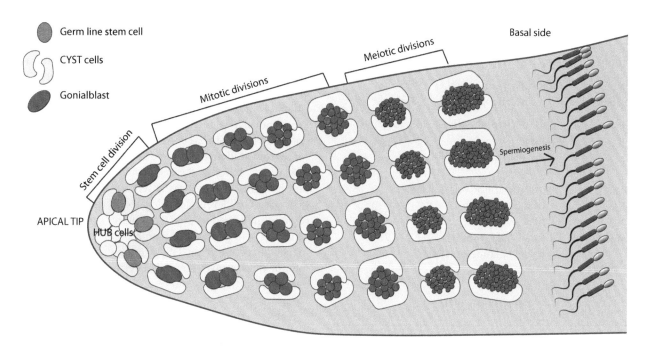

Figure 15.6 The *Drosophila* stem cell niche. At the apical tip near testis wall, hub cells (yellow) are localized. Hub cells are surrounded by germ line stem cells (brown) and cyst stem cells (blue). Stem cell division results in two populations, cells near the hub retain stem cell characteristics and distal cells become gonialblast (red) or cyst cell. Gonialblasts undergo further mitotic and meiotic divisions to give rise to spermatid population.

of stem cells are connected through cell adhesion molecules. As shown in Figure 15.6, the hub cells are located at the apical tip, near the testis wall and attached through integrins (55), and germline stem cells are in contact with hub cells by adherens junctions such as E-cadherin (56). Studies on their removal have suggested the importance of adhesion molecules in maintaining stem cell niche. Similarly, if one would talk about the physical distance, cells lying near the hub cells maintain stem cell characteristics, and those that move a little bit away from niche differentiate.

15.5.3 Role of JAK-STAT in maintenance of stem cell niche

In the stem cell niche environment, one cell influences the behavior of another through diffusible signaling molecules, which on receptor interaction initiates a cascade of events in the target cell. The JAK-STAT signaling pathway is known to maintain the stem cell population to ensure gamete production throughout the reproductive life. As previously described, the JAK-STAT pathway is well understood in *Drosophila* because of simple genetics offering a single copy of JAK-STAT components (57) and the availability of easy genetic tools (58). In the stem cell niche microenvironment of *Drosophila* testis, different cells communicate through ligand-receptor interaction. The hub cells secrete a ligand called Unpaired (Upd) (16), which is recognized by the receptor Domeless of germline stem cells or somatic stem cells lying in close proximity to the hub cells (20,21). This ligand-receptor interaction initiates a downstream signaling

cascade, which involves the activation of receptor-associated hopscotch (22), a homolog of JAK and a transcription activator STAT92E localized in the cytoplasm, which enters the nucleus to activate transcription of the target genes (23,24).

Drosophila hub cells are the source of Upd, which activates the JAK-STAT pathway in adjacent cells surrounding the hub (39). Depletion of Hop and Stat92E from the testis show complete loss of the stem cell population, while ectopic expression of Upd in testis apex resulted in stem cell population renewal. The loss of stem cell population can be suppressed with Hop mutation, which indicates that Upd and Hop work in a coordinated manner and have a role in stem cell renewal (39). STAT92E activation and STAT92E depletion studies suggested the role of JAK-STAT signaling is stem cell renewal (59). Further studies identified the molecular target of STAT92E in cyst stem cells, i.e., *Zfh1* (60) and chinmo (61). Another group contradicted the previous observations that CysSCs provide a signal for the maintenance of GSCs (62).

15.5.4 Integration of signaling pathways for stem cell maintenance

There is another candidate pathway for stem cell renewal such as the BMP signaling pathway, which is a major class of TGF-β pathway (36,63,64). The BMP pathway is discussed in other chapters in this book. The major players of the pathway are represented in Table 15.6.

These players act in a coordinated way to transduce the signal to gene response elements inside the nucleus. Here

Table 15.6 List of known components of the bone morphogenetic protein (BMP) signaling pathway in *Drosophila melanogaster*

Basic components	Identified components in *Drosophila*	References
Ligand	dpp (decapentaplegic) Screw gbb (glass bottom boat 60A)	(65,66,67,68)
Receptor	Type I-Tkv (thick veins), Sax (Saxophone) Type II-punt	(69,70)
Smad proteins	R-smad-Mad (Mothers of decapentaplegic) Co-smad-Medea Anti-smad-Dad (daughters against DPP)	(71,72,73)

the ligand-receptor interaction results in the phosphorylation of R-smad (receptor regulator class of smad) localized in the cell cytoplasm, which associates with Co-smad (common mediator class of smad). This signal-dependent association of R-smad and Co-smad translocates them to the nucleus to bind BMP gene response elements and regulate gene function (74). In *Drosophila*, the BMP pathway is known for stem cell maintenance and transit cell proliferation of differentiating cells in testis. In *Drosophila* testis, the ligands for BMP pathway are expressed in hub cells and somatic cyst cells that are in close association with GSCs. Gbb and Dpp are two different ligands that are known to mediate BMP signaling (36). To test the involvement of Gbb and Dpp in the maintenance of GSCs, their mutants were generated. In *Gbb* mutant testis, there was a loss of GSCs

population with no effect on cell proliferation, whereas *Dpp* mutations had little effect on GSC maintenance. Gbb/Dpp signaling activates pMAD, which on association with Co-smad, regulates responsive genes. The responsive gene of the Gbb/Dpp pathway includes anti-smad, i.e., *Dad*, which is a negative regulator of the Gbb/Dpp pathway, but the responsive genes that regulate GSCs maintenance are not known. Another cue regarding the pathway function came from studying another transcription factor, Bam (Bag of Marbles). In testis, *Bam* was transcribed only in differentiating germ cells and was absent in GSCs and gonialblast (63). Bam-GFP levels were elevated in the *Gbb* mutant and remain unaffected in the *Dpp* mutant, suggesting that Gbb signaling is important for Bam repression and Dpp signaling has little effect on GSCs' maintenance. Further *Bam* mutant studies have shown that germ cells have lost control over mitotic divisions and result in clusters with more than 16 germ cells (75).

These two pathways might be interconnected as they are regulating the same function. This interconnection was first identified by Leatherman and Dinardo (59). They found that STAT-depleted germline stem cells have a high accumulation of phospho-smad and BMP target gene *Dad,* which indicate strong BMP activation. These levels were higher as compared to the wild-type germ stem cells. The conclusion derived from these observations is that a higher level of STAT in CysSC may result in higher BMP ligand activation which then interacts with their receptors on GSCs. Similar observations were obtained from sustained Zfh1 expression—a STAT responsive gene in CysSCs. Therefore, Zfh1 might be an intermediary molecule interconnecting both pathways (59). On the basis of these studies, Figure 15.7 represents the current working model for interconnection between stem cell maintaining pathways.

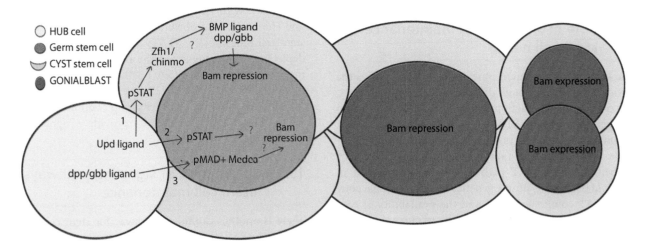

Figure 15.7 Integration of cell signaling pathways for stem cell maintenance in the *Drosophila* testis niche. HUB cells (yellow) secreting Upd ligand, which activates JAK-STAT signaling in cyst stem cell (blue) and germline stem cells (brown) (1) and (2), respectively. The target gene in cyst stem cells is *zfh1* and *chinmo*, which might act as intermediates and regulate BMP ligand expression in cyst stem cells, whereas the target in germ line stem cells is not known. BMP signaling pathway in germ line stem cells (3) is activated by BMP ligands either provided by the hub cells or cyst stem cells, which might repress Bam expression in germline stem cells, but the mechanism of repression is still unknown.

15.6 JAK-STAT PATHWAY IN HUMAN SPERM CAPACITATION

The JAK-STAT pathway and its family members have been extensively studied in the hematopoietic system and in embryonic development, but the identification of JAK-STAT members in human spermatozoa and its inducers in the human reproductive tract suggested a new role for the JAK-STAT pathway. However, JAK-STAT in sperm may not play a role in gene regulation, as sperm are transcriptionally and translationally inactive (76). Nevertheless, various sperm functions including sperm motility, capacitation and acrosome reaction are known to be mediated by hormones, cytokines and growth factors (41,77–80), where JAK-STAT could play a role.

In mammals, there are four JAK family members; out of these TYK2 (81), JAK1 (41) and JAK2 (80) were found in human spermatozoa. The phosphorylation of JAK proteins, in response to ligand-receptor interactions, induces the activation of STAT proteins. Initially, STAT1 and STAT4 were detected in human spermatozoa (81). Another study by Lachance and Leclerc also detected STAT3, STAT5 and STAT6 in human spermatozoa (76). The STAT proteins in addition to acting as transcription factors are known to interact with tubulin binding proteins, thus facilitating protein-protein interactions (82). However, the latter needs further exploration.

JAK-STAT signaling may be one of the many pathways that are required by sperm in acquiring the ability to fertilize the ovum. The process of capacitation involves various biochemical and physiological changes, which involve an increase in membrane fluidity, Ca^{2+} concentration and protein tyrosine phosphorylation (83). Since both capacitation and the JAK-STAT pathway involve an increase in protein tyrosine phosphorylation, the extent of protein tyrosine phosphorylation of JAK and STAT proteins of capacitated spermatozoa in response to various cytokines was assessed. It was found that STAT1 and STAT4 in human spermatozoa undergo tyrosine phosphorylation in response to interferons (IFNα and IFNγ) and interleukin-12 (IL-12) (81). These results supported the existence of the JAK-STAT pathway in human spermatozoa.

The process of capacitation takes place in the female reproductive tract, which must be triggered by molecules present in the female reproductive tract (84). IL-6, an endometrial secretion, is a well-investigated cytokine, inducing capacitation (41). IL-6 concentration is found to be higher in preovulatory periods than in the luteal phase (85), and both JAK1 and Tyk2 are known to be activated in the presence of IL-6 (86). Localization studies showing the IL-6 receptor in the tail region (41), which also has JAK2 (80), suggests JAK2 tyrosine phosphorylation. This was also supported by *in vitro* capacitation experiments showing maximum tyrosine phosphorylation in the tail region (80).

Progesterone is another inducer of capacitation (87), which is also known to activate JAK-STAT signaling in human spermatozoa (80). Progesterone induces the phosphorylation of JAK1/2 and STAT1 (80) and dephosphorylation of STAT4 (81). Progesterone is also known to increase calcium influx, which is a rapid response to progesterone exposure, and a delayed response includes tyrosine phosphorylation. Thus, the JAK-STAT pathway seems to be a late-acting pathway in progesterone signaling (80). How progesterone activates the pathway remains unknown. Nevertheless, the presence of JAK-STAT components in spermatozoa gave a clue about the functions of the JAK-STAT pathway beyond transcriptional activation.

15.7 JAK-STAT PATHWAY IN SPERM MOTILITY

The cytokines are present in the human reproductive tract (88) and are known activators of JAK-STAT signaling (6), but their exact mechanism of action remains unknown. There are some cytokines that are known to affect sperm motility.

Leptin: Leptin is a 16 kDa peptide hormone that is encoded by *ob* gene and is recognized by OB-R leptin receptor. Due to the homology of leptin with cytokine type I family members and OB-R receptor with cytokine family I receptors, they are also known to activate JAK-STAT signaling inside the cell (89). The identification of leptin in human seminal plasma and leptin receptor on the tail of human spermatozoa suggested their role in sperm function (90). Initial studies by Glander et al. (2002) have shown a negative correlation of seminal plasma leptin with sperm motility (91). The negative correlation between leptin levels and sperm motility was further supported by a study on asthenozoospermic patients, which have a higher level of seminal leptin as compared to the control group (92). In contrast to these studies, Lampiao and Plessis showed that leptin enhances sperm motility alone and in combination with insulin after 1 hour of incubation (93). The exact mechanism of Leptin action on human spermatozoa remains unknown, and further studies are required to figure out the exact effect of leptin on sperm motility.

Cytokines: Human spermatozoa were incubated in the presence of IFNγ and TNFα, which had a negative effect on sperm viability and motility (78). Similarly, IGF-I (insulin growth factor I) also reduced sperm motility parameters, i.e., curvilinear velocity and amplitude of lateral head movement (79). The role of IGF-I signaling in spermatogenesis and male infertility is discussed in detail in Chapter 6. A lot remains to be understood about the role of cytokines on sperm motility and to find if their effects are mediated by the JAK-STAT pathway.

15.8 CONCLUSIONS AND FUTURE DIRECTIONS

The major studies available on JAK-STAT signaling in mammals and *Drosophila* have helped in understanding the molecular details of how ligands promote their effect on the target cells. Considering both the model organisms, it can be concluded that the JAK-STAT pathway plays various roles from sexual development to the maturation of gametes to achieve fertilization competence. The JAK-STAT pathway regulates sexual development and germline stem cell maintenance in *Drosophila*. The presence of JAK-STAT components in spermatozoa and the presence of cytokines in the male reproductive tract suggest a major role in sperm functions. The involvement of cytokines such as IFNs and IGF-1 in reducing sperm motility has been studied, but their exact mechanisms of action remain unknown. Similarly, contradicting findings are available on correlation between the leptin levels and sperm motility. The levels of these cytokines in the male reproductive tract could help in developing male infertility markers and in developing ways to treat male infertility.

Progesterone is a known inducer of capacitation, and the JAK-STAT pathway components such as JAK1/2 and STAT1 are present in human spermatozoa. Because of the availability of fewer studies, it is hard to conclude that increased tyrosine phosphorylation during capacitation is because of the JAK-STAT pathway only. Further, the effects of phosphorylated STATs on human spermatozoa remain unknown. Their presence in spermatozoa gave a new direction toward understanding other functions of STAT molecules in regulating male fertility. There is not much data available to directly connect JAK-STAT signaling functions to spermatozoal functions and fertility. Since this is a major pathway mediated by cytokines, which are more related to immune functions, most of the knockouts for JAK-STAT components were lethal or had immune problems. Hence, they could not help in understanding the tissue-specific role of these cytokines. There are no studies that can link the levels of cytokines, impairment of STAT functions or polymorphisms to infertility.

Studies on the germline stem cell maintenance helped in further exploration of other target stem cell niche maintained by the JAK-STAT pathway, such as intestinal, hematopoietic and neuronal niche in *Drosophila* and only hematopoietic and neuronal systems in mammals (94). Thus, the JAK-STAT pathway regulates different stem cell populations, and further exploration of a mammalian niche would help in the advancement of mammalian stem cell technology. The role of JAK-STAT signaling in post-implantation development is evident through knockout studies. The absence of its components manifests their role in neuronal, cardiac and hematopoietic lineage defects. In germline development, PGCs are the precursors to adult germ cells and gametes. *In vitro* experiments have shown that PGCs can be induced in the presence of LIF, BMP8b, EGF and SCF (stem cell factor), but no *in vivo* study has been undertaken to prove the role of JAK-STAT in the germline development (95). Nonetheless, the JAK-STAT pathway is not a solo player here. This works in a complex integration with other signaling pathways. The understanding of this molecular web would help in better projecting the role of this pathway and other key players in spermatogenesis and male fertility.

ACKNOWLEDGMENTS

Poonam Mehta would like to thank the University Grants Commission (UGC) for graduate fellowship. The authors are thankful to the CSIR-CDRI for providing institutional support.

REFERENCES

1. Igaz P, Toth S, Falus A. Biological and clinical significance of the JAK-STAT pathway; lessons from knockout mice. *Inflamm Res.* 2001 Sep 1;50(9):435–41.
2. Schindler CW. Series introduction: JAK-STAT signalling in human disease. *J Clin Invest.* 2002 May 1;109(9):1133–7.
3. O'Shea JJ, Gadina M, Schreiber RD. Cytokine signalling in 2002: New surprises in the JAK/STAT pathway. *Cell.* 2002 Apr 19;109(2): S121–31.
4. Luo H, Dearolf CR. The JAK/STAT pathway and *Drosophila* development. *BioEssays.* 2001 Dec;23(12):1138–47.
5. Hombría JC, Brown S. The fertile field of *Drosophila* JAK/STAT signalling. *Curr Biol.* 2002 Aug 20;12(16):R569–75.
6. Schindler C, Darnell Jr JE. Transcriptional responses to polypeptide ligands: The JAK-STAT pathway. *Annu Rev Biochem.* 1995 Jul;64(1):621–52.
7. Darnell JE, Kerr IM, Stark GR. Jak-STAT pathways and transcriptional activation in response to IFNs and other extracellular signalling proteins. *Science.* 1994 Jun 3;264(5164):1415–21.
8. Schindler C, Plumlee C. Inteferons pen the JAK–STAT pathway. In: Watson CJ, Brown S (Eds). *Seminars in Cell and Developmental Biology* (Vol. 19, No. 4). New York, NY: Academic Press; 2008 Aug 1, pp. 311–8.
9. Rawlings JS, Rosler KM, Harrison DA. The JAK/STAT signalling pathway. *J Cell Sci.* 2004 Mar 15;117(8):1281–3.
10. Heim MH. The JAK-STAT pathway: Cytokine signalling from the receptor to the nucleus. *J Recept Signal Transduct Res.* 1999 Jan 1;19(1–4):75–120.
11. Taniguchi T. Cytokine signalling through nonreceptor protein tyrosine kinases. *Science.* 1995 Apr 14;268(5208):251–5.
12. Yeh TC, Pellegrini S. The Janus kinase family of protein tyrosine kinases and their role in signalling. *Cell Mol Life Sci.* 1999 Sep 1;55(12):1523 34.
13. Schindler C, Levy DE, Decker T. JAK-STAT signalling: From interferons to cytokines. *J Biol Chem.* 2007 Jul 13;282(28):20059–63.
14. Greenhalgh CJ, Hilton DJ. Negative regulation of cytokine signalling. *J Leukoc Biol.* 2001 Sep 1;70(3):348–56.
15. Arbouzova NI, Zeidler MP. JAK/STAT signalling in *Drosophila*: Insights into conserved regulatory and cellular functions. *Development.* 2006 Jul 15;133(14):2605–16.

16. Harrison DA, McCoon PE, Binari R, Gilman M, Perrimon N. *Drosophila* unpaired encodes a secreted protein that activates the JAK signalling pathway. *Genes Dev.* 1998 Oct 15;12(20):3252–63.

17. Agaisse H, Petersen UM, Boutros M, Mathey-Prevot B, Perrimon N. Signalling role of hemocytes in *Drosophila* JAK/STAT-dependent response to septic injury. *Dev Cell.* 2003 Sep 1;5(3):441–50.

18. Gilbert MM, Weaver BK, Gergen JP, Reich NC. A novel functional activator of the *Drosophila* JAK/STAT pathway, unpaired 2, is revealed by an *in vivo* reporter of pathway activation. *Mech Dev.* 2005 Jul 1;122(7–8):939–48.

19. Hombría JC, Brown S, Häder S, Zeidler MP. Characterisation of Upd2, a *Drosophila* JAK/STAT pathway ligand. *Dev Biol.* 2005 Dec 15;288(2):420–33.

20. Brown S, Hu N, Hombría JC. Identification of the first invertebrate interleukin JAK/STAT receptor, the *Drosophila* gene domeless. *Curr Biol.* 2001 Oct 30;11(21):1700–5.

21. Chen HW, Chen X, Oh SW, Marinissen MJ, Gutkind JS, Hou SX. mom identifies a receptor for the *Drosophila* JAK/STAT signal transduction pathway and encodes a protein distantly related to the mammalian cytokine receptor family. *Genes Dev.* 2002 Feb 1;16(3):388–98.

22. Binari R, Perrimon N. Stripe-specific regulation of pair-rule genes by hopscotch, a putative Jak family tyrosine kinase in *Drosophila*. *Genes Dev.* 1994 Feb 1;8(3):300–12.

23. Hou XS, Melnick MB, Perrimon N. Marelle acts downstream of the *Drosophila* HOP/JAK kinase and encodes a protein similar to the mammalian STATs. *Cell.* 1996 Feb 9;84(3):411–9.

24. Yan R, Small S, Desplan C, Dearolf CR, Darnell Jr JE. Identification of a Stat gene that functions in *Drosophila* development. *Cell.* 1996 Feb 9;84(3):421–30.

25. Aaronson DS, Horvath CM. A road map for those who don't know JAK-STAT. *Science.* 2002 May 31;296(5573):1653–5.

26. Hirano T, Nakajima K, Hibi M. Signalling mechanisms through gp130: A model of the cytokine system. *Cytokine Growth Factor Rev.* 1997 Dec 1;8(4):241–52.

27. Darnell JE. STATs and gene regulation. *Science.* 1997 Sep 12;277(5332):1630–5.

28. Decker T, Kovarik P. Transcription factor activity of STAT proteins: Structural requirements and regulation by phosphorylation and interacting proteins. *Cell Mol Life Sci.* 1999 Sep 1;55(12):1535–46.

29. Gupta S, Yan H, Wong LH, Ralph S, Krolewski J, Schindler C. The SH2 domains of Stat1 and Stat2 mediate multiple interactions in the transduction of IFN-α signals. *EMBO J.* 1996 Mar;15(5):1075–84.

30. Vinkemeier U, Cohen SL, Moarefi I, Chait BT, Kuriyan J, Darnell Jr JE. DNA binding of *in vitro* activated Stat1 α, Stat1 β and truncated Stat1: Interaction between NH2-terminal domains stabilizes binding of two dimers to tandem DNA sites. *EMBO J.* 1996 Oct;15(20):5616–26.

31. Xu D, Qu CK. Protein tyrosine phosphatases in the JAK/STAT pathway. *Front Biosci.* 2008 May 1; 13:4925.

32. Kiu H, Nicholson SE. Biology and significance of the JAK/STAT signalling pathways. *Growth Factors.* 2012 Apr 1;30(2):88–106.

33. Kile BT, Alexander WS. The suppressors of cytokine signalling (SOCS). *Cell Mol Life Sci.* 2001 Oct 1;58(11):1627–35.

34. Zhang Y, Kalderon D. Hedgehog acts as a somatic stem cell factor in the *Drosophila* ovary. *Nature.* 2001 Mar;410(6828):599.

35. López-Schier H, Johnston DS. Delta signalling from the germ line controls the proliferation and differentiation of the somatic follicle cells during *Drosophila* oogenesis. *Genes Dev.* 2001 Jun 1;15(11):1393–405.

36. Kawase E, Wong MD, Ding BC, Xie T. Gbb/Bmp signalling is essential for maintaining germline stem cells and for repressing bam transcription in the *Drosophila* testis. *Development.* 2004 Mar 15;131(6):1365–75.

37. Duchek P, Somogyi K, Jékely G, Beccari S, Rørth P. Guidance of cell migration by the *Drosophila* PDGF/VEGF receptor. *Cell.* 2001 Oct 5;107(1):17–26.

38. Wawersik M, Milutinovich A, Casper AL, Matunis E, Williams B, Van Doren M. Somatic control of germline sexual development is mediated by the JAK/STAT pathway. *Nature.* 2005 Jul;436(7050):563.

39. Tulina N, Matunis E. Control of stem cell self-renewal in *Drosophila* spermatogenesis by JAK-STAT signalling. *Science.* 2001 Dec 21;294(5551):2546–9.

40. Kiger AA, Jones DL, Schulz C, Rogers MB, Fuller MT. Stem cell self-renewal specified by JAK-STAT activation in response to a support cell cue. *Science.* 2001 Dec 21;294(5551):2542–5.

41. Laflamme J, Akoum A, Leclerc P. Induction of human sperm capacitation and protein tyrosine phosphorylation by endometrial cells and interleukin-6. *Mol Hum Reprod.* 2005 Feb 1;11(2):141–50.

42. Cline and TW, Meyer BJ. Vive la difference: Males vs females in flies vs worms. *Annu Rev Genet.* 1996 Dec;30(1):637–702.

43. Jinks TM, Polydorides AD, Calhoun G, Schedl P. The JAK/STAT signalling pathway is required for the initial choice of sexual identity in *Drosophila melanogaster*. *Mol Cell.* 2000 Mar 1;5(3):581–7.

44. Zeidler MP, Perrimon N. Sex determination: Co-opted signals determine gender. *Curr Biol.* 2000 Sep 14;10(18):R682–4.

45. Avila FW, Erickson JW. *Drosophila* JAK/STAT pathway reveals distinct initiation and reinforcement steps in early transcription of Sxl. *Curr Biol.* 2007 Apr 3;17(7):643–8.

46. Spradling A, Fuller MT, Braun RE, Yoshida S. Germline stem cells. *Cold Spring Harbor Perspect Biol.* 2011 Jul 26:a002642.

47. Takahashi K, Tanabe K, Ohnuki M, Narita M, Ichisaka T, Tomoda K, Yamanaka S. Induction of pluripotent stem cells from adult human fibroblasts by defined factors. *Cell.* 2007 Nov 30;131(5):861–72.

48. Hardy RW, Tokuyasu KT, Lindsley DL, Garavito M. The germinal proliferation center in the testis of *Drosophila melanogaster*. *J Ultrastruct Res*. 1979 Nov 1;69(2):180–90.

49. Yamashita YM, Mahowald AP, Perlin JR, Fuller MT. Asymmetric inheritance of mother versus daughter centrosome in stem cell division. *Science*. 2007 Jan 26;315(5811):518–21.

50. Fuller M. Spermatogenesis. In: Bate M, Arias AM (Eds), *The Development of Drosophila*. Cold Spring Harbor, NY: Cold Spring press;1993:71–147.

51. Demarco RS, Eikenes ÅH, Haglund K, Jones DL. Investigating spermatogenesis in *Drosophila melanogaster*. *Methods*. 2014 Jun 15;68(1):218–27.

52. Michel M, Kupinski AP, Raabe I, Bökel C. Hh signalling is essential for somatic stem cell maintenance in the *Drosophila* testis niche. *Development*. 2012 Aug 1;139(15):2663–9.

53. Amoyel M, Sanny J, Burel M, Bach EA. Hedgehog is required for CySC self-renewal but does not contribute to the GSC niche in the *Drosophila* testis. *Development*. 2013 Jan 1;140(1):56–65.

54. Zhang Z, Lv X, Jiang J, Zhang L, Zhao Y. Dual roles of Hh signalling in the regulation of somatic stem cell self-renewal and germline stem cell maintenance in *Drosophila* testis. *Cell Res*. 2013 Apr;23(4):573.

55. Tanentzapf G, Devenport D, Godt D, Brown NH. Integrin-dependent anchoring of a stem-cell niche. *Nat Cell Biol*. 2007 Dec;9(12):1413.

56. Voog J, D'Alterio C, Jones DL. Multipotent somatic stem cells contribute to the stem cell niche in the *Drosophila* testis. *Nature*. 2008 Aug;454(7208):1132.

57. Bausek N. JAK-STAT signalling in stem cells and their niches in *Drosophila*. *JAKSTAT*. 2013 Jul 15;2(3):e25686.

58. Tolwinski NS. Introduction: *Drosophila*—A model system for developmental biology. *J Dev biol*. 2017;5(3):9.

59. Leatherman JL, DiNardo S. Germline self-renewal requires cyst stem cells and stat regulates niche adhesion in *Drosophila* testes. *Nat Cell Biol*. 2010 Aug;12(8):806.

60. Leatherman JL, DiNardo S. Zfh-1 controls somatic stem cell self-renewal in the *Drosophila* testis and nonautonomously influences germline stem cell self-renewal. *Cell Stem Cell*. 2008 Jul 3;3(1):44–54.

61. Flaherty MS, Salis P, Evans CJ, Ekas LA, Marouf A, Zavadil J, Banerjee U, Bach EA. chinmo is a functional effector of the JAK/STAT pathway that regulates eye development, tumor formation, and stem cell self-renewal in *Drosophila*. *Dev Cell*. 2010 Apr 20;18(4):556–68.

62. Lim JG, Fuller MT. Somatic cell lineage is required for differentiation and not maintenance of germline stem cells in *Drosophila* testes. *Proc Natl Acad Sci USA*. 2012 Oct 18:201215516.

63. Shivdasani AA, Ingham PW. Regulation of stem cell maintenance and transit amplifying cell proliferation by TGF-β signalling in *Drosophila* spermatogenesis. *Curr Biol*. 2003 Dec 2;13(23):2065–72.

64. Schulz C, Kiger AA, Tazuke SI, Yamashita YM, Pantalena-Filho LC, Jones DL, Wood CG, Fuller MT. A misexpression screen reveals effects of bag-of-marbles and TGFβ class signalling on the *Drosophila* male germ-line stem cell lineage. *Genetics*. 2004 Jun 1;167(2):707–23.

65. Spencer FA, Hoffmann FM, Gelbart WM. Decapentaplegic: A gene complex affecting morphogenesis in *Drosophila melanogaster*. *Cell*. 1982 Mar 1;28(3):451–61.

66. Arora K, Levine MS, O'Connor MB. The screw gene encodes a ubiquitously expressed member of the TGF-β family required for specification of dorsal cell fates in the *Drosophila* embryo. *Genes Dev*. 1994 Nov 1;8(21):2588–601.

67. Wharton KA, Thomsen GH, Gelbart WM. *Drosophila* 60A gene, another transforming growth factor β family member, is closely related to human bone morphogenetic proteins. *Proc Natl Acad Sci USA*. 1991 Oct 15;88(20):9214–8.

68. Doctor JS, Jackson PD, Rashka KE, Visalli M, Hoffman FM. Sequence, biochemical characterization, and developmental expression of a new member of the TGF-β superfamily in *Drosophila melanogaster*. *Dev Biol*. 1992 Jun 1;151(2):491–505.

69. Brummel TJ, Twombly V, Marques G, Wrana JL, Newfeld SJ, Attisano L, Massagué J, O'Connor MB, Gelbart WM. Characterization and relationship of Dpp receptors encoded by the saxophone and thick veins genes in *Drosophila*. *Cell*. 1994 Jul 29;78(2):251–61.

70. Letsou A, Arora K, Wrana JL, Simin K, Twombly V, Jamal J et al. *Drosophila* Dpp signalling is mediated by the punt gene product: A dual ligand-binding type II receptor of the TGFβ receptor family. *Cell*. 1995 Mar 24;80(6):899–908.

71. Sekelsky JJ, Newfeld SJ, Raftery LA, Chartoff EH, Gelbart WM. Genetic characterization and cloning of mothers against dpp, a gene required for decapentaplegic function in *Drosophila melanogaster*. *Genetics*. 1995 Mar 1;139(3):1347–58.

72. Tsuneizumi K, Nakayama T, Kamoshida Y, Kornberg TB, Christian JL, Tabata T. Daughters against dpp modulates dpp organizing activity in *Drosophila* wing development. *Nature*. 1997 Oct;389(6651):627.

73. Wisotzkey RG, Mehra A, Sutherland DJ, Dobens LL, Liu X, Dohrmann C, Attisano L, Raftery LA. Medea is a *Drosophila* Smad4 homolog that is differentially required to potentiate DPP responses. *Development*. 1998 Apr 15;125(8):1433–45.

74. Raftery LA, Sutherland DJ. TGF-β family signal transduction in Drosophila development: From Mad to Smads. *Dev Biol*. 1999 Jun 15;210(2):251–68.

75. Gonczy P, Matunis E, DiNardo S. bag-of-marbles and benign gonial cell neoplasm act in the germline to restrict proliferation during *Drosophila* spermatogenesis. *Development*. 1997 Nov 1;124(21):4361–71.

76. Lachance C, Leclerc P. Mediators of the Jak/STAT signalling pathway in human spermatozoa. *Biol Reprod*. 2011 Dec 1;85(6):1222–31.

77. Naz RK, Kaplan P. Interleukin-6 enhances the fertilizing capacity of human sperm by increasing capacitation and acrosome reaction. *J Androl*. 1994 May 6;15(3):228–33.

78. Estrada LS, Champion HC, Wang R, Rajasekaran M, Hellstrom WJ, Aggarwal B, Sikka SC. Effect of tumour necrosis factor-α (TNF-α) and interferon-γ (IFN-γ) on human sperm motility, viability and motion parameters. *Int J Androl*. 1997 Aug;20(4):237–42.

79. Miao ZR, Lin TK, Bongso TA, Zhou X, Cohen P, Lee KO. Effect of insulin-like growth factors (IGFs) and IGF-binding proteins on *in vitro* sperm motility. *Clin Endocrinol*. 1998 Aug;49(2):235–9.

80. Sagare-Patil V, Modi D. Progesterone activates Janus Kinase 1/2 and activators of transcription 1 (JAK1-2/STAT1) pathway in human spermatozoa. *Andrologia*. 2013 Jun 1;45(3):178–86.

81. D'Cruz OJ, Vassilev AO, Uckun FM. Members of the Janus kinase/signal transducers and activators of transcription (JAK/STAT) pathway are present and active in human sperm. *Fertil Steril*. 2001 Aug 1;76(2):258–66.

82. Ng DC, Lin BH, Lim CP, Huang G, Zhang T, Poli V, Cao X. Stat3 regulates microtubules by antagonizing the depolymerization activity of stathmin. *J Cell Biol*. 2006 Jan 16;172(2):245–57.

83. Jin SK, Yang WX. Factors and pathways involved in capacitation: How are they regulated? *Oncotarget*. 2017 Jan 10;8(2):3600.

84. Austin CR. The 'capacitation' of the mammalian sperm. *Nature*. 1952 Aug;170(4321):326.

85. Angstwurm MW, Gärtner R, Ziegler-Heitbrock HL. Cyclic plasma IL-6 levels during normal menstrual cycle. *Cytokine*. 1997 May 1;9(5):370–4.

86. Heinrich PC, Behrmann I, Müller-Newen G, Schaper F, Graeve L. Interleukin-6-type cytokine signalling through the gp130/Jak/STAT pathway. *Biochem J*. 1998 Sep 1;334(2):297–314.

87. Foresta C, Rossato M, Mioni R, Zorzi M. Progesterone induces capacitation in human spermatozoa. *Andrologia*. 1992 Jan 2;24(1):33–5.

88. Srivastava MD, Lippes J, Srivastava BS. Cytokines of the human reproductive tract. *Am J Reprod Immunol*. 1996 Sep;36(3):157–66.

89. Frühbeck G. Intracellular signalling pathways activated by leptin. *Biochem J*. 2006 Jan 1;393(1):7–20.

90. Jope T, Lammert A, Kratzsch J, Paasch U, Glander HJ. Leptin and leptin receptor in human seminal plasma and in human spermatozoa. *Int J Androl*. 2003 Dec;26(6):335–41.

91. Glander HJ, Lammert A, Paasch U, Glasow A, Kratzsch J. Leptin exists in tubuli seminiferi and in seminal plasma. *Andrologia*. 2002 Sep;34(4):227–33.

92. Guo J, Zhao Y, Huang W, Hu W, Gu J, Chen C, Zhou J, Peng Y, Gong M, Wang Z. Sperm motility inversely correlates with seminal leptin levels in idiopathic asthenozoospermia. *Int J Clin Exp Med*. 2014;7(10):3550.

93. Lampiao F, Du Plessis SS. Insulin and leptin enhance human sperm motility, acrosome reaction and nitric oxide production. *Asian J Androl*. 2008 Sep;10(5):799–807.

94. Stine RR, Matunis EL. JAK-STAT signalling in stem cells. In: Hime G, Abud H (Eds.), *Transcriptional and Translational Regulation of Stem Cells*. Dordrecht: Springer; 2013, pp. 247–267.

95. Onishi K, Zandstra PW. LIF signalling in stem cells and development. *Development*. 2015 Jul 1;142(13):2230–6.

16

PI3K signaling in spermatogenesis and male infertility

ARCHANA DEVI AND GOPAL GUPTA

HIGHLIGHTS

- The phosphoinositide-3 kinase (PI3K) pathway is an important regulator of the balance between spermatogonial stem cell (SSC) self-renewal and differentiation.
- Various downstream signaling molecules help in maintaining the balance between SSC self-renewal and differentiation through a common PI3K/Akt pathway.
- PI3K signaling is also an important regulator of sperm motility and postejaculation events.
- Defects in PI3K signaling may result in asthenozoospermia and infertility.

16.1 INTRODUCTION

Spermatogenesis is the transformation of undifferentiated diploid spermatogonial stem cells (SSCs) into highly differentiated haploid spermatozoa over a precisely defined period of time within the seminiferous tubule of the testis (1). It is a strictly controlled, continuous and fundamental process required for male fertility. The undifferentiated diploid spermatogonia lie at the periphery of the seminiferous tubules of testes in an ordered fashion (2). Spermatogenesis is initiated with the diploid spermatogonia, which after a defined number of mitotic divisions undergo differentiation to form primary spermatocytes that divide to form secondary spermatocyte after the first meiotic division and round spermatids after the second meiotic division. Thus, each diploid spermatogonium gives rise to four haploid spermatids. This is followed by spermiogenesis, where spermatids undergo massive differentiation to form highly specialized sperm cells, which get released into the seminiferous tubule lumen (3).

Mammalian spermatogenesis is a highly systematized stem cell system that relies on the SSCs for maintaining spermatogenic lineage (4). Moreover, these SSCs, like all other stem cells, have the ability to maintain a balance between self-renewal and differentiation at every mitotic division to keep their stem cell pool constant, and in parallel maintain the continuous production of millions of sperm every day (5,6). During the course of spermatogenesis, the developing germ cells establish a close association with the neighboring somatic cells, called Sertoli cells that facilitate their progression to spermatozoa by controlling the environmental milieu (3).

SSCs dwell within the specialized microenvironment in the testis called niche (7), which have a highly organized architecture made of seminiferous epithelium, basement membrane, Sertoli cells and the interstitial cells (8). Sertoli cells, the key component of the niche, play a predominant role by providing physical anchorage and nutrition to the developing germ cells and providing growth factors to control proliferation and differentiation of SSCs (9,10). In addition, the basement membrane and integrins play an important role by providing physical support and emanating stimuli from the surrounding vascular network and interstitial cells for the undifferentiated spermatogonia (11).

A coordinated balance between the extrinsic or intrinsic factors mediates self-renewal and differentiation of the SSCs (12). The extrinsic factors are produced by different components of the niche (13,14), which ensure niche homeostasis through the modulation of intrinsic signals of SSCs such as kinases, second messengers and transcription factors (15). Tight regulation of the balance between self-renewal and differentiation of SSCs is crucial, as too many daughter cells undergoing differentiation may result in depletion of the stem cell population, while uncontrolled stem cell self-renewal may lead to tumorigenesis (16). The PI3K/Akt signaling pathway plays an important role in maintaining the SSC homeostasis (17), by maintaining a balance between self-renewability and differentiation of SSCs (18). Additionally, it is also involved in mobilization/homing, senescence and apoptosis. An overview of the role of PI3K/Akt signaling pathway in spermatogenesis, especially the role of glial cell line-derived neurotrophic factor (GDNF) and SCF/c-Kit mediated PI3K/Akt pathway in proliferation and differentiation of SSCs is presented herewith (19,20). In addition, the role of AKT signaling in sperm motility is discussed.

16.2 PHOSPHATIDYLINOSITOL 3-KINASE (PI3K)

Phosphatidylinositide 3-kinase (PI3K) is a family of dimeric enzymes comprising catalytic and regulatory subunits. PI3K phosphorylates phosphoinositides, acidic phospholipids in cell membranes at the 3-hydroxyl group. Additionally, this enzyme is known to have serine-threonine kinase activity (21). Somatic cells widely express PI3Ks, which regulate multiple cellular functions like survival, cell growth, proliferation and metabolism (22). Furthermore, PI3Ks have been grouped into three classes (I, II, III) on the basis of their substrate specificity, structural characteristics and mechanism of activation (23). All mammalian PI3Ks share a conserved domain structure but differ in catalytic activities and substrate preferences. Class-I PI3Ks are heterodimers and comprise a regulatory and a catalytic subunit (p110 subunit, encoded by PI3KCA gene). However, unlike the class-I PI3Ks, the regulation and signal transduction by extracellular ligands of class-II PI3Ks (PI3K-C2α, PI3K-C2β and PI3K-C2γ) and the class III PI3K (vps34) are less understood or might be involved in the modulation of such signaling directly or indirectly (24,25). Furthermore, depending on the type of regulatory subunits (p85, encoded by the PIK3R1 gene) or p84/p101 for class IA and IB present in the complex, they have been further subdivided into class IA (PI3Kα, PI3Kβ and PI3Kδ) and IB (PI3Kγ) (see Figure 16.1). Class IA PI3Ks are activated by receptor tyrosine kinases (RTKs), and class IB PI3Ks are activated by the G-protein-coupled receptors. In the PI3K pathway, the main function of the p85

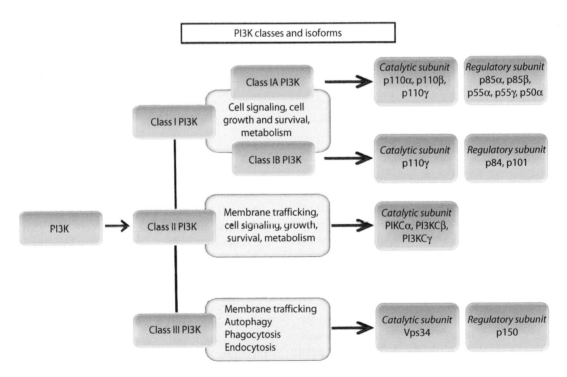

Figure 16.1 Phosphatidylinositol 3-kinase (PI3K) classes, functions and catalytic/regulatory subunits.

subunit is to bind and stabilize the p110 catalytic subunit. The upstream adaptor proteins or receptor tyrosine kinases activate class-I PI3K protein kinase and reduce the inhibitory activity on p110, which subsequently induces activation of downstream effector molecules (26).

At the plasma membrane, the class-I PI3Ks couple to the cell surface receptors, and upon activation, phosphorylate phosphatidylinositol 4,5-bisphosphate (PI [4,5] P2), which gives rise to short-lived second messenger phosphatidylinositol 3,4,5 trisphosphate (PI [3,4,5] P3) (27). PIP3 induces the recruitment of pleckstrin homology (PH) domain-containing effector proteins such as protein kinases, adaptor proteins and regulators of small GTPases, at the localized site of accumulation.

Protein kinase B (PKB)/Akt is a serine/threonine-specific kinase and a key class-I PI3K effector, which plays a pivotal role in the regulation of cell survival, cell cycle, glucose metabolism, protein synthesis and migration. There is no direct role of PIP3 in the activation of (PKB)/Akt. It allows recruitment of Akt/PKB to the plasma membrane and its subsequent phosphorylation on Thr^{308} by the phosphoinositide-dependent kinase-1 (PDK1) (22). Additionally, PDK2 phosphorylates AKT on Ser^{473}, which results in its full activation, followed by its migration to the nucleus and regulation of various cellular functions through phosphorylation of several downstream targets (22) (see Figure 16.2). Activated AKT also leads to the activation of the mTOR complex (21,28–30).

16.3 CATALYTIC SUBUNIT (p110) ROLE IN MALE FERTILITY

Several factors decide the cellular function to be mediated by the PI3K signaling cascade, e.g., stimulus type, PI3K isoform and the nature of second messenger lipid (31). The class-I PI3K p110α and p110β isoforms are expressed in many mammalian tissues and play important roles in intracellular signaling pathways, while the expression of the p110δ subunit is limited to the leukocytes (32). Both p110α and p110β isoforms are capable of sustaining cell proliferation and survival, with the former being important in glucose metabolism and insulin signaling and the latter being crucial for DNA synthesis/replication and cell mitosis (33). Both the isoforms play roles in sustaining male fertility.

16.3.1 p110α isoform in spermatogenesis

The role of p110α in spermatogenesis was studied in mutant mice with kinase-dead knock-in allele of p110α. The homozygous p110α$^{D933A/D933A}$ mice died at the embryonic stage, while the heterozygous p110α$^{D933A/WT}$ males were subfertile. Their testicular size was significantly lower than the wild type, and 40% mutant mice displayed atrophy of the seminiferous tubules at 35 days of age, which got reversed at ~56 days of age. It was found that p110α contributes to c-Kit signaling in adult mice testes (34). Leptin, an important hormone in reproductive physiology, is produced by adipose

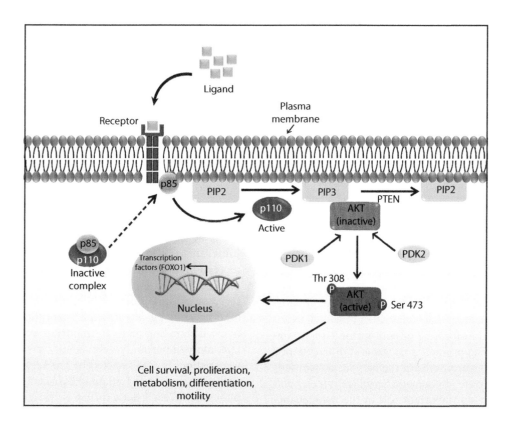

Figure 16.2 The molecular mechanism of PI3K signaling in male germ cells.

tissue and is adversely affected by the deletion of p110α in adipose tissue (35). Hyperleptinemia caused by increased adiposity results in disrupted PI3K signaling, delayed onset of puberty and infertility, in male mice (36). In Sertoli cells, the role of p110α isoform has not been identified (34). *In vitro*, selective inhibition of p110α isoform by PIK75 inhibited the proliferation of SSCs by inhibiting GDNF-mediated Akt activation, though this needs validation *in vivo* (37). In some cell types, a highly selective and potent inhibitor for p110α isoform, A66, has demonstrated that p110α alone is sufficient to inhibit growth factor signaling (38).

16.3.2 p110β isoform in spermatogenesis

The role of PI3K isoform p110β in spermatogenesis was studied in mutant knock-in mice with homozygous mice expressing a catalytically inactive p110β (*Pik3cb*$^{K805R/K805R}$). This mutation resulted in testicular hypertrophy, inhibited spermatogenesis, caused oligozoospermia and caused sub-fertility. Pre- and postmeiotic germ cell proliferation and viability were adversely affected. The study revealed the role of PI3K isoform p110β in c-Kit–mediated spermatogonial proliferation via activation of Akt by SCF in c-Kit positive cells. Similarly, the inhibition of p110β *in vitro* by pharmacological inhibitor supported the requirement of p110ß for c-Kit–mediated spermatogonial expansion and differentiation (37). In another mutant mouse model mimicking constitutive pharmacological inactivation of p110β, the homozygous p110β kinase-dead male mice that survived embryonic lethality were completely infertile, while their nonreproductive functions were unaffected (34). The inhibition of p110β specifically blocked the maturation of spermatogonia to spermatocytes through inhibition of the expression of Sertoli cell–specific androgen receptor target gene, Rhox5, which is crucial for spermatogenesis (34). However, the p110δ isoform apparently had no role in spermatogenesis.

16.4 REGULATION OF SELF-RENEWAL AND DIFFERENTIATION OF SPERMATOGONIAL STEM CELLS

16.4.1 Self-renewal of SSCs

SSCs have the capability of both self-renewal and differentiation. The decision of SSCs to self-renew or undergo differentiation is the fate-determining step and is precisely regulated by the stem cell niche factors (39). SSC self-renewal provides the basis for incessant spermatogenesis in males. GDNF is a member of the transforming growth factor-β superfamily and is reported to promote survival and differentiation of several types of neuron cells in the nervous system (40). In testis, GDNF secreted by somatic Sertoli cells (neighboring the SSCs) plays an important role in the maintenance of SSCs through their self-renewal, both *in vitro* and *in vivo* (19). Mutant mice with decreased expression of GDNF exhibited the depletion of SSC reserves, while overexpression

of GDNF accumulated undifferentiated spermatogonia and did not express c-Kit, the marker for spermatogonial differentiation. GDNF-overexpressing mice often encountered testicular tumors at old age (10). The effect of GDNF is mediated through a multicomponent receptor complex, which consists of GFRα1 (GDNF family receptor–α1) and RET (transmembrane tyrosine kinase receptor). GDNF binds to Ret through Gfrα1, which functions as a glycosylphosphatidylinositol-anchored docking acceptor. The depletion of GDNF, GFRα1 or Ret results in germ cell loss and defects in SSC self-renewal (41). Subsequent studies indicated that Akt is rapidly phosphorylated on addition of GDNF to germline stem (GS) cell culture system *in vitro*, while the addition of an inhibitor of PI3K (LY294002) blocked GS self-renewal. Conditional activation of myristoylated Akt could also induce GS proliferation in the absence of GDNF, and on transplantation into the testes of infertile mice, these cells supported spermatogenesis and produced offsprings (18). PI3K inhibitor LY294002 blocked Akt phosphorylation in SSCs treated with GDNF, which directly indicated that GDNF utilizes the PI3K/Akt signaling to control SSCs survival and self-renewal (19), especially in view of the fact that overexpression of an activated form of Akt could mediate GDNF-independent SSC self-renewal (18).

16.4.2 SSC differentiation

It is well documented that vitamin A deficiency compromises spermatogenesis that can be restored by retinoid supplementation in rat and mice. Vitamin A–deficient male mice show the presence of only undifferentiated spermatogonia and Sertoli cells in their seminiferous tubules. The effect of vitamin A deficiency and vitamin A replacement on spermatogenesis was studied in mice (42). Retinoic acid (RA) encourages differentiation of undifferentiated spermatogonia and their entry into meiosis by utilizing PI3K/Akt signaling. A study has found that RA utilizes the PI3K/AKT/mTOR signaling pathway to induce the expression of Kit, whose mRNAs are present but not translated in undifferentiated spermatogonia. Fundamentally, it has been suggested that RA initially stimulates PI3K/Akt signaling to synthesize the Kit receptor, which binds with Kit ligands and assures maintenance of mTORC1 activation when RA is deficient or absent in later stages of differentiation. Inhibiting mTORC1 activation resulted in translational repression of Kit mRNAs followed by the accumulation of undifferentiated spermatogonia (43,44). c-KIT is a type III receptor tyrosine kinase whose activation depends on the binding of its ligand stem cell factor (SCF). The activation of c-Kit signaling plays an important role in deciding cell fate, most importantly, cell viability, proliferation and differentiation. SCF is secreted by the Sertoli cells and binds with Kit receptor to initiate PI3K/Akt signaling that phosphorylates p70S6 kinase (p70S6 K) via a mammalian target of rapamycin (mTOR) in spermatogonia (45). By inactivation of the proapoptotic factor BAD, SCF/c-KIT/PI3K/AKT also ensures cell survival. Conversely, in Leydig cells, Kit mediates testosterone biosynthesis via activation of PI3K signaling (46). SCF may be necessary for differentiation, but not for the proliferation of spermatogonial stem cells (47).

16.5 FOXO1: MOLECULAR SWITCH BETWEEN SELF-RENEWAL AND DIFFERENTIATION

The transcription factors, FOXOs are the downstream effectors of PI3K/Akt signaling and are considered as pivotal regulators of cell survival and proliferation (48). Especially, FOXO1 is a known marker of SSCs and is essential for their self-renewal or differentiation for continual spermatogenesis. PI3K signaling ensures the balance between SSCs renewal and differentiation through maintaining the stability of Foxo1 and its subcellular localization (49). The transcriptional activity of FOXO1 is regulated by its phosphorylation by Akt, which is the downstream kinase of PI3K. Phosphorylated FOXO1 has low affinity toward DNA but increased binding affinity for 14–3–3 protein. This newly formed 14–3–3-FOXO complex is released from the nucleus, resulting in the inhibition of FOXO1-mediated transcription (50). As PI3K signaling regulates *Foxo1* stability and subcellular localization, Foxos become pivotal effectors of PI3K-Akt signaling in SSCs. Conditional inactivation of *Foxo1* in the male germ line caused male infertility (51). Additionally, conditional inactivation of 3-phosphoinositide–dependent protein kinase 1 (Pdk1), which is downstream to PI3K, promoted continued SSC self-renewal, whereas the ablation of phosphatase and tensin homolog (*Pten*) promoted SSC differentiation (51). Hence, the model proposed for the switch from SSC self-renewal to differentiation explains that the transcription factor FOXO1 present in the nucleus of SSCs promotes *Ret* mRNA transcription and expression of the protein on the cell surface. GDNF binds to Ret/Gfrα1 receptor complex and activates PI3K/AKT signaling to phosphorylate FOXO1. The phosphorylation of FOXO1 reduces its DNA binding affinity and increases affinity for 14–3–3 protein. The newly formed 14–3–3-FOXO complex then moves from nucleus to cytoplasm causing inhibition of FOXO1-mediated Ret transcription and commitment of SSCs for differentiation (51).

16.6 PI3K/AKT IN SPERM MOTILITY

The role of PI3K is not limited only up to the production of spermatozoa, but is also important in the acquisition of sperm motility. Post-spermatogenesis spermatozoa further mature while passing through the epididymis to acquire motility and fertilizing ability. Several modifications are reported to be responsible for the attainment of motility by the sperm during their journey in the epididymis, including remodeling of the plasma membrane. For initiation of motility, some intracellular mediators regulate flagellar activity through cell signaling involving phosphorylation cascades. One such important phosphorylation cascade is phosphatidylinositol-3-kinase (PI3K) signaling. The

presence of PI3K signaling in human spermatozoa has been confirmed, revealing a highly specific pattern of subcellular localization (52). The catalytic subunit p110 is localized in the acrosomal region, the neck and the principal piece of the sperm tail, but not in the midpiece that houses the mitochondria. Moreover, the activated regulatory subunit p85 (phospho-Tyr467 and phospho-Tyr199) is also mainly located in the principal piece of the sperm tail and is absent from the midpiece. By contrast, the majority of PTEN exists in phosphorylated form and is localized in the equatorial segment of the sperm head. This distant localization of PI3K and phosphorylated PTEN is unique in spermatozoa and suggests that PI3K can freely convert PIP2 to PIP3 without any interference from PTEN activity (52). To identify the role of PI3K in sperm motility, two structurally unrelated inhibitors (LY294002 and wortmannin) were used by several investigators. In human spermatozoa, negative regulation of PI3K is positively correlated with sperm motility (53–55). The intracellular cAMP level and tyrosine phosphorylation of the PKA anchoring protein, AKAP3, were increased after PI3K inhibition. It stimulated PKA binding to AKAP3 in the sperm tail through the regulatory subunit. These results suggest that PI3K negatively controls the cAMP/PKA pathway for the regulation of human sperm motility (53,54,56). Similarly, in boar sperm, the PI3K pathway negatively regulated sperm motion parameters. On treating boar sperm with LY294002, total and progressive motility were unaffected, but significant increases in other motility parameters like VCL, VAP and VSL were observed (57). However, in hamster sperm, PI3K inhibition decreased the hyperactivation of sperm during capacitation (55).

16.7 PI3K IN HUMAN INFERTILITY

Human fertility is critically dependent on proper PI3K signaling. The expression of Foxo1, the main regulator of the PI3K/Akt signaling pathway that plays a critical role in the maintenance of stem cell population and male fertility, is seen in SSC across the species, including human (58). Asthenozoospermia, which is a leading cause of male infertility, is caused by low sperm motility. A study of sperm samples from asthenozoospermia patients has revealed that their sperm has high RNASET2 content, which causes significant inhibition of PI3K activity and motility loss (59). Human sperm motility requires a concerted effort of several pathways, including the PI3K signaling pathway (60). Inhibition of PI3K activity results in spermatozoa switching to apoptotic cascade, which is characterized by quick motility loss, mitochondrial ROS generation, activation of caspases, localization of phosphatidylserine to the cell surface, cytoplasmic vacuolization and DNA damage (52). PI3K signaling also plays a critical role in the capacitation of ejaculated sperm. Activation of PI3K is by PKA-mediated phosphorylation pathway through degradation of PKCα, which keeps PI3K inactivated. This cascade leads to actin polymerization, which is necessary for hyperactivated motility that follows capacitation (61). Estradiol, which is known to influence post-ejaculation events of human spermatozoa like capacitation and acrosome reaction, requires the activation of the PI3K/Akt pathway via interaction of ER-α with the p55 regulatory subunit of PI3K and ER-β with Akt1 (62). Similarly, PI3K/Akt pathway activation is also required for the progesterone-induced hyperactivation of capacitated sperm and is inhibited by PI3K inhibitor wortmannin that reduces tyrosine phosphorylation and progressive motility but does not affect acrosome reaction (63). However, PI3K inhibitor LY294002 had no direct effect on human sperm/oocyte interaction (64).

16.8 CONCLUSION

Phosphoinositide 3-phosphate kinase (PI3K) signaling plays a very crucial role in spermatogenesis by controlling SSC homeostasis and sustaining continual production of spermatozoa by way of maintaining a balance between SSC self-renewal and differentiation. This step is vital for spermatogenesis, and defects in PI3K signaling in testis may result either in increased differentiation and depletion of SSC causing male infertility or uncontrolled SSC proliferation causing testicular cancer. GDNF secreted by the Sertoli cells initiates the PI3K/Akt signaling in the spermatogonial cells located in the testicular niche. Akt phosphorylates the transcription factor Foxo-1, which is located in the nucleus and promotes the transcription of *Ret* mRNA and expression of the protein on the cell surface for binding of GDNF to Ret/Gfrα1 receptor complex and activation PI3K/AKT signaling. Phospho-Foxo-1 loses affinity for DNA and gains affinity toward 14-3-3 protein. The Foxo-14-3-3 protein complex is released from the nucleus to switch off the Foxo-1 mediated Ret transcription. Apparently, localization of Foxo-1 in the nucleus favors SSC differentiation, and its release into the cytoplasm promotes SSC self-renewal. However, the process is not that simple and is under the regulation of a number of cofactors and signaling molecules like retinoic acid, PTEN, Pkd1 kinase, mTOR, c-Kit and SCF.

REFERENCES

1. Sharma R, Agarwal A. Spermatogenesis: An overview. In: *Sperm Chromatin*. New York, NY: Springer; 2011, pp. 19–44.
2. Okabe M, Ikawa M, Ashkenas J. Male infertility and the genetics of spermatogenesis. *Am J Hum Genet*. 1998 Jun 1;62(6):1274–81.
3. Hess RA, de Franca LR. Spermatogenesis and cycle of the seminiferous epithelium. In: Cheng CY (Ed.), *Molecular Mechanisms in Spermatogenesis*. New York, NY: Springer; 2009, pp. 1–15.
4. Yoshida S. Stem cells in mammalian spermatogenesis. *Dev Growth Differ*. 2010 Apr;52(3):311–7.
5. Aponte PM. Spermatogonial stem cells: Current biotechnological advances in reproduction and regenerative medicine. *World J Stem Cells*. 2015 May 26;7(4):669.
6. Song HW, Wilkinson MF. Transcriptional control of spermatogonial maintenance and differentiation. In: *Seminars in Cell and Developmental Biology* (Vol. 30). Academic Press; 2014 Jun 1, pp. 14–26.
7. Nóbrega RH, Greebe CD, Van De Kant H, Bogerd J, de França LR, Schulz RW. Spermatogonial stem cell niche and spermatogonial stem cell transplantation in zebrafish. *PLOS ONE*. 2010 Sep 20;5(9):e12808.
8. Oatley JM, Brinster RL. The germline stem cell niche unit in mammalian testes. *Physiol Rev*. 2012 Apr;92(2):577–95.
9. Caires K, Broady J, McLean D. Maintaining the male germline: Regulation of spermatogonial stem cells. *J Endocrinol*. 2010 May 1;205(2):133–45.
10. Meng X, Lindahl M, Hyvönen ME, Parvinen M, de Rooij DG, Hess MW, Raatikainen-Ahokas A, Sainio K, Rauvala H, Lakso M, Pichel JG. Regulation of cell fate decision of undifferentiated spermatogonia by GDNF. *Science*. 2000 Feb 25;287(5457):1489–93.
11. Yoshida S, Sukeno M, Nabeshima YI. A vasculature-associated niche for undifferentiated spermatogonia in the mouse testis. *Science*. 2007 Sep 21;317(5845):1722–6.
12. Mei XX, Wang J, Wu J. Extrinsic and intrinsic factors controlling spermatogonial stem cell self-renewal and differentiation. *Asian J Androl*. 2015 May;17(3):347.
13. Shinohara T, Orwig KE, Avarbock MR, Brinster RL. Remodeling of the postnatal mouse testis is accompanied by dramatic changes in stem cell number and niche accessibility. *Proc Natl Acad Sci USA*. 2001 May 22;98(11):6186–91.
14. Spradling A, Drummond-Barbosa D, Kai T. Stem cells find their niche. *Nature*. 2001 Nov 1;414(6859):98.
15. Kostereva N, Hofmann MC. Regulation of the spermatogonial stem cell niche. *Reprod Domest Anim*. 2008 Jul;43:386–92.
16. Yamashita YM, Fuller MT. Asymmetric stem cell division and function of the niche in the *Drosophila* male germ line. *Int J Hematol*. 2005 Dec 1;82(5):377.
17. Feng LX, Ravindranath N, Dym M. Stem cell factor/c-kit up-regulates cyclin D3 and promotes cell cycle progression via the phosphoinositide 3-kinase/p70 S6 kinase pathway in spermatogonia. *J Biol Chem*. 2000 Aug 18;275(33):25572–6.
18. Lee J, Kanatsu-Shinohara M, Inoue K, Ogonuki N, Miki H, Toyokuni S, Kimura T, Nakano T, Ogura A, Shinohara T. Akt mediates self-renewal division of mouse spermatogonial stem cells. *Development*. 2007 May 15;134(10):1853–9.
19. Oatley JM, Avarbock MR, Brinster RL. Glial cell line-derived neurotrophic factor regulation of genes essential for self-renewal of mouse spermatogonial stem cells is dependent on Src family kinase signaling. *J Biol Chem*. 2007 Aug 31;282(35):25842–51.
20. Cao LH, Zhang QL, Lin XH. Spermatogonial stem cell self-renewal and differentiation. *Reprod Dev Med*. 2017 Jul 1;1(3):171.

21. Lien EC, Dibble CC, Toker A. PI3K signaling in cancer: Beyond AKT. *Curr Opin Cell Biol.* 2017 Apr 1;45:62–71.

22. Song G, Ouyang G, Bao S. The activation of Akt/PKB signaling pathway and cell survival. *J Cell Mol Med.* 2005 Jan 1;9(1):59–71.

23. Yu X, Long YC, Shen HM. Differential regulatory functions of three classes of phosphatidylinositol and phosphoinositide 3-kinases in autophagy. *Autophagy.* 2015 Oct 3;11(10):1711–28.

24. Vanhaesebroeck B, Whitehead MA, Piñeiro R. Molecules in medicine mini-review: Isoforms of PI3K in biology and disease. *J Mol Med.* 2016 Jan 1;94(1):5–11.

25. Kissel H, Timokhina I, Hardy MP, Rothschild G, Tajima Y, Soares V, Angeles M, Whitlow SR, Manova K, Besmer P. Point mutation in kit receptor tyrosine kinase reveals essential roles for kit signaling in spermatogenesis and oogenesis without affecting other kit responses. *EMBO J.* 2000 Mar 15;19(6):1312–26.

26. Yang Y, Li M, Li Y. High expression of PIK3R1 (p85α) correlates with poor survival in patients with metastatic breast cancer. *Int J Clin Exp Pathol.* 2016 Jan 1;9(12):12797–806.

27. Manning BD, Toker A. AKT/PKB signaling: Navigating the network. *Cell.* 2017 Apr 20;169(3):381–405.

28. Hemmings BA, Restuccia DF. Pi3k-pkb/akt pathway. *Cold Spring Harbor Perspect Biol.* 2012 Sep 1;4(9):a011189.

29. Matsuda S, Nakanishi A, Wada Y, Kitagishi Y. Roles of PI3K/AKT/PTEN pathway as a target for pharmaceutical therapy. *Open Med Chem J.* 2013;7:23.

30. Jason SL, Cui W. Proliferation, survival and metabolism: The role of PI3K/AKT/mTOR signalling in pluripotency and cell fate determination. *Development.* 2016 Sep 1;143(17):3050–60.

31. Katso R, Okkenhaug K, Ahmadi K, White S, Timms J, Waterfield MD. Cellular function of phosphoinositide 3-kinases: Implications for development, immunity, homeostasis, and cancer. *Annu Rev Cell Dev Biol.* 2001 Nov;17(1):615–75.

32. Bi L, Okabe I, Bernard DJ, Nussbaum RL. Early embryonic lethality in mice deficient in the p110β catalytic subunit of PI 3-kinase. *Mamm Genome.* 2002 Mar 1;13(3):169–72.

33. Li B, Sun A, Jiang W, Thrasher JB, Terranova P. PI-3 kinase p110β: A therapeutic target in advanced prostate cancers. *Am J Clin Exp Urol.* 2014;2(3):188.

34. Guillermet-Guibert J, Smith LB, Halet G, Whitehead MA, Pearce W, Rebourcet D et al. Novel role for p110β PI 3-kinase in male fertility through regulation of androgen receptor activity in Sertoli cells. *PLOS Genet.* 2015 Jul 1;11(7):e1005304.

35. Moschos S, Chan JL, Mantzoros CS. Leptin and reproduction: A review. *Fertil Steril.* 2002 Mar 1;77(3):433–44.

36. Nelson VL, Negrón AL, Reid I, Thomas JA, Yang L, Lin RZ, Acosta-Martínez M. Loss of PI3K p110α in the adipose tissue results in infertility and delayed puberty onset in male mice. *BioMed Res Int.* 2017;2017.

37. Ciraolo E, Morello F, Hobbs RM, Wolf F, Marone R, Iezzi M et al. Essential role of the p110β subunit of phosphoinositide 3-OH kinase in male fertility. *Mol Biol Cell.* 2010 Mar 1;21(5):704–11.

38. Jamieson S, Flanagan JU, Kolekar S, Buchanan C, Kendall JD, Lee WJ et al. A drug targeting only p110α can block phosphoinositide 3-kinase signalling and tumour growth in certain cell types. *Biochem J.* 2011 Aug 15;438(1):53–62.

39. Schmidt JA, Avarbock MR, Tobias JW, Brinster RL. Identification of glial cell line-derived neurotrophic factor-regulated genes important for spermatogonial stem cell self-renewal in the rat. *Biol Reprod.* 2009 Jul 1;81(1):56–66.

40. Arenas E, Trupp M, Åkerud P, Ibáñez CF. GDNF prevents degeneration and promotes the phenotype of brain noradrenergic neurons *in vivo*. *Neuron.* 1995 Dec 1;15(6):1465–73.

41. Naughton CK, Jain S, Strickland AM, Gupta A, Milbrandt J. Glial cell-line derived neurotrophic factor-mediated RET signaling regulates spermatogonial stem cell fate. *Biol Reprod.* 2006 Feb 1;74(2):314–21.

42. Van Pelt AM, de Rooij DG. Synchronization of the seminiferous epithelium after vitamin A replacement in vitamin A-deficient mice. *Biol Reprod.* 1990 Sep 1;43(3):363–7.

43. Busada JT, Chappell VA, Niedenberger BA, Kaye EP, Keiper BD, Hogarth CA, Geyer CB. Retinoic acid regulates Kit translation during spermatogonial differentiation in the mouse. *Dev Biol.* 2015 Jan 1;397(1):140–9.

44. Busada JT, Niedenberger BA, Velte EK, Keiper BD, Geyer CB. Mammalian target of rapamycin complex 1 (mTORC1) Is required for mouse spermatogonial differentiation in vivo. *Dev Biol.* 2015 Nov 1;407(1):90–102.

45. Cardoso HJ, Figueira MI, Correia S, Vaz CV, Socorro S. The SCF/c-KIT system in the male: Survival strategies in fertility and cancer. *Mol Reprod Dev.* 2014 Dec;81(12):1064–79.

46. Rothschild G, Sottas CM, Kissel H, Agosti V, Manova K, Hardy MP, Besmer P. A role for kit receptor signaling in Leydig cell steroidogenesis. *Biol Reprod.* 2003 Sep 1;69(3):925–32.

47. Ohta H, Yomogida K, Dohmae K, Nishimune Y. Regulation of proliferation and differentiation in spermatogonial stem cells: The role of c-kit and its ligand SCF. *Development.* 2000 May 15;127(10):2125–31.

48. Hay N. Interplay between FOXO, TOR, and Akt. *Biochim Biophys Acta.* 2011 Nov 1;1813(11):1965–70.

49. Zhang X, Tang N, Hadden TJ, Rishi AK. Akt, FoxO and regulation of apoptosis. *Biochim Biophys Acta.* 2011 Nov 1;1813(11):1978–86.

50. Prasad SB, Yadav SS, Das M, Govardhan HB, Pandey LK, Singh S, Pradhan S, Narayan G. Down regulation of FOXO1 promotes cell proliferation in cervical cancer. *Journal of Cancer.* 2014;5(8):655.

51. Goertz MJ, Wu Z, Gallardo TD, Hamra FK, Castrillon DH. Foxo1 is required in mouse spermatogonial stem cells for their maintenance and the initiation of spermatogenesis. *J Clin Invest.* 2011 Sep 1;121(9):3456–66.

52. Koppers AJ, Mitchell LA, Wang P, Lin M, Aitken RJ. Phosphoinositide 3-kinase signalling pathway involvement in a truncated apoptotic cascade associated with motility loss and oxidative DNA damage in human spermatozoa. *Biochem J.* 2011 Jun 15;436(3):687–98.

53. Luconi M, Marra F, Gandini L, Filimberti E, Lenzi A, Forti G, Baldi E. Phosphatidylinositol 3-kinase inhibition enhances human sperm motility. *Hum Reprod.* 2001 Sep 1;16(9):1931–7.

54. Luconi M, Carloni V, Marra F, Ferruzzi P, Forti G, Baldi E. Increased phosphorylation of AKAP by inhibition of phosphatidylinositol 3-kinase enhances human sperm motility through tail recruitment of protein kinase A. *J Cell Sci.* 2004 Mar 1;117(7):1235–46.

55. NagDas SK, Winfrey VP, Olson GE. Identification of ras and its downstream signaling elements and their potential role in hamster sperm motility. *Biol Reprod.* 2002 Oct 1;67(4):1058–66.

56. Du Plessis SS, Franken DR, Baldi E, Luconi M. Phosphatidylinositol 3-kinase inhibition enhances human sperm motility and sperm–zona pellucida binding. *Int J Androl.* 2004 Feb;27(1):19–26.

57. Aparicio IM, Gil MC, Garcia-Herreros M, Pena FJ, Garcia-Marin LJ. Inhibition of phosphatidylinositol 3-kinase modifies boar sperm motion parameters. *Reproduction.* 2005 Mar 1;129(3):283–9.

58. Tarnawa ED, Baker MD, Aloisio GM, Carr BR, Castrillon DH. Gonadal expression of Foxo1, but not Foxo3, is conserved in diverse Mammalian species. *Biol Reprod.* 2013 Apr 25;88(4):103.

59. Xu Y, Fan Y, Fan W, Jing J, Xue K, Zhang X, Ye B, Ji Y, Liu Y, Ding Z. 2018. RNASET2 impairs the sperm motility via PKA/PI3K/calcium signal pathways. *Reproduction,* 155(4), pp. 383–392.

60. Parte PP, Rao P, Redij S, Lobo V, D'Souza SJ, Gajbhiye R, Kulkarni V. Sperm phosphoproteome profiling by ultra-performance liquid chromatography followed by data independent analysis (LC-MS(E)) reveals altered proteomic signatures in asthenozoospermia. *J Proteomics.* 2012 Oct 22;75(18):5861–71.

61. Ickowicz D, Finkelstein M, Breitbart H. Mechanism of sperm capacitation and the acrosome reaction: Role of protein kinases. *Asian J Androl.* 2012 Nov;14(6):816–21.

62. Aquila S, Sisci D, Gentile M, Middea E, Catalano S, Carpino A, Rago V, Andò S. Estrogen receptor (ER)-α and ER-β are both expressed in human ejaculated spermatozoa: Evidence of their direct interaction with phosphatidylinositol-3-OH kinase/Akt pathway. *J Clin Endocrinol Metab.* 2004 Mar;89(3):1443–51.

63. Sagare-Patil V, Vernekar M, Galvankar M, Modi D. Progesterone utilizes the PI3K-AKT pathway in human spermatozoa to regulate motility and hyperactivation but not acrosome reaction. *Mol Cell Endocrinol.* 2013 Jul 15;374(1–2):82–91.

64. Barbonetti A, Zugaro A, Sciarretta F, Santucci R, Necozione S, Ruvolo G, Francavilla S, Francavilla F. The inhibition of the human sperm phosphatidylinosytol 3-kinase by LY294002 does not interfere with sperm/oocyte interaction. *Int J Androl.* 2006 Aug;29(4):468–74.

Spermatogenesis, heat stress and male infertility

JOHN J. PARRISH

HIGHLIGHTS

- Apoptosis and germ cell death are a normal part of spermatogenesis.
- Apoptosis of spermatocytes and spermatids increases during heat stress.
- Heat stress upregulates the heat stress factors (HSFs) HSF1 and HSF2 leading to prosurvival effects in testicular somatic cells and apoptosis in meiotic germ cells.
- Androgen production decreases and androgen receptor is downregulated in heat stress, impacting the blood-testis barrier (BTB) and support of meiosis.
- Unifying theories of heat stress now explain discrepancies in mild to severe heat stress in animal models.
- Both contraceptive research and improvement of sperm production have exploited research in heat stress.

17.1 INTRODUCTION

The production of sperm occurs within the testes of mammals. In most mammals, the testis is held in the scrotal sacks outside of the body cavity and thus is maintained 2°C–8°C below body temperature. In some mammals such as elephants, porpoises and whales, the testis is within the body cavity, and spermatogenesis may occur at higher temperatures near the core body temperature. Little is known about how spermatogenesis is regulated in such abdominal testes. This review focuses on mammals with external testes.

Once puberty is reached, spermatogenesis occurs continuously to produce sperm until a gradual decrease occurs in old age. Within the testes are two general spaces: the seminiferous tubules, which contain germ cells, and the Sertoli cells, which are somatic cells. The seminiferous tubules are surrounded by a basement membrane and contractile myoid cells. Outside the seminiferous tubule is the interstitial space containing Leydig cells, blood vessels, lymphatics and nerve cells. Myoid and Leydig cells are again somatic cells.

Germ cells go through mitosis as spermatogonia; meiosis as primary spermatocytes, secondary spermatocytes and round spermatids; and then spermiogenesis, which consists of a morphological change to form the spermatozoa (reviewed in [1]). The general sequence is that type A_1 spermatogonia divide mitotically three times to form 2 A_2, 4 A_3 and finally 8 A_4 spermatogonia, dividing again mitotically to form 16 intermediate spermatogonia and then 32 B spermatogonia, and finally 64 primary spermatocytes. The primary spermatocytes must then cross a junctional barrier known as the blood-testis barrier (BTB) that is composed of a tight junction, desmosomes, gap junction and ectoplasmic specializations (2). The basal compartment is between the BTB and the basement membrane, the adluminal compartment is between the BTB and lumen and then the lumen is in the center of the seminiferous tubule. Following mitosis in the basal compartment, meiosis occurs in the adluminal compartment in which the primary spermatocytes divide to form 128 secondary spermatocytes and then divide again to form 256 round spermatids. A modification to the round spermatids occurs to transform them into spermatozoa with no further divisions in the process of spermiogenesis. The spermatozoa are then released into the lumen in spermiation. As a developing type A spermatogonia goes through these divisions producing the various daughter germ cells, it is associated with a single Sertoli cell that controls and coordinates the events of spermatogenesis. There is also a coordination along the length of seminiferous tubules consisting of waves and cycles that ensure a steady production of sperm. As a normal part of spermatogenesis, there is an overproduction of germ cells that if allowed to continue would disrupt the BTB and function of the seminiferous tubule. The processes of apoptosis and autophagy are thus normal events that limit the eventual number of spermatozoa produced (1,3–5). In porcine spermatogenesis, only 10%–30% of the potential spermatozoa are produced (1,6,7), while approximately 25% reach this point in rodent and human spermatogenesis (3).

Stressors are now known to exploit the decretory processes of apoptosis and autophagy during spermatogenesis (4). Many stressors disrupt thermoregulation of the testis, such as increased environmental temperatures, cryptorchidism, febrile disease, fever as a result of vaccination or obesity (4,8,9). In humans, this may also be as a result of lifestyle choices, but in livestock, it is human intervention from designs of housing, environmental controls or other management factors. The end result of these heat stressors is a decrease in the number and quality of sperm produced.

There have been many studies examining the molecular mechanisms of spermatogenesis (1–3,10,11). The goal has been to either understand the mechanisms that might be exploited for contraception or how to increase the number and quality of sperm produced. The former has focused on research related to rodent, nonhuman primate and even humans. The latter is work principally with livestock species such as porcine, bovine, ovine and even equine. The work with heat stress is converging on a unified theory of how apoptosis and other cell death pathways play a role in normal, pathological and environmental regulation of spermatogenesis.

17.2 HEAT STRESS

Studies in a variety of species come to the same conclusion about heat stress. First there is a decrease in the amount of sperm produced (1,4,10,12,13). This is associated with increased apoptosis of primary spermatocytes through round spermatids (14,15). Interestingly, even sperm that survive this apoptosis may have damaged DNA and are of lower fertility (16,17). Animal models have used increased environmental temperatures, mild local scrotal heating, experimental induced cryptorchidism or even short-term higher temperatures applied to the scrotum (1,18). Human exposure to testicular heat stress is usually via lifestyle choices, job-related conditions or pathological conditions (4). The intensity and/or duration of the heat exposure impact the severity of the response to spermatogenesis observed. For example,

scrotal insulation can produce a rise in testicular temperatures close to body temperature and is similar to experimental cryptorchidism. Scrotal insulation for 48 hours can produce an immediate effect on testicular histology, abnormal sperm produce 3–5 weeks later, but following the normal length of spermatogenesis there is complete recovery to pretreatment levels of germ cell differentiation and production of sperm (1,16,17). A common approach in rodents that has also been applied to some livestock species is a short-term increase for 30–120 minutes in scrotal temperatures to 41°C–43°C, well above body temperature (12,19,20). This is a more severe procedure with spermatogenesis often completely disrupted, although in some cases, recovery can occur with very short heat exposure (12). Increasing environmental temperatures into the range of 35°C–37°C for several hours a day followed by returning animals to normal conditions of 21°C–23°C can also produce similar changes but requires exposure for most of the length of spermatogenesis and a range from 3 to 6 weeks to achieve consistent results (18,21). Changing environmental temperatures were intended to mimic changes seen during warmer months of the year, but just measuring semen or testicular tissue response to animals under summer conditions produces variable results, as conditions do not remain constant and may or may not increase in a particular year (1).

Most of our detailed knowledge of heat stress mechanisms of damage in the testis comes from rodent models. While both testicular and epididymal germ cells are sensitive to heat stress, we focus on the testicular cells. Germ cells and, in particular, primary spermatocytes undergo apoptosis, and if they survive will often contain damaged DNA and poor fertility when ejaculated as spermatozoa (22–24). This is also true in the bull (16,17). Both intrinsic and extrinsic pathways of apoptosis occur in response to heat stress in primary spermatocytes and round spermatids (4), as well as disruption to the BTB, which then also impact survival of primary and secondary spermatocytes, and spermatids (12). The intrinsic mechanisms of apoptosis involve the mitochondria, heat shock factors and heat shock proteins, while the extrinsic effects are from Sertoli cells and involve secretion of Fas ligand (FasL) from Sertoli cells and binding to Fas receptors on germ cells that then activate the apoptotic process involving caspases (5). Both the extrinsic and intrinsic pathways also involve the p53 system that triggers proapoptotic events in the mitochondria and translocation to the nuclease and cell cycle stasis and death by binding and regulating DNA expression (5). Heat also results in the disruption of Sertoli cell–Sertoli cell junctional complexes of the BTB that are essential for meiosis to occur in the adluminal space (2,5,12).

While we now know much about the control of spermatogenesis by the BTB and Sertoli cells (2) and that heat induces a variety of molecular changes to the testes (4), the specific sequence of heat stress events remains unclear. Part of the problem is that there are heat effects on both somatic and germ cells. The impact on Sertoli cells to provide control and support of the BTB and the Leydig cells to produce testosterone that have an effect on Sertoli cells is critical

(12,25,26). Another problem is that different models of inducing heat stress are used, for example, 30–120 minutes of 41°C–43°C (or lower) increases in temperature by periodic increases in environmental temperatures, experimental cryptorchid simulation or scrotal insulation.

Early studies found a decrease in testicular weight following heat stress that was associated with evidence of apoptosis upon histological evaluation using histochemical staining or terminal deoxynucleotidyl transferase-mediated dUDP nick-end labeling (14,15). The initial cells to be affected by heat stress were primary spermatocytes of the first meiotic division and then round spermatids (1). Both short-term and mild heat stress can experience recovery of germ cells, but if the heat stress is continued, then germ cells may not recover suggesting that possibly stem cell spermatogonia can be impacted (1,27).

17.3 INTERACTIONS OF HEAT SHOCK PROTEINS AND HEAT SHOCK FACTORS

Germ cells like somatic cells use heat shock proteins (HSPs) to act as molecular chaperones under normal circumstances and are essential for normal spermatogenesis by ensuring correct assembly and transport of proteins (28). An example of such a HSP is HSP70, the most abundant HSP. Under heat stress, heat shock factors (HSFs), a series of transcription factors, are activated (11). The HSF1 has a dual role to first stabilize and protect somatic cells (heat-resistant cells) but then to trigger apoptosis in germ cells such as primary spermatocytes (heat-sensitive cells) (11). Rather than to preserve germ cells following heat stress, HSF1 appears to trigger germ cell removal, perhaps due to damaged DNA. Widlak and Vydra (11) suggest that this may be due to the overproduction of sperm, and it may be better to just destroy these cells rather than chance the possibility of damaged DNA interfering with fertilization, embryo or fetal development. Even with this removal, we have observed that some sperm produced after heat stress do indeed have damaged DNA and reduced ability to sustain embryo development after fertilization (16,17).

The role of HSFs is complex. In HSF1 knockout mice, among other defects, male mice produce 20% less sperm and more sperm with abnormal head morphology (29–31). In HSF2 knockout mice, there were much fewer sperm produced due to increased apoptosis of primary spermatocytes. However, double knockout mice were completely infertile due to lack of postmeiotic cells, suggesting synergistic roles of HSF1 and HSF2 (32). Other HSFs are expressed in the testis, but roles remain unclear in terms of spermatogenesis. Interestingly, HSF1 and HSF2 regulate expression of some genes that escape postmeiotic sex chromosome repression and allow expression of these genes in round spermatids and particularly in chromatin packaging changes during spermiogenesis (33). The HSF1/HSF2 complex and associated proteins are essential to normal spermatogenesis.

In somatic cells, activation of HSF1 leads to increased HSPs that protect cells, allowing them to survive heat stress.

In these somatic cells, the set point for activation of HSF1 is 41°C, but in the testis it is activated at 35°C–38°C (34). Surprisingly, somatic cells of the testes including Leydig and Sertoli cells have profiles of HSF1 activation similar to the general somatic cells of the organism (34). In contrast to somatic cells, germ cell activation of HSF1 does not lead to transcription of antiapoptotic pathway proteins (35–37) and often leads to downregulation of heat shock proteins (38) and upregulation of apoptosis (39,40).

Cells sense heat stress by the activation of a variety of cell signaling mechanisms that can include mitogen-activated protein kinases (MAPK), the extracellular signal-regulated kinase (ERK), c-Jun N-terminal kinase and p38, as well as protein kinases A, B and C, Rac1, and CaMKII (5,41). Many of these pathways are initiated by changes in lipids at the level of the plasma membrane (41). All of these signaling mechanisms can impact HSF1, but responses vary by temperature exposure. It is reasonable then to expect that responses to heat stress of cryptorchidism or mild heat stress (37°C–38°C) will be different than responses to acute heat stress at 41°C–43°C. This correlates well with the rapid testis response to 41°C–43°C in which the heat-sensing factors MAPK and p38 were shown to be activated within 6 hours of heat stress and then triggered a reduction in the components of the BTB, inhibiting further meiosis (12). Specific evidence of apoptosis has also been reported (24,42). Even earlier, 0.5–2 hours after heat stress, redistribution of apoptotic regulators is occurring (10,43,44). Recently, acute heat stress has also been shown to change the expression of a series of miRNA and protein acetylation, which have a variety of downstream effects (42,45). In contrast to acute heat stress, longer-term and lower temperatures of cryptorchidism, scrotal insulation or mild environmental temperatures produce a much slower response. Apoptosis increases over 2–4 days following mild heat exposure but uses similar pathways (1,18,21,46–48).

While HSF1 is stable following heat stress, HSF2 degrades rapidly, and its degradation increases with temperature (49) leading to fewer HSF1/HSF2 complexes at higher temperatures such as 41°C (19). As the complexes decrease, HSF1 is released to bind to regulatory components of DNA that promote apoptosis in spermatocytes (11). Thus, at 43°C, a rapid decrease in HSF2 leads to free HSF1 that triggers quick apoptosis responses.

In somatic cells, HSF1 again triggers cell survival, but in spermatocytes and spermatids, it causes proapoptotic events and initiates capase-3 dependent apoptosis (50). Thus, HSF1 has been proposed to be a gatekeeper, and its activation in germ cells triggers the removal of damaged cells rather than their repair or survival (4,11,36).

17.4 EFFECTS OF MODERATE HEAT STRESS

Because moderate heat stress near body temperature (37°C–38°C) for multiple days to weeks occurs at a much slower pace than acute heat stress, more events may come into play to trigger DNA damage (51). It may be this slow response is more important to understand, as this is what would occur due to daily increases in environmental temperature changes or lifestyle results associated with obesity (4). For example, let's consider reactive oxygen species (ROS) generation. During heat stress, there is an increase in ROS production by the testis (52–54), and this can trigger apoptosis (55,56). While the testis has naturally occurring antioxidants to combat ROS, the effect of heat stress is predominately an increase in ROS (20,57) but has sometimes been associated with decreases in naturally occurring antioxidants (20). Mitigation of moderate heat stress has thus been attempted by increasing antioxidants in the testis (20,52) with often very good results due to blocking increases in ROS and downstream events of apoptosis. However, in addition to direct increases in ROS, there are also downstream events of DNA damage, or the DNA damage might be due to the activation of other pathways (5,20). If examining heat stress for mechanisms of potential contraception, there is no need to repair ROS damage. For livestock, we are interested in preventing heat stress damage to spermatogenesis and production of mature sperm. While treatment with antioxidants reduces impacts of heat stress and increases the speed of recovery (20), it is not clear this should be an approach used. Do we wish to save some sperm that already have damaged DNA and therefore reduced fertility? Antioxidants may be of greater benefit when used under normal environmental conditions to increase sperm production.

Moderate heat stress has also been shown to cause an increase in Leydig cell numbers and a decrease in testosterone (20). The role of testosterone in heat stress has been fraught with conflicting reports (26,58–60). The increase in Leydig cell numbers in heat stress may be due to the prosurvival activation of HSF1 as seen in other somatic cells (34). High heat exposure led to Leydig cell hyperplasia and decreased testosterone production due to effects on cyclins and the steroidogenic enzymes CYP17 and Star (26), which could be mediated by HSF1 activation. The exact mechanisms impacting Leydig cells under moderate heat stress remain unclear and require measurement of intratesticular testosterone to be sure. Heat stress also results in a decrease of the androgen receptor (AR) activation in Sertoli cells leading to disruption of the BTB (61). Part of the effect of heat stress on the AR of Sertoli cells is the upregulation of HSP70 likely via upregulation of HSF1 (18). The high amounts of HSP70 interact with AR and can inhibit testosterone binding. Surprisingly, supplementation of moderate heat stressed mice with antioxidants prevented Leydig cell hyperplasia, decreases in testosterone and other apoptotic changes to spermatocytes, suggesting a powerful role of ROS in this process (20). Despite the previous conflicting response of heat stress on testosterone production and circulating levels, we now conclude that heat stress does lead to decreased testosterone at least within the testis. Further, the effect of heat stress on the AR only enhances this effect leading to disruption of the Sertoli cell support of spermatogenesis. The end result of decreased testosterone support for

spermatogenesis is activation of apoptosis by some of the same mechanisms as activated by HSF1 in other aspects of heat stress (5).

During moderate heat stress such as scrotal insulation, although apoptosis occurs, not all the damaged sperm are removed. There are still motile sperm ejaculated that have damaged DNA and fail to support proper embryo development after fertilization (16,17). For example, ejaculated sperm following scrotal insulation express increased FasL, DNA damage via TUNEL assay, increased mitochondrial damage suggestive of increased ROS production and failure to support embryo development *in vitro* following *in vitro* fertilization; all in agreement with sperm DNA damage (16,17). A role of autophagy remains unclear (4). Further examination of such animal models and how sperm escape apoptotic removal could provide insight into why males differ in fertility even without sperm motility or morphological defects.

17.5 DISCUSSION AND FUTURE DIRECTIONS

Spermatogenesis is clearly complex, and understanding the molecular mechanisms has been difficult due to the research goals of either development of contraceptives or improved sperm production. A unified idea of mechanisms is now coming to light by the utilization of heat stress models. Both HSF1 and HSF2 are needed for normal spermatogenesis, and in particular, for meiosis and nuclear changes associated with spermiogenesis. Upon heat stress, a variety of membrane-bound sensors upregulate cell signaling molecules that activate HSF1 and HSF2 leading to increased HSF1 activity in spermatocytes and early spermatids. Release of HSPs, in particular, HSP70 and its transcription, lead to germ cell apoptosis via intrinsic pathways. In Leydig and Sertoli cells, HSF1 activation initiates prosurvival pathways resulting in increased Leydig cell numbers but with decreases in testosterone production. In Sertoli cells, there is downregulation of AR likely due to upregulation of HSF1 and HSP70. The negative effects of decreased androgen response lead to disruption of the BTB and decreased support of meiosis by Sertoli cells. Sertoli cells also secrete FasL that triggers extrinsic apoptosis of germ cells.

Following the initial events of heat stress, one of the downstream consequences is the increase in ROS due either to increased production or to decreased antioxidants. The location is within spermatocytes and spermatids in the testis, which is different than what most andrologists are concerned with—production of ROS in ejaculated sperm. The increased ROS will lead to DNA damage and can be reduced by adding antioxidants, but the approach may be questionable since DNA damage can occur in apoptosis due to other pathways and events. Should we save sperm that perhaps still have DNA damage by other pathways? The production of ROS is just one of many pathways activated via heat stress to trigger apoptosis that should also be considered (4,5,11,42,45,51).

Understanding how HSF1 and HSF2 respond to temperatures in the testis has clarified both speed and downstream events of different heat stress animal and cellular models. We still need to bring together researchers examining contraception action and maximizing germ cell production/survival to understand how molecular models and events affect spermatogenesis.

17.6 CONCLUSION

Using heat stress animal models has led to a better understanding of the mechanism and events within spermatogenesis. A unified concept of how heat impacts the testis has also brought together divergent areas of research dealing with contraception and improvement in semen quality from rodents, nonhuman primates, primates and livestock species. Previous research has been hard to reconcile in the past, as the research has focused on various aspects of spermatogenesis. Now the total efforts can be used to address the various end goals of the different types of research.

REFERENCES

1. Parrish JJ, Willenburg KL, Gibbs KM, Yagoda KB, Krautkramer MM, Loether TM, Melo FCSA. Scrotal insulation and sperm production in the boar. *Mol Reprod Dev.* 2017;84:969–78.
2. Cheng CY, Mruk DD. The blood-testis barrier and its implications for male contraception. *Pharmacol Rev.* 2012;64:16–64.
3. Shukla KK, Mahdi AA, Rajender S. Apoptosis, spermatogenesis and male infertility. *Front Biosci (Elite Ed)* 2012;4:746–54.
4. Durairajanayagam D, Agarwal A, Ong C. Causes, effects and molecular mechanisms of testicular heat stress. *Reprod Biomed Online.* 2015;30:14–27.
5. Xu YR, Dong HS, Yang WX. Regulators in the apoptotic pathway during spermatogenesis: Killers or guards? *Gene.* 2016;582:97–111.
6. França LR, Avelar GF, Almeida FFL. Spermatogenesis and sperm transit through the epididymis in mammals with emphasis on pigs. *Theriogenology.* 2005;63:300–18.
7. Costa DS, Faria FJ, Fernandes CA, Silva JC, Auharek SA. Testis morphometry and kinetics of spermatogenesis in the feral pig (*Sus scrofa*). *Anim Reprod Sci.* 2013;142:63–70.
8. Agarwal A, Desai NR, Ruffoli R, Carpi A. Lifestyle and testicular dysfunction: A brief update. *Biomed Pharmacother.* 2008;62:550–3.
9. Skakkebaek NE, Rajpert-De Meyts E, Buck Louis GM, Toppari J, Andersson A-M, Eisenberg ML et al. Male reproductive disorders and fertility trends: Influences of environment and genetic susceptibility. *Physiol Rev* 2016;96:55–97.
10. Rockett JC, Mapp FL, Garges JB, Luft JC, Mori C, Dix DJ. Effects of hyperthermia on spermatogenesis, apoptosis, gene expression, and fertility in adult male mice. *Biol Reprod.* 2001;65:229–39.
11. Widlak W, Vydra N. The role of heat shock factors in mammalian spermatogenesis. *Adv Anat Embryol Cell Biol.* 2017;222:45–65.
12. Cai H, Ren Y, Li XX, Yang JL, Zhang CP, Chen M, Fan CH, Hu XQ, Gao HF, Liu YX. Scrotal heat stress causes a transient alteration in tight junctions and induction of TGF-β expression. *Inter J Androl.* 2011;344:352–62.
13. Rao M, Zhao X-L, Yang J, Hu S-F, Lei H, Xia W, Zhu C-H. Effect of transient scrotal hyperthermia on sperm parameters, seminal plasma biochemical markers, and oxidative stress in men. *Asian J Androl.* 2015;17:668–75.
14. Yin Y, Hawkins KL, DeWolf WC, Morgentaler A. Heat stress causes testicular germ cell apoptosis in adult mice. *J Androl.* 1997;18:159–65.
15. Lue YH, Lasley BL, Laughlin LS, Swerdloff RS, Hikim AP, Leung A, Overstreet JW, Wang C. Mild testicular hyperthermia induces profound transitional spermatogenic suppression through increased germ cell apoptosis in adult cynomolgus monkeys (*Macaca fascicularis*). *J Androl.* 2002;223:799–805.
16. Parrish J, Schindler J, Willenburg K, Enwall L, Kaya A. Quantitative sperm shape analysis: What can this tell us about male fertility. *24th Meeting of the National Association of Animal Breeders*, Columbia MO. 2012;74–80.
17. Parrish JJ, Ostermeier C, Schindler J, Willenburg K, Enwall L, Kaya A. Quantifying sperm nuclear shape with Fourier harmonic analysis and relationship to spermatogenesis and fertility. *Association for Applied Animal Andrology 2014 meeting.* 2014;30–49. In. International Veterinary Information Service. http://www.ivis.org/proceedings/aaaa/2014/3.pdf
18. Shen H, Fan X, Zhang Z, Xi H, Ji R, Liu Y, Yue M, Li Q, He J. Effects of elevated ambient temperature and local testicular heating on the expressions of heat shock protein 70 and androgen receptor in boar testes. *Acta Histochem.* 2019; 121(3):297–302.
19. Korfanty J, Stokowy T, Widlak P, Gogler-Piglowska A, Handschuh L, Podkowiński J, Vydra N, Naumowicz A, Toma-Jonik A, Widlak W. Crosstalk between HSF1 and HSF2 during the heat shock response in mouse testes. *Int J Biochem Cell Biol.* 2014;57:76–83.
20. Badr G, Abdel-Tawab HS, Ramadan NK, Ahmed SF, Mahmoud MH. Protective effects of camel whey protein against scrotal heat-mediated damage and infertility in the mouse testis through YAP/Nrf2 and PPAR-gamma signaling pathways. *Mol Reprod Dev.* 2018;85:505–18.
21. Costa GMJ, Lacerda SMSN, Figueiredo AFA, Leal MC, Rezende-Neto JV, França LR. Higher environmental temperatures promote acceleration of spermatogenesis *in vivo* in mice (*Mus musculus*). *J Therm Biol.* 2018;77:14–23.
22. Perez-Crespo M, Pintado B, Gutierrez-Adan A. Scrotal heat stress effects on sperm viability, sperm DNA integrity, and the offspring sex ratio in mice. *Mol Reprod Dev.* 2008;75:40–7.

23. Yaeram J, Setchell BP, Maddocks S. Effect of heat stress on the fertility of male mice *in vivo* and *in vitro*. *Reprod Fertil Dev.* 2006;18:647–53.

24. Kanter M, Aktas C, Erboga M. Heat stress decreases testicular germ cell proliferation and increases apoptosis in the short term: An immunohistochemical and ultrastructural study. *Toxicol Industrial Health.* 2013:29:99–113.

25. Kanter M, Aktas C. Effects of scrotal hyperthermia on Leydig cells in long-term: A histological, immunohistochemical and ultrastructural study in rats. *J Mol Histol.* 2009;40:123–30.

26. Li Z, Tian J, Cui G, Wang M, Yu D. Effects of local testicular heat treatment on Leydig cell hyperplasia and testosterone biosynthesis in rat testes. *Reprod Fertil Dev.* 2016;28:1424–32.

27. Gasinska A, Hill S. The effect of hyperthermia on the mouse testis. *Neoplasma.* 1990;37:357–66.

28. Legare C, Thabet M, Sullivan R. Expression of heat shock protein 70 in normal and cryptorchid human excurrent duct. *Mol Hum Reprod.* 2004;10:197–202.

29. Xiao X, Zuo X, Davis AA, McMillan DR, Curry BB, Richardson JA, Benjamin IJ. HSF1 is required for extra-embryonic development, postnatal growth and protection during inflammatory responses in mice. *EMBO J.* 1999;18:5943–52.

30. Salmand PA, Jungas T, Fernandez M, Conter A, Christians ES. Mouse heat shock factor 1 (HSF1) is involved in testicular response to genotoxic stress induced by doxorubicin. *Biol Reprod.* 2008;79:1092–101.

31. Abane R, Mezger V. Roles of heat shock factors in gametogenesis and development. *FEBS J.* 2010;277:4150–72.

32. Wang G, Ying Z, Jin X, Tu N, Zhang Y, Phillips M, Moskophidis D, Mivechi NF. Essential requirement for both hsf1 and hsf2 transcriptional activity in spermatogenesis and male fertility. *Genesis.* 2004;38:66–80.

33. Akerfelt M, Vihervaara A, Laiho A, Conter A, Christians ES, Sistonen L, Henriksson E. Heat shock transcription factor 1 localizes to sex chromatin during meiotic repression. *J Biol Chem.* 2010;285:34469–76.

34. Sarge KD. Male germ cell-specific alteration in temperature set point of the cellular stress response. *J Biol Chem.* 1995;270:18745–8.

35. Huang L, Mivechi NF, Moskophidis D. Insights into regulation and function of the major stress-induced hsp70 molecular chaperone *in vivo*: Analysis of mice with targeted gene disruption of the hsp70.1 or hsp70.3 gene. *Mol Cell Biol.* 2001;21:8575–91.

36. Izu H, Inouye S, Fujimoto M, Shiraishi K, Naito K, Nakai A. Heat shock transcription factor 1 is involved in quality-control mechanisms in male germ cells. *Biol Reprod.* 2004;70:18–24.

37. Kus-Liśkiewicz M, Polańska J, Korfanty J, Olbryt M, Vydra N, Toma A, Widlak W. Impact of heat shock transcription factor 1 on global gene expression profiles in cells which induce either cytoprotective or pro-apoptotic response following hyperthermia. *BMC Genomics.* 2013;14:456–78.

38. Widlak W, Vydra N, Malusecka E, Dudaladava V, Winiarski B, Scieglińska D, Widlak P. Heat shock transcription factor 1 down-regulates spermatocyte-specific 70kDa heat shock protein expression prior to the induction of apoptosis in mouse testes. *Genes Cells Devoted Mol Cell Mech.* 2007a;12:487–99.

39. Widlak W, Winiarski B, Krawczyk A, Vydra N, Malusecka E, Krawczyk Z. Inducible 70kDa heat shock protein does not protect spermatogenic cells from damage induced by cryptorchidism. *Int J Androl.* 2007b;30:80–7.

40. Korfanty J, Stokowy T, Chadalski M, Toma-Jonik A, Vydra N, Widlak P, Wojtaś B, Gielniewski B, Widlak W. SPEN protein expression and interactions with chromatin in mouse testicular cells. *Reproduction.* 2018;156:195–206.

41. Balogh G, Péter M, Glatz A, Gombos I, Török Z, Horváth I, Harwood JL, Vígh L. Key role of lipids in heat stress management. *FEBS Lett.* 2013;587:1970–80.

42. Rao M, Zeng Z, Tang L, Cheng G, Xia W, Zhu C. Next-generation sequencing-based microRNA profiling of mice testis subjected to transient heat stress. *Oncotarget. Dec* 2017;8:111672–82.

43. Yamamoto CM, Sinha Hikim AP, Huynh PN, Shapiro B, Lue Y, Salameh WA, Wang C, Swerdloff RS. Redistribution of Bax is an early step in an apoptotic pathway leading to germ cell death in rats, triggered by mild testicular hyperthermia. *Biol Reprod.* 2000;63:1683–90.

44. Hikim APS, Lue Y, Yamamoto CM, Vera Y, Rodriguez S, Yen PH, Soeng K, Wang C, Swerdloff RS. Key apoptotic pathways for heat-induced programmed germ cell death in the testis. *Endocrinology.* 2003;144:3167–75.

45. Xie C, Shen H, Zhang H, Yan J, Liu Y, Yao F, Wang X, Cheng Z, Tang TS, Guo C. Quantitative proteomics analysis reveals alterations of lysine acetylation in mouse testis in response to heat shock and X-ray exposure. *Biochim Biophys Acta Proteins Proteom.* 2018;1866:464–72.

46. Barqawi A, Trummer H, Meacham R. Effect of prolonged cryptorchidism on germ cell apoptosis and testicular sperm count. *Asian J Androl.* 2004;6:47–51.

47. Chaki SP, Misro MM, Ghosh D, Gautam DK, Srinivas M. Apoptosis and cell removal in the cryptorchid rat testis. *Apoptosis Int J Program Cell Death.* 2005;10:395–405.

48. Tao S-X, Guo J, Zhang X-S, Li Y-C, Hu Z-Y, Han C-S, Liu Y-X. Germ cell apoptosis induced by experimental cryptorchidism is mediated by multiple molecular pathways in *Cynomolgus* Macaque. *Front Biosci J Virtual Library.* 2006;11:1077–89.

49. Ahlskog JK, Björk JK, Elsing AN, Aspelin C, Kallio M, Roos-Mattjus P, Sistonen L. Anaphase-promoting complex/cyclosome participates in the acute response to protein-damaging stress. *Mol Cell Biol.* 2010;30:5608–20.

50. Vydra N, Malusecka E, Jarzab M, Lisowska K, Glowala-Kosinska M, Benedyk K, Widlak P, Krawczyk Z, Widlak W. Spermatocyte-specific expression of constitutively active heat shock factor 1 induces HSP70i-resistant apoptosis in male germ cells. *Cell Death Differ.* 2006;13:212–22.

51. Yadav SK, Pandey A, Kumar L, Devi A, Kushwaha B, Vishvkarma R, Maikhuri JP, Rajender S, Gupta G. The thermo-sensitive gene expression signatures of spermatogenesis. *Reprod Biol Endocrinol.* 2018;16:56–78.

52. Ahotupa M, Huhtaniemi I. Impaired detoxification of reactive oxygen and consequent oxidative stress in experimentally cryptorchid rat testis. *Biol Reprod.* 1992;46:1114–8.

53. Ikeda M, Kodama H, Fukuda J, Shimizu Y, Murata M, Kumagai J, Tanaka T. Role of radical oxygen species in rat testicular germ cell apoptosis induced by heat stress. *Biol Reprod.* 1999;61:393–9.

54. Kim B, Park K, Rhee K. Heat stress response of male germ cells. *Cell Mol Life Sci.* 2013;70: 2623–36.

55. Agarwal A, Hamada A, Esteves SC. Insight into oxidative stress in varicocele-associated male infertility: Part 1. *Nat Rev Urol.* 2012;9:678–90.

56. Paul C, Teng S, Saunders PT. A single, mild, transient scrotal heat stress causes hypoxia and oxidative stress in mouse testes, which induces germ cell death. *Biol Reprod.* 2009;80:913–9.

57. Peltola V, Huhtaniemi I, Ahotupa M. Abdominal position of the rat testis is associated with high level of lipid peroxidation. *Biol Reprod.* 1995;53:1146–50.

58. Wettemann RP, Desjardins C. Testicular function in boars exposed to elevated ambient temperature. *Biol Reprod.* 1979;20:235–41.

59. Lue YH, Hikim AP, Swerdloff RS, Im P, Taing KS, Bui T, Leung A, Wang C. Single exposure to heat induces stage-specific germ cell apoptosis in rats: Role of intratesticular testosterone on stage specificity. *Endocrinology.* 1999;140:1709–17.

60. Rasooli A, Jalali MT, Nouri M, Mohammadian B, Barati F. Effects of chronic heat stress on testicular structures, serum testosterone and cortisol concentrations in developing lambs. *Animal Reproduction Sci.* 2010;117:55–9.

61. Li XX, Chen SR, Shen B, Yang JL, Ji SY, Wen Q et al. The heat-induced reversible change in the blood-testis barrier (BTB) is regulated by the androgen receptor (AR) via the partitioning-defective protein (Par) polarity complex in the mouse. *Biol Reprod.* 2013;89:1–10.

Index

Printed and bound by CPI Group (UK) Ltd, Croydon, CR0 4YY

17/10/2024

01775698-0017